P9-BZE-238

# AT.
# TEAS®

## Strategies, Practice & Review with 2 Practice Tests

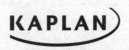

KAPLAN

PUBLISHING

New York

Bridgeport Public Library
925 Broad St.
Bridgeport, CT 06604

Special thanks to the team that made this book possible: Gina Allison, Erika Blumenthal, Joel Boyce, Chanti Burnette, Matthew Callan, Irene Cheung, Dorothy Cummings, Lola Dart, Marilyn Engle, Paula Fleming, Bootsie, Dan Frey, Lauren Hanson, Justine Harkness, Allison Harm, Jack Hayes, Cinzia Iacono Pelletier, Stephanie Jolly, Ashley Kapturkiewicz, Jennifer Land, Karen Lilyquist, Edwina Lui, Heather Maigur, Maureen McMahon, Nou Moua, Alex Ricken, Christine Ricketts, Gordon Spector, Bruce Symaka, Lo'Rita Vargas, Pedro Villanueva, Dan Wittich, Jessica Yee, and many others.

ATI TEAS® and ATI Test of Essential Academic Skills™ are registered trademarks of Assessment Technologies Institute, LLC, which neither sponsors nor endorses this product.

This publication is designed to provide accurate information in regard to the subject matter covered as of its publication date, with the understanding that knowledge and best practice constantly evolve. The publisher is not engaged in rendering medical, legal, accounting, or other professional service. If medical or legal advice or other expert assistance is required, the services of a competent professional should be sought. This publication is not intended for use in clinical practice or the delivery of medical care. To the fullest extent of the law, neither the Publisher nor the Editors assume any liability for any injury and/or damage to persons or property arising out of or related to any use of the material contained in this book

© 2017 Kaplan, Inc.

Published by Kaplan Publishing, a division of Kaplan, Inc.
750 Third Avenue
New York, NY 10017

All rights reserved. The text of this publication, or any part thereof, may not be reproduced in any manner whatsoever without written permission from the publisher.

10 9 8 7 6 5 4 3 2

ISBN: 978-1-5062-1115-2

Kaplan Publishing books are available at special quantity discounts to use for sales promotions, employee premiums, or educational purposes. For more information or to purchase books, please call the Simon & Schuster special sales department at 866-506-1949.

# CONTENTS

# FOREWORD

Congratulations! If you have picked up this book, you are considering applying to a nursing or allied health school. This is an exciting step! Your career in healthcare will provide you with many rewarding experiences and opportunities.

I speak from personal experience. Early in my career as a nurse, I was caring for a client newly diagnosed with stage 4 lung cancer. The care team had addressed his symptoms: cough, shortness of breath, fatigue, and weight loss among others. The physician had discussed the treatment plan. The social worker had offered her services. Thanks to my education, I understood the diagnosis and prognosis—the science behind the malignancy. I understood that simple remedies would not eliminate the chronic cough. I understood that the dyspnea and fatigue were inevitable and that treatment options were limited.

I also understood that no one had taken the time to *be* with the client—to sit quietly and give support, to ask questions and listen. In your role as a care provider, you will have the opportunity to offer client-centered care. You will give people respect, sensitivity, and open communication. Caring for this man during his journey did not feel like work. It was the most rewarding effort I had ever undertaken.

Because their students will someday be entrusted with the well-being of other people, healthcare programs want strong students. This only makes sense: your degree program will culminate in caring for clients who will depend on you for their health and maybe their life. We do not make or sell things. Instead, it is people and families, young and old, well and sick, who get our attention. I teach in a two-year RN program, so I fully appreciate the importance of well-prepared students. Nursing and allied healthcare programs are rigorous. I have high standards, as will your instructors. This is why school admissions can be very competitive.

To weigh the qualifications of applicants, many schools require candidates to take ATI's Test of Essential Academic Skills (TEAS®). The TEAS measures competencies in reading, math, science, and language use. Your TEAS score quantifies your academic preparedness and test-taking skills, and it is an important indicator of your potential to succeed in school.

Your nursing or allied health program will challenge you in ways that other classes have not. A lot of information will be thrown at you. You will do more academic reading than you have ever done before, and studying will require more than memorization. You must use your understanding of the knowledge of your field to recognize important facts you encounter in real-life situations and then draw sound conclusions. Especially as you move to the clinical setting, you will be making critical decisions for your clients based on information you gather.

You will also need to use math. If you want to determine the correct dose of medication for a client, you will need to be able to set up and compute proportions. You cannot trust the computer to do this—you are responsible. In any healthcare career, you are committing to lifelong learning, which means reading and evaluating research studies. Therefore, an understanding of statistics is key. Your career may take you into managing your own business or being a consultant, and then arithmetic and algebra skills will be important to you as a businessperson.

Healthcare practice requires science—anatomy and physiology, biology, and chemistry—to understand your clients' medical conditions. You may need to understand the implications of fluid balance, interpret laboratory and radiology tests, and know what effect medications can have in the body. With a good scientific education, your assessment of the client, interpretation of data, and selection of interventions will be based on evidence-based practice, not on what "feels right."

You will need strong communication skills in school and throughout your career as you speak and write to clients and colleagues. Using the correct word is critical to say what you mean to say, and you will be judged on your use of grammar. In emails and in phone conversations, your confidence and expertise must come through so people view you as someone they can depend on.

I say these things not to make you nervous and question your decision, but to emphasize the need to prepare for the TEAS. The TEAS gives you an opportunity to show schools your academic skills and ability to think like a healthcare professional. It gives you a chance to demonstrate that you are prepared for the courses ahead of you so you can gain admission to the program of your choice.

Getting into your school is just the first step toward a lifetime of opportunities. Indeed, my nursing education opened doors I didn't even imagine when I was filling out my applications. While my initial jobs were in clinical settings, I have held titles such as Nurse Manager, Clinical Reimbursement Specialist, and Subject Matter Expert. Because of my healthcare expertise and skills, I have been able to pursue consulting, business ownership, training, nursing education, and publication writing and editing. The opportunities in healthcare were so exciting and my love of learning so deep that after earning my RN, I pursued additional credentials. Today, I proudly add PhD and APRN, CNP after my name. Who knows what you will be doing in 10, 20, or 30 years? There are so many possibilities!

I encourage you to get the most that you can from this Kaplan TEAS book so that you can get into the program of your choice. Being a healthcare professional is about helping people—you will make a lasting difference in the lives of others. It is also a personally rewarding career, limited only by your imagination.

Kaplan is the premier test preparation company in the world, and we have gathered an expert team to write *ATI TEAS® Strategies, Practice, and Review*. It is important to become comfortable with both the content and structure of the exam to ensure you obtain a TEAS score that reflects your abilities. This book will be help you succeed on this important test so this part of your application will be strong. Flip through the book. Get a sense of its content and structure. Take the full-length diagnostic test and use the Study Guide to plan your review. Use the lessons to understand how the TEAS will test certain material. Use the glossary to make flashcards of key terms you need to memorize. Apply your knowledge to the practice questions in the book and in the online Qbank and review the explanations. Analyze your results: What went well and what did not? Refocus your study plan based on your analysis. Finally, take the full-length test online to find out how far you have come.

Understand that pursuing a degree in nursing or an allied healthcare field is a huge commitment. Dive right in! Develop your time management skills. Seek learning opportunities. Make friends. Reach out for support. Take care of yourself. Your program is meant to be demanding—but others have come through it, and you can also. Be prepared to be successful!

Karen Lilyquist, PhD, MSN, APRN, CNP
NCLEX Instructor, Kaplan Test Prep

# WELCOME TO YOUR TEAS® STUDIES!

Thank you for choosing Kaplan to help you study for the ATI TEAS®. We are honored to be part of your preparation for a career in healthcare. You will soon join the millions of nurses and other professionals who make a significant positive difference in the lives of others.

## YOUR KAPLAN RESOURCES

Your Kaplan book contains:

- A full-length diagnostic test with an explanation of every question
- Tools to help you plan your studies
- Lessons that cover all of the skills and concepts on the test
  - Kaplan Methods for every question type
  - Worked examples that show the expert approach
  - Key terms in bold and a glossary with definitions of every key term
  - Key takeaway summaries
  - Practice questions with explanations

Your Student Homepage offers:

- An additional full-length, online test with an explanation of every question
- A 50-question Qbank for additional practice. The Qbank is a collection of questions you can use to create customized practice sets.

## GETTING STARTED

- Go to **kaptest.com/booksonline** to register your book.
- Take the diagnostic test in Part One of this book.
- Learn, practice, and review.
- Log in to your Student Homepage at **kaptest.com** to get more practice using your Qbank and to take a full-length online practice test.

## Register Your Book

To access your Student Homepage, visit **kaptest.com/booksonline**. Choose "TEAS" from the list of tests at the top and answer the questions that appear.

Once you have created your username and password, you'll be able to log in to your resources at **kaptest.com**. When you're ready to use your full-length online test and Qbank, click **Sign In** at the upper right of the page and enter your username and password. Then click on your TEAS product to open it.

## Take the Diagnostic Test

You'll find the diagnostic test in Part One of this book. Taking the diagnostic test will help you learn about the format and content of the TEAS. Your results will help you decide where to focus your studying. Set aside about 4 uninterrupted hours to take your diagnostic test. The test has four sections, and the timing for each is given in the test. You may take a 10-minute break after the second section of the test.

Also plan to set aside time to check your answers. Use the Study Planner at the end of Part One to evaluate your strengths and what areas you need to study most. Finally, begin your preparation for the TEAS by studying the explanation given for each question.

## Learn, Practice, and Review

After you take the diagnostic test, you may feel confident that you can tackle most TEAS questions and only need to review a few areas or practice some skills a little more. Alternatively, you may want to study and practice much more in order to approach the test with confidence.

No matter what your performance is on the diagnostic test, you can and will improve if you set aside time to study for the TEAS. Block out study time on your calendar, just as you would write down any other appointment. These blocks of time are appointments with yourself, so keep them!

A great deal of research shows that we learn better in shorter, more frequent study sessions. Therefore, plan to study at least three days a week for one to three hours, rather than one or two days a week for four or more hours.

Also, consider how much time you have between now and when you will take the TEAS. Estimate how many hours you need to study to master the material. Divide the number of hours of study by the number of weeks. This is the number of hours you need to study each week. Then divide that number by the number of days you will study each week. This is the number of hours per day you need to study. Here's an example:

Taking the TEAS in 4 weeks, need to study about 40 hours, and can study 4 days a week

Calculate hours per week:
40 hours ÷ 4 weeks = 10 hours/week

Calculate hours per day:
10 hours/week ÷ 4 days/week = 2.5 hours/day

This person will block out 2.5 hours on 4 days each week for the next 4 weeks to prepare for the TEAS.

Finally, every time you sit down to study, set a goal for that session. Examples of goals are "Complete two Reading lessons and understand the explanation of every practice question," or "Memorize the path of blood through the body and be able to diagram it." Setting a goal at the beginning of your study session sets you up to feel great when you have achieved it at the end of the session.

| The one-month plan, for a light brush-up . . . | The two- or three-month plan, for an in-depth review . . . | If you need to (re)learn much of the material from scratch . . . |
|---|---|---|
| Devote one week to each of the four content areas. Read the appropriate lessons and do the practice questions at the end of each. Depending on the results of your diagnostic test, you may want to spend just a few days on one content area and more than a week on another.<br><br>At the end of the month, take the online practice test. Are there still areas where you would like to do better? If so, revisit those lessons to make sure you have mastered them by Test Day. | Use the results of your diagnostic test to identify several areas you need to study most. Spend two weeks on each of those areas, reading the appropriate lessons and doing the practice questions. Make flashcards of the key terms that appear in bold in these lessons, using the definitions in the glossary. Then go back to the diagnostic test and review the questions that address those areas: Could you get all the questions right now?<br><br>Once you feel you've made significant improvement in your areas of greatest need, move on to a comprehensive review of all the lessons in the book.<br><br>Once you've completed your comprehensive review, take the online practice test. Are there still areas where you would like to do better? If so, revisit those lessons to make sure you have mastered them by Test Day. | Give yourself plenty of time to work through this book, lesson by lesson. Make flashcards of the key terms that appear in bold in the lessons, using the definitions in the glossary. Periodically review earlier lessons to refresh your memory of them.<br><br>After you have spent several months studying, go back to review the questions on the diagnostic test. Could you get most of them right now? If there are areas where you still need more work, return to those lessons and study them until you feel confident with the material.<br><br>Once you feel you have made significant improvement in each of the four content areas, take the online practice test. Are there still areas where you would like to do better? If so, revisit those lessons to make sure you have mastered them by Test Day. |

## Use Your Online Resources

The Qbank in your Student Homepage allows you to get focused practice in particular content areas. A great way to use this resource is to create a practice set of five questions in one topic, try your best on them, and then review the explanations thoroughly. If you missed a question, review the explanation until you understand the correct answer. Then do the question again. Of course, you already know the answer. However, actually doing the question correctly will reinforce the memory in your brain, helping you to retain the knowledge so you will know it on Test Day. If you miss more than one or two questions out of five on a topic, then review the relevant lesson(s) in your book to increase your mastery.

In addition to the full-length diagnostic test in this book, you have a full-length practice test online. You may be taking the TEAS online, so taking a practice test in the same format is great preparation. In any case, taking a practice test after studying the lessons in this book will help you gauge your progress and identify any areas where you need further study so you are ready for the TEAS.

### Want More?

Your Kaplan book covers all the concepts and skills you need to master to succeed on the TEAS, and the online full-length test on your Student Homepage will help you gauge your readiness for the test. For over 500 additional practice questions, check out Kaplan's **ATI TEAS® Qbank**.

## MANAGING STRESS

You have a lot riding on the TEAS. However, you're also doing the work you need to do to reach your goals. Unfortunately, sometimes just knowing that you're working hard won't make your test anxiety go away. Thus, here are some stress management tips from our long experience of helping students prepare for standardized tests.

**Clock in and out:** Once you've set up a study schedule for yourself, treat it like a job. That is, imagine clocking yourself in and out of TEAS studies according to that schedule. Do your best to stick to your schedule, and when you're not "clocked in," don't let yourself think about the TEAS. That will help you release your stress about the test in between study sessions.

**Don't punish yourself:** If you get tired or overwhelmed or discouraged when studying, don't respond by pushing yourself harder. Instead, step away and engage in a relaxing activity like going for a walk, watching a movie, or playing with your cat or dog. Then, when you're ready, return to your studies with fresh eyes.

**Breathe:** Remember to take deep breaths, consciously using your diaphragm to breathe "into your stomach." This breathing technique will help your muscles to relax, and when your body relaxes, your mind relaxes as well.

**Set small, manageable goals:** Each week, set manageable goals for your TEAS progress. Then reward yourself when you've achieved them. Examples of small goals might be:

- This week, memorize and practice the Kaplan Method for Science until I no longer have to think about what the steps of the Method are.

- This week, do 20 math questions and practice each until I can move confidently and efficiently from the information provided to the correct answer.

- This week, review all the spelling rules that the TEAS is likely to test until I can identify words that use them and words that are common exceptions.

**Keep yourself healthy:** Good health, adequate rest, and regular interactions with friends and family make it easier to cope with the challenges of studying. Stay on a regular sleep schedule as much as possible during your studies, eat well, continue to exercise, and spend time with those you care about and those who help you feel good about yourself. Also, don't fuel your studies with caffeine and sugar. Those substances may make you feel alert, but they can also damage focus.

**Remind yourself why you are doing this:** If you feel tempted to pass up a planned study session because you're tired or something comes up that feels like a higher priority, remind yourself how important a good score on the TEAS is. Success on this test will open the doors to an important educational credential and many career opportunities after that. If you planned to study for 90 minutes and don't think you can study for that long, then study for 30 minutes. You will make progress toward the score you want, and you will feel better about yourself than if you "blow it off." You may even be surprised at how fast the 30 minutes go by and decide that you can study longer after all.

**Keep the right mindset:** Most importantly, keep telling yourself that you *can* do this. Don't fall into the trap of thinking that you're not "allowed" to feel confident yet. That's a self-punishing attitude that will only hurt you. Rather, remember that confidence breeds success. So let yourself be confident about your abilities. You're obviously ambitious and intelligent, so walk into the TEAS knowing that about yourself.

**If you get discouraged, make a list:** If you start to wonder if you'll ever reach your TEAS goals, stop what you're doing and make a list of everything you're good at. List *every specific skill* that you are bringing to the TEAS. Here are some examples:

- Finding the main point of a passage
- Using commas correctly in lists
- Identifying what a math question is asking for
- Comparing two fractions to find which one is larger
- Naming the organ systems of the human body
- Explaining how oxygen reaches tissues in the body

Post that list of things you're good at somewhere you'll see it every day and add to it as you continue to study. It will be a long list in no time! We at Kaplan recommend making this list because many people focus too heavily on their weaknesses while preparing for a standardized test. But if you only focus on your weaknesses, you aren't seeing an objective picture. There *are* TEAS skills you're good at. Keep that in mind and focus on building on those strengths.

## ALSO IMPORTANT . . .

- Think about what school(s) you will apply to. What are your criteria for a program? Consider the degrees offered, geographic location, cost, campus culture, and other factors.
- Research the colleges and universities that offer the kind of program you're interested in. Visit their websites to learn more about the admissions process and talk to an admissions officer about the school's acceptance criteria for prospective students.
- Talk to alumni of your target programs to learn about how their education has prepared them for their careers and what surprises and challenges they have encountered.

By researching the school(s) you'll apply to, you will be able to choose a school that is a good fit for you and your goals. You'll experience much less stress as you work toward your degree than you would if you are not in a school that meets your needs.

## THE ROAD TO TEST DAY

You've read this book. You know what to expect on the TEAS. You've studied a lot. Your Test Day is approaching. How can you make sure you do your best?

### The Week Before Test Day

**Rest:** Make sure you're on a regular sleep schedule.

**Rehearse:** Find out where you will be taking the test and consider doing a "dry run." Drive or commute to the test site around the same time of day as your test will be. You don't want to be surprised by traffic or road construction on Test Day. You also don't want to get delayed or stressed out trying to figure out where to park, which way to go after you get off the bus, or where the restrooms are.

**Review:** Do a high-level review. Flip through the lessons and rework a few practice problems here and there to reinforce all of the good habits you've developed in your preparation. (Redoing practice problems you've already done is fine: you can actually learn a lot that way about how to approach those types of questions more efficiently in the future.)

**Stop:** Two days before the test, stop studying—no studying at all! You're not likely to learn anything new in those two days, and you'll get a lot more out of walking into the test feeling rested.

**Relax:** The evening before the test, do something fun (but not crazy or tiring). Maybe you could have a nice dinner (without alcohol), watch a movie, catch up on housework (a clean house is relaxing for some people), or play a game.

**Go to bed:** Go to bed early enough to get a full night's sleep (7–8 hours) before the day of the exam.

## On Test Day Itself

**Warm up:** Before you take the test, do a TEAS warm-up. This will help your brain get ready to function at its best. Don't take any practice materials into the testing center, but do a few easy practice questions at home or work before you leave for the test.

**Don't let nerves derail you:** You have every reason to feel confident. You have prepared for this test! But if you do find yourself getting nervous or losing focus, sit back in your seat and place your feet flat on the floor. Then take a few deep breaths and close your eyes or focus them on something other than the computer screen or test booklet for a moment. Remind yourself that you have studied diligently and are ready for the TEAS. When you're ready, reengage with the test.

**Keep moving:** Don't let yourself get bogged down on any one question. You can come back to questions that you aren't sure about, so skip questions whenever they threaten to slow you down or to steal time from the other questions. There is no penalty for a wrong answer on the TEAS, so make sure to answer every question before time is called, even if you have to guess on some questions. Also, remember to use the multiple-choice format to your advantage: if you can eliminate one or two answer choices as incorrect, you have greatly increased your chances of guessing correctly.

**Don't assess yourself:** This is very important. As you're testing, don't let yourself stop and think about how you *feel* you're doing. Taking a standardized test hardly ever *feels* good. Your own impressions of how it's going are totally unreliable. So, instead of focusing on that, remind yourself that you're prepared and that you are going to succeed, even if you feel discouraged as the test is underway.

**After the test, celebrate!** You've prepared, practiced, and performed like a champion. Now that the test is over, it's time to congratulate yourself on a job well done. Celebrate responsibly with friends and family and enjoy the rest of your day, knowing you just took an important step toward reaching your goals.

## GOOD LUCK!

We at Kaplan wish you the very best in your studies, on the TEAS, and in your career as a healthcare professional. If you have feedback or questions about this book, please email us at TEASfeedback@kaplan.com.

# ABOUT THE TEAS

## WHAT IS THE TEAS?

The ATI TEAS was developed to evaluate the academic readiness of applicants to health science programs, such as nursing programs. *TEAS* stands for Test of Essential Academic Skills. *ATI* is the name of the testmaker and stands for Assessment Technologies Institute.

More programs accept TEAS scores than any other health science admissions test, but some programs want applicants to submit scores from other tests. Therefore, before studying for the TEAS and taking the test, check with the schools you're interested in to make sure they accept a TEAS score.

### What Does the TEAS Test?

The questions you will see on the TEAS assess knowledge and skills that have been identified by health science schools as relevant to assessing your readiness to begin a college program of study. The material tested is typically taught in grades 7–12. The TEAS tests material in four content areas as follows:

| Content Area | Number of Questions (Number of Scored Questions) | Time Limit |
|---|---|---|
| *Reading* | 53 (47) | 64 minutes |
| *Mathematics* | 36 (32) | 54 minutes |
| Break | | 10 minutes |
| *Science* | 53 (47) | 63 minutes |
| *English and language usage* | 28 (24) | 28 minutes |
| **Total** | **170 (150)** | **219 minutes** |

The 20 unscored questions are experimental questions included to test their validity. You will not know whether a question is scored or unscored, so do your best on every question.

There is no penalty for wrong answers on the TEAS, so make sure to answer every question. Even if you need to guess, you might get the question right. If you can eliminate one or two answer choices as clearly incorrect, then you increase your chances of guessing correctly.

This book is organized to correspond to the content areas of the test. Part One contains a diagnostic test and answers and explanations for every question on the test, as well as a Study Guide to help you use your test results. After that are the following sections:

- Part Two: Reading
- Part Three: Mathematics
- Part Four: Science
- Part Five: English and Language Usage

Part Six provides answers and explanations for every practice question you find at the end of each lesson in Parts Two through Five. Part Seven contains a glossary of key terms.

## How Is the ATI TEAS Different From the TEAS V?

The retirement date for the TEAS V was August 31, 2016. Since this date, prospective health science students have been taking the ATI TEAS. There are three key differences between the old and new editions of the test:

- A calculator is now permitted on the *Mathematics* section. If you are taking the test on a computer, a four-function calculator is embedded in the onscreen test interface. If you are taking the pencil-and-paper version of the test, the proctor will give you a four-function calculator. You may not bring your own calculator to the test.

- The four content areas of the test have not changed. However, the specific competencies emphasized in each have been realigned in response to the feedback of educators about the skills that entry-level health science students should possess.

- The previous test reported all scores as a percentage. The ATI TEAS reports your composite score as a number and continues to report your content area scores as percentages.

# TEAS LOGISTICS

Learning all you can about the TEAS will help you have a smooth experience on Test Day, and you'll be able to submit your applications to schools efficiently. Just as preparing for the questions you will see on the test is important, so too is preparing to register and take the test.

## How to Register for the Test

Be sure to register early because seating for each test administration is limited. One way to register for the TEAS is to go to the testmaker's website at **atitesting.com**. You will need to create an account and be logged in to the site to register for the test. Click on the Online Store and select Register for... TEAS. You will be asked where you want to take the test. Then you will be asked for billing information. The fee for the test varies depending on the testing site you choose, but is generally between $50 and $100.

You can also register to take the test at a PSI (formerly Pearson Vue) test center. You will pay for the test and receive a registration number at **atitesting.com** and then go to **psiexams.com** or call 1-800-733-9267 to schedule the exam. Visit ATI's website to read detailed instructions for this option. The fee to take the test at a PSI test center is $115.

Another way to register is to contact the school to which you plan to apply and ask for a list of TEAS testing locations. Many nursing and allied health programs administer the TEAS on campus, and registration for the test is sometimes available through the school.

If you register for the test through ATI, your registration is final. To change your test date, you will need to register again and pay the test fee again. If you register through PSI, then to reschedule, you must contact PSI two days before your scheduled test date. If you registered for the test through a school and want to change your test date, contact the school to find out what the policy is.

When you register for the TEAS, you can request that the school at which you are taking your test receive your score at no additional cost. If you want to submit your score to other schools, go to the testmaker's website at **atitesting.com** and use the Online Store to order your transcript(s). The fee is $27 per transcript.

If you want to request accommodations for a disability, contact ATI at 800-667-7531.

## Test Administration

On the day of your test, arrive at least 15 minutes early so the proctor can verify your identity and get you checked in. Proctors will monitor you throughout the test, and they will intervene if they observe disruptive behavior.

Bring the following items to the testing site:

- Government-issued identification with a current photograph, your signature, and your permanent address. Examples include a driver's license or state ID card, military ID, US passport, or US permanent resident card (green card).
    - Not acceptable: Student ID card, credit card
- Two sharpened No. 2 pencils with attached erasers
    - Not acceptable: Pens, highlighters, mechanical pencils, separate erasers
- Your ATI assessment ID. You receive this in a confirmation email when you register for the test.
- If your test will be online, you will need to know your ATI account username and password so you can log in.

Your testing site may issue specific instructions about Test Day. Read the instructions carefully and follow them so you are not denied admittance when you show up to take your test.

Do *not* bring these items to the test:

- Electronic or Internet-enabled devices of any kind. These include cell or smart phones, portable music players, tablets, and digital or smart watches. Leave these in your car or at home. Do not bring a calculator—one will be provided to you.
- Clothing and accessories such as a jacket, hat, or sunglasses. The proctor may inspect any article of clothing.
    - Exception: The proctors have discretion to permit items of religious apparel to be worn.
- Other personal items such as a purse, backpack, or bag of any kind
- Food and beverages
    - Exception: Items documented as medically necessary

The following items will be provided to you by the proctor:

- A four-function calculator, if you are taking the paper-and-pencil version of the test. If your test is on the computer, then the calculator will be onscreen.
- Scratch paper. You may not write on this paper before the test begins or during your break, and you must return all scratch paper to the proctor at the end of the test.

Note that during the test, if you need to leave for any reason, you must raise your hand and be excused by the proctor. While you are out of the room, the timer will continue to count down; any time you miss cannot be made up. If you need the proctor's assistance for any other reason, such as a technical malfunction with your computer, raise your hand. Finally, if you find the test setting uncomfortable or inadequate, report your concern to the proctor before leaving the room at the end of the test.

## Your Scores

You will receive a composite score reflecting your overall performance and a sub-score for each content area. If you take the test online, you will see your scores immediately upon completion of the test. If you take the paper-and-pencil version, your scores will show up in your ATI online account within 48 hours of ATI's receiving the test from the testing site. In addition to your scores, the report will identify topics on which you missed questions. You can access your score report at the testmaker's website at any time by logging in.

Some schools require a certain composite score for admission, while others require you to meet a minimum score in each content area. Some schools do not have any specific cutoff scores for admission. Be sure to check with the program(s) to which you are applying to find out the requirements.

Be aware that some schools with a cutoff score require applicants to achieve the minimum score within a certain number of test administrations. For example, a school may require applicants to obtain the minimum score by taking the TEAS no more than twice. In this case, if you did not achieve the cutoff score after taking the test twice but did get a score above the threshold the third time you took the test, your application would still not meet that school's criteria for admission.

Finally, just because a school gives a minimum score or scores for admission, that does not mean that every applicant who meets or exceeds that score(s) is accepted. Other aspects of your application are generally considered as well. In the same way, a school that does not have a minimum TEAS score may nonetheless mostly accept students with high scores. Again, research the schools to which you are applying to find out what they seek in a successful candidate.

*Note:* All information in this section "About the TEAS" is current as this book goes to press. Check the ATI website at **atitesting.com** for the most up-to-date information.

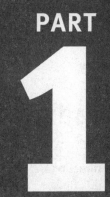

# TEAS Diagnostic Test

This diagnostic test is designed to help guide you in your preparation for the TEAS. You will learn several things from taking this test.

## What's on the TEAS?

The test you are about to take is designed to be very similar to the TEAS. This test is the same length as the TEAS. The questions are in the same multiple-choice format, and the knowledge and skills tested reflect those you will need to do well on Test Day. By the end of this test, you will have a very good idea of what to expect on Test Day in each of the four content areas tested: *Reading*, *Mathematics*, *Science*, and *English language and usage*.

Furthermore, following the diagnostic test are comprehensive answers and explanations of every question. Read all the explanations—of the questions you got right as well as those you got wrong. When you got a question correct, the explanation will validate and reinforce your approach, or it might reveal a strategy that would have gotten you to the right answer more quickly and confidently. When you missed a question, the explanation will teach you what you need to know to get a similar question right on Test Day.

## What Is It Like to Take the TEAS?

The TEAS is a 3.5-hour test. It's a long test! To evaluate your current mental endurance, take this diagnostic test under test-like conditions. Set aside a block of 4 hours when you won't be interrupted and find a quiet space. You won't be allowed to eat or drink during the test, so reserve refreshments for your breaks. Shut down email, social media, and other distractions.

If you find that fatigue interferes with your ability to do your best toward the end of the test, then plan to build up your mental endurance gradually, studying for longer and longer periods of time until you can focus on test material for several hours. Once you have used these pages to study, take the online test included with this book and see if your endurance has improved.

## What Are My Strengths? Where Are My Opportunities?

After you take this diagnostic test, use the Answers and Explanations immediately following the test to check your answers. Then use the Study Planner charts to analyze what content and skills you already feel comfortable with and which areas you need to study more. Use this analysis to plan how you will use this book.

# Reading

**Directions** You have 64 minutes to answer 53 questions. Do not work on any other section of the test during this time.

**Questions 1–2 are based on the following passage.**

The first detective stories, written by Edgar Allan Poe and Arthur Conan Doyle, emerged in the mid-nineteenth century, at a time when there was enormous public interest in science. The newspapers of the day continually publicized the latest scientific discoveries, and scientists were acclaimed as the heroes of the age. Poe and Conan Doyle shared this fascination with the methodical, logical approach used by scientists in their experiments and instilled their detective heroes with outstanding powers of scientific reasoning.

Granted, public knowledge and attitudes about science at the time were not the same as today's, and Doyle's lifelong interest in ghost hunting might appear malapropos for a rationalist. These apparent quirks aside, the spirit of science is hardly better exemplified or better known than in Doyle's stories, especially in the methods and attitude of his fictional detective, Sherlock Holmes.

1. According to the passage, Poe and Conan Doyle were similar in that

    (A) they both enjoyed gothic horror.
    (B) they wrote about heroes whose rational approach mirrored that of real-life scientists.
    (C) they wrote true accounts of police detective work for newspapers.
    (D) they were scientists.

2. The word "malapropos" means that an object or behavior is

    (A) scientific.
    (B) appropriate.
    (C) endearingly quirky.
    (D) out of place.

J. R. Sorensen, a critic of the judicial system, wrote, "In each of the last three years, a court in this country has awarded a settlement in excess of $300 million. This is a travesty of justice, and it unfairly burdens the court system, setting precedent as well as incentive for more and more suits of this kind."

3. What would Sorensen likely suggest to alleviate the strain on the courts?

    (A) There should be fewer lawsuits.
    (B) Courts should stop awarding such excessive settlements.
    (C) Lawsuits should name more than one defendant.
    (D) Larger out-of-court settlements should be awarded to ensure they meet victims' needs.

For do-it-yourself types, the cost of getting regular oil changes seems unnecessary. After all, the steps are fairly easy as long as you exercise basic safety precautions. First, make sure that the car is stationary and on a level surface. Always use the emergency brake to ensure that the car does not roll on top of you. Next, locate the drain plug for the oil under the engine. Remember to place the oil drain pan under the plug before you start. When the oil is drained fully, wipe off the drain plug and the plug opening and then replace the drain plug. Next, simply place your funnel in the engine and pour in new oil. Be sure to return the oil cap when you are done. Finally, run the engine for a minute and then check the dipstick to see if you need more oil in your engine.

4. After draining the old oil from the engine, you should

    (A) replace the oil cap.
    (B) run the engine for a moment and check the dipstick.
    (C) wipe off and replace the drain plug.
    (D) engage the emergency brake.

**Questions 5–10 are based on the following passage.**

Does true happiness come from within or from without? Do we achieve fulfillment when life circumstances happen to satisfy our desires, as the modern utilitarian view maintains? Or, on the contrary, is it as the ancient Stoics and Buddhists claim, that we become happy only through renouncing material wants and cultivating a positive perception and attitude?

In his landmark work, *The Happiness Hypothesis*, psychologist Jonathan Haidt shows that the source of happiness is neither internal nor external—or, more accurately, that it is both. Having embarked upon an ambitious project of cataloging the world's wisdom and then looking for scientific results that verify ancient proverbs, Haidt establishes that true happiness comes from "between," requiring a mix of internal and external conditions. Some of those conditions are within you, like your perspective and personality. Other conditions are external. Just as plants need sun, water, and good soil to thrive, people need love, work, and a connection to something larger to be happy.

5. The main idea of the passage is that

(A) Buddhism and utilitarianism both fail to explain or create happiness.
(B) ancient proverbs and philosophies contain wisdom that science has only recently acknowledged.
(C) even if a person has the best attitude in the world, there will be a limit to his or her emotional endurance.
(D) happiness requires a combination of the right internal attitude as well as external life circumstances.

6. According to the passage, which belief system states that people's happiness comes from the state of the world?

(A) Utilitarianism
(B) Experimental psychology
(C) Buddhism
(D) Stoicism

7. Why did the author of the passage describe utilitarianism in the second sentence?

(A) To support the main purpose of the passage by explaining the utilitarian perspective on happiness
(B) To provide an example of how a person can experience happiness from "between"
(C) To offer evidence against the idea that happiness is under internal control
(D) To provide an example of a belief system in which happiness is held to be influenced by external factors

8. What is the author's main goal in writing this passage?

(A) To argue that both internal attitude and life circumstances play a role in a person's happiness
(B) To explain that there are many views on how to achieve happiness, dating back thousands of years
(C) To argue that, while psychologists like Jonathon Haidt think they have figured out happiness, achieving happiness is not as simple as they claim
(D) To compare and contrast ancient Buddhist and Stoic beliefs on the topic of happiness

9. Suppose a new study revealed that the happiest people tend to have few attachments to material objects and want little besides what they already possess. What effect would this evidence have if the author included it in the passage?

(A) It would weaken the claim that happiness comes from "within."
(B) It would challenge the claim that happiness comes from "without."
(C) It would strengthen the claim that happiness comes from "without."
(D) It would support the claim that happiness comes from "between."

10. With which of the following statements would the author of the passage most likely NOT agree?

(A) Social services that provide food and housing to refugees and foster their sense of belonging make the world a happier place.
(B) Because there is more than one way to be happy, even someone in difficult circumstances can find joy with the right outlook.
(C) People who appreciate what they have tend to be happier than those who always seek to complain.
(D) Even a person who has everything can be unhappy, and their loved ones may not be able to help.

**K** | 3

11. Start with the figure below. Follow the instructions to rearrange its parts.

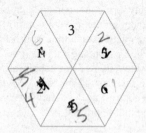

1. Switch the positions of numbers 1 and 6.
2. Switch the positions of numbers 2 and 5.
3. Switch the positions of numbers 4 and 5.

The shape now looks like which of the following?

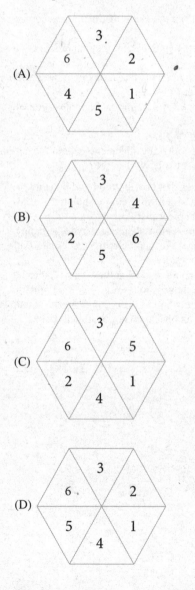

Many people strongly dislike snakes, finding them unappealing to look at and uncomfortable to touch. On the contrary, snakes are fascinating creatures, with their iridescent scales and elegant movements.

12. Which word best describes the author's attitude toward snakes?

(A) Disgusted
(B) Appreciative
(C) Uninterested
(D) Fearful

Dear Grandma,

Thanks so much for the birthday card! I love it. The flowers are so pretty. It's just like your garden. When the snow melts here in the Rockies, I'll come visit you and we can plant flowers together.

I love you!

13. Based on the information in this letter, the writer's birthday is most likely in

(A) January.
(B) May.
(C) August.
(D) September.

**"Akira Kurosawa," a paper by Jack Schroeder for English 410 (first draft)**

The Japanese filmmaker Akira Kurosawa (1910–1988) is renowned as one of the greatest directors in film history. He directed thirty films in his almost sixty-year career, and among his movies are classics like *Rashomon*, *Seven Samurai*, and *Yojimbo*. His first feature work was an action movie, but he later turned to William Shakespeare for inspiration, freely adapting the Bard's plays for his own films: *Throne of Blood* (*Macbeth*), *The Bad Sleep Well* (*Hamlet*), and *Ran* (*King Lear*). His films are highly regarded for their epic scope, striking visuals, and Kurosawa's keen interest in every aspect of filmmaking, including scriptwriting, casting, editing, and even set design. In 1990, he accepted a Lifetime Achievement from the Academy of Motion Picture Arts and Sciences…

**English 410: Advanced Topics in Shakespeare Adaptation**

This seminar will examine the influence of Shakespeare's plays and poetry on works in other media, including fiction, cinema, music, and the visual arts. Students will be expected to conduct independent research into adaptations of Shakespeare's work and bring their findings to class.

**STUDENT SURVEY! FREE MOVIE NIGHT!**

The University Student Association has received funding for extracurricular activities. We have decided to organize a weekly film night but want to hear from you! What kind of films would you like to see in our new series? Please email us your suggestions for movies we should include. Hope to hear from you!

___ Silent Comedies

___ Hollywood Horror

___ Classic International Japanese and German Cinema

___ English Spy Movies

14. Jack Schroeder is very concerned about getting high grades. Given the paper he is currently writing for English 410, which of the following is he most likely to do in response to the student survey?

(A) State his preference for Hollywood Horror because he wants to see *Throne of Blood*.
(B) Contact the Student Association and name some movies by Akira Kurosawa the Association should show.
(C) Choose English Spy Movies because he hopes there's still room in a very popular course on the spy novels of Ian Fleming and John le Carré.
(D) Ignore the petition because he will be too busy reading Shakespeare plays to watch movies.

**Questions 15–16 are based on the following story.**

For red-blooded American boys, baseball is a rite of passage. It's something passed on from father to son that creates a bond both between and within generations of men. Toby knew this because his father had explained it to him. Today's game was the final game of the season, but it was also the final league game, period, for this young man. Soon after his 16th birthday, he would be headed to the military academy as a fresh cadet, and his time for recreational sports would be finished.

As the sky cleared and sun at last rushed into the room, Toby smiled, knowing that the game would proceed as scheduled. It had to, if only because his father would be there and it would be the last opportunity he would have to see Toby play. Now the birds began to appear here and there. Toby had a special feeling about today. He got out his baseball glove and waited for his dad to arrive to take him to the game.

15. What were the author's intentions in writing this passage?

(A) To tell a story about a significant life milestone
(B) To inform the reader about the cultural and historical significance of baseball
(C) To argue for the importance of rituals in moving into new stages of life
(D) To share an opinion about baseball's cultural relevance

16. The mood of the character in the passage is

(A) sad.
(B) careless.
(C) uneasy.
(D) eager.

**Questions 17–18 are based on the following statements.**

The school board is considering the amount of homework students should be assigned and has solicited input from parents. The following statements were submitted to the board.

## More Homework!

Don't get me wrong. I don't exactly have fond memories of spending my evenings struggling through my high school chemistry work, but did I learn the subject better by putting the time in? You bet I did. And I didn't become a chemist, but as a small-business owner putting in those late nights when I just have to get my books up-to-date, or make the work schedule, or just clean up after a particularly busy day, I'm thankful that my parents didn't let me shirk my duties way back when. Being self-employed means no one's going to stand there and make you get your work done, so you better have the wherewithal to do what needs to be done without someone on your back. You learn this by challenging yourself and doing the work you signed up for.

## We're Really Starting Young with the Life Sentences Now

We're turning ourselves into a society with no boundaries and no work-life balance (the very fact that we have a term to describe this concept tells you that it's no longer a given), and we're starting younger and younger. My third-grade daughter is sitting at the kitchen table with me until nine o'clock at night trying to get her social studies homework done. Why? What happens if she's limited to the 36 hours per week she spends with her teacher? Will she know not quite enough about Jamestown to ever be successful in life? Is this what we're trading our quality time for each night? I don't want my kid to get an ulcer before she's even out of grade school, just to prepare her for the theoretical point in life when this ridiculous amount of work might actually become necessary rather than contrived.

17. What do the two authors disagree about?
    (A) They disagree over whether career success is important in life.
    (B) They disagree over how heavy the student workload actually is.
    (C) They disagree over whether the benefit of completing homework is worth the effort.
    (D) They disagree over whether quality time with one's family is worthwhile.

18. Which of the following statements, if true, would weaken both arguments in this passage?
    (A) A study shows that students who took heavier course loads and participated in more academic extracurricular activities showed a decreased ability to work independently in their later careers.
    (B) A survey of students in kindergarten through grade 12 found that most considered their academic load to be minimal and unchallenging.
    (C) In a state-wide survey, young children consistently listed "learning together" as one of the most enjoyable and important things they did with their parents.
    (D) A comparative study of syllabi shows that, on average, the academic workload at the college level has remained stable.

The English language is an amalgam of several other languages, but relies most heavily on Latin. Over time, new English words have often been created from Latin prefixes and roots. Thus, the word *ambidextrous* combines the Latin root *ambi*, meaning "both," and *dexter*, meaning "right-handed." Literally, this means "right-handed on both sides," but we interpret it as meaning being capable of using both hands equally well.

19. The word "ambidextrous" is used in the paragraph in order to
    (A) provide a supporting detail for the main idea.
    (B) introduce the primary topic.
    (C) illustrate a word that is always interpreted literally.
    (D) give an example of a Latin word.

Dear Janelle,

Sorry for taking so long to get back to you but it's so busy this time of year, as you know. To answer your question, the Marketing Department has decided to implement the new direct marketing campaign via social media because we feel that social media users tend to be the demographic—younger, cosmopolitan, educated—that our new app is designed to serve. It's an exciting opportunity for our group as a whole. The decision has already been made, but I thank you for your input.

Best,
Asafa

20. What is the author's purpose in writing this memo?
    (A) She is explaining the basis for a marketing decision.
    (B) She is ignoring Janelle's input.
    (C) She is apologizing for an unfortunate outcome.
    (D) She is suggesting that Janelle make more use of social media.

**Questions 21–23 are based on the following passage.**

The history of astronomy is very much the history of what became visible to human beings and when. The four brightest moons of Jupiter were the first objects in the solar system discovered with the use of the telescope. Their discovery played a central role in Galileo's famous argument in support of the Copernican model of the solar system, in which the planets are described as revolving around the sun. For several hundred years, scientific understanding of these moons was slow to develop. But spectacular close-up photographs sent back by the 1979 *Voyager* missions forever changed our perception of these moons, as did improved observations from the powerful Hubble Space Telescope.

Of course, there's a reason these moons were the first to be discovered—after Earth's own moon, of course. The table below shows the brightness (apparent magnitude) of different solar system objects as seen from Earth. There are nearer planetary satellites; indeed, Mars has two moons. However, distance is only one variable affecting brightness. Size is also very important. Note that on this scale, the higher the number, the fainter the object appears.

| Name of Moon (Planet It Orbits) | Apparent Magnitude |
| --- | --- |
| Luna (Earth's moon) | −12.6 |
| Ganymede (Jupiter) | 4.8 |
| Calipso (Jupiter) | 5.6 |
| Phobos (Mars) | 11.3 |
| Charon (Pluto) | 15.6 |

21. The main idea of the passage is that

   (A) the four moons of Jupiter provided strong evidence of Copernicus's solar system model.
   (B) the four moons of Jupiter provided strong evidence of Galileo's solar system model.
   (C) The telescope completely changed our understanding of the universe.
   (D) astronomy has advanced based on our ability to perceive different celestial objects.

22. Given the information in the passage, it's reasonable to assume that

   (A) the four moons of Jupiter would be brighter than Earth's moon if they were closer.
   (B) the planets were all discovered before their moons because the planets are larger.
   (C) the more powerful the telescope, the fainter the objects it can be used to discover.
   (D) an astronomer can use an object's brightness to determine how far away it is.

23. Based on the passage, which is the most reasonable value for the apparent magnitude of the sun?

   (A) −26.7
   (B) −5.4
   (C) 6.9
   (D) 31.2

Chef Marion: "You should add salt to water you wish to boil. Because salty water has a higher boiling point than unsalted water, you can cook at a higher temperature with it. Also, some foods, like pasta, taste better when cooked in salted water."

24. Which of the following is an opinion Chef Marion offers?

   (A) Food is healthier when cooked in unsalted water.
   (B) Added salt raises the temperature of boiling water.
   (C) Some foods taste better when cooked in salted water.
   (D) Salted water enables food to be cooked more quickly.

When painting a room, initially decide on the general color desired, for example, some shade of blue. Buy a small amount of several blue shades to test out at home. Paint a small patch of wall with each color. After letting the paint dry, determine which blue you prefer, buy an adequate amount of that color, and paint the entire room.

25. Which of the following is NOT a step in painting a room?

   (A) Painting small areas with blue and other colors
   (B) Choosing colors from dry samples
   (C) Deciding on the general color for the room
   (D) Buying small amounts of paint

**Questions 26–27 are based on the following passage.**

The English-born fashion designer Charles Frederick Worth is widely considered the inventor of haute couture, establishing new benchmarks for quality of construction and luxuriousness of materials. At his Paris salon, he created grand clothes for European royalty, including the Empress Eugénie. Despite his illustrious clientele and painstaking craftsmanship, his clothing was also suitable for everyday life. Yet, his importance goes beyond making beautiful dresses. Because of his relentless self-promotion—by the 1870s, his name was familiar not only to the wealthy women who could afford his creations but also to the readers of the newly popular women's magazines—he was the forerunner of today's superstar fashion designers. Thus, the structure of the fashion industry today owes a great deal to this nineteenth-century entrepreneur.

26. According to the passage, which of the following contributes to a piece of clothing being considered haute couture?

    (A) Its suitability for everyday life
    (B) Its appeal to European royalty
    (C) Its quality of construction and luxuriousness of materials
    (D) Its creator's relentless self-promotion

27. Which of the following statements, if true, would strengthen the author's argument?

    (A) Worth has a prominent entry in an encyclopedia of fashion throughout history.
    (B) Many fashion designers today seek to be well-known among people who cannot afford their clothes.
    (C) Worth's clothes for the Empress Eugénie are still considered a model for designers who receive commissions from European royal families.
    (D) Worth was not only famous during his lifetime but ran a highly profitable business.

What a week it had been! When Jason arrived late to work on Friday, he told his boss there had been a big accident on Maple Street and the police had shut down all the lanes. There was a detour, but unfortunately larger trucks could not take that route and had to backtrack several blocks instead. When Jason had finally arrived in the parking lot at work, he could only find spaces for compact cars. Jason's boss accepted the explanation, this time. At least Jason could sleep in the next morning.

28. Which of the following was NOT implied by Jason's story?

    (A) Jason had been late to work earlier in the week.
    (B) Jason drove down Maple on his way in to work.
    (C) Jason drives a larger truck.
    (D) Jason had to backtrack several blocks.

The Most Excellent Order of the British Empire, or MBE, is the order of chivalry of the British constitutional monarchy. In 1917, King George V identified a need to fill a gap in the British honors system, specifically to recognize those who had served in noncombat roles in the Great War (what would come to be known as the First World War). The war had lasted much longer than expected, and there was no way to acknowledge the contributions that civilians had made to the war effort at home or that military personnel had made in support positions. Soon after its foundation, the order was divided into military and civil divisions, and these days it continues to fulfill its original purpose in new ways, rewarding people for their contributions to public service, the arts and science, sports, and charity and welfare organizations.

29. Which of the following identifies the structure of the passage?

    (A) Biographical narrative
    (B) Compare and contrast
    (C) Opinion and rationale
    (D) Problem and solution

Total national expenditures on healthcare exceed those on transportation and related infrastructure, the justice system (including law enforcement), and even agriculture and food distribution. Could healthcare cost less than it does? Some people argue that high costs are inevitable because doctors have student loans to pay and pharmaceutical companies have a responsibility to their shareholders. However, it is worth looking at the largest costs to see whether a savings of a few percent might be possible. Considering the cost breakdown below, not much savings could be found in, for example, syringes, cotton swabs, and other disposable (nondurable) medical products. On the other hand, reducing the top two or three categories by a few percentage points could have a significant impact.

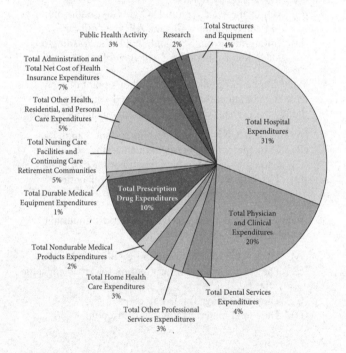

30. Which of the following cost-saving measures would the author of the passage be least likely to support?

(A) A pooling of hospitals' and clinics' procurement of surgical tools, such as laser scalpels, so these instruments are purchased at lower cost

(B) A self-service medical portal that lowers the incidence of unnecessary hospital and physician visits

(C) Incentives to encourage pharmaceutical companies to make the most commonly prescribed drugs available as less expensive generics

(D) A more efficient system of rural hospitals that would reduce the number of buildings and amount spent on overhead

Dear Editor,

Last week, this newspaper reported on the mayor's misguided plan to open two new municipally sponsored daycare centers. The mayor cites a lack of affordable child care as the reason that many parents, predominantly mothers, are not able to return to work. He promises that the daycare centers would improve the economy by providing high-paying jobs for daycare workers while also allowing skilled workers to return to work. Does he not realize that the average hourly wage in this county is barely $16, with many citizens earning much less, while he is promising daycare workers $14? Why should mothers go back to work for a net gain of $2 an hour, while other people raise their children? One parent, not necessarily a female parent, should stay at home to raise children until they're old enough to go to school. This is a goal worth investing in.

31. What is the flaw in the main argument of this letter to the editor?

(A) The $2 net gain calculation assumes equal hours for the parent and daycare worker.

(B) It assumes that one daycare worker will be required for each parent who wants to return to work.

(C) The mayor assumes that all parents are skilled workers.

(D) The author clearly has a personal opinion about whether parents should stay home with their children.

Jim was always smiling, so his friends complimented him on his sunny disposition.

32. Which of the following would be the best word to substitute for "sunny" in the above sentence?

(A) Rude
(B) Pleasant
(C) Grave
(D) Wooden

Thomas: "Our study group should concentrate on the respiratory system because that area of study made up a major portion of last year's anatomy and physiology final."

Martina: "Should we really waste valuable time on the respiratory system? Everyone knows our professor is new to the faculty and is an expert in the cardiovascular system."

33. Which word best describes Martina's tone?

    (A) Challenging
    (B) Encouraging
    (C) Understanding
    (D) Puzzled

## Questions 34–38 are based on the following passage.

In the young American democracy, public libraries were prized. Open to all without restriction, requiring no fees, and lending their collections freely, they were deemed important sources of knowledge to inform a literate and thoughtful citizenry. Though often funded by taxes, libraries benefited most significantly from their greatest private supporter, steel tycoon Andrew Carnegie. A self-educated Scottish immigrant, Carnegie spent $60 million to fund libraries. Though a ruthless businessman who refused to accede to workers' demands for higher pay, he believed that knowledge, not money, was the currency of value (as perhaps only a very wealthy man can believe). Carnegie lived by his statement that "the man who dies rich dies in disgrace." His first commissioned library was in his home town of Allegheny, Pennsylvania, followed by others in Pittsburgh. The Carnegie library in Washington, D.C., the city's oldest, bears over its entrance the motto "Dedicated to the diffusion of knowledge." Before he died in 1919, Carnegie built 1,689 libraries throughout the United States, which served hard-scrabble farmers and miners as well as middle-class and affluent patrons.

34. Which of the following provides the best summary of the passage?

    (A) A self-educated man, Andrew Carnegie lived by a motto that required him to give away most of his money.
    (B) As a ruthless tycoon, Carnegie believed that the accumulation of wealth was the most important endeavor in the young democracy.
    (C) Public libraries, which are important resources for educating people in a democracy, benefited greatly from Andrew Carnegie's library funding.
    (D) Andrew Carnegie subscribed to the idea that free libraries, open to all, are the foundation of a thriving democracy.

35. The primary purpose of the author's reference to the Washington, D.C., library is

    (A) to serve as an example of Carnegie's support for libraries.
    (B) to provide evidence for Carnegie's desire to beautify the nation's capital.
    (C) to explain the importance of libraries to a young nation.
    (D) to underscore the need for free access to public buildings.

36. Which of the following presents events in Andrew Carnegie's life in the correct order?

    (A) Becomes wealthy; returns to Scotland; builds the Washington, D.C., library
    (B) Immigrates from Scotland; becomes wealthy; builds the Allegheny library
    (C) Builds the Washington, D.C., library; builds libraries in Pennsylvania; builds the Allegheny library
    (D) Immigrates from Scotland; builds the Washington, D.C., library; builds the Allegheny library

37. What can be inferred about the author's point of view from the comment that Carnegie prized knowledge over money "as perhaps only a very wealthy man can believe"?

    (A) Knowledge is always more important than money.
    (B) Carnegie was hypocritical in amassing wealth.
    (C) Carnegie misunderstood the importance of money.
    (D) The very wealthy can afford to downplay the importance of money.

38. According to the passage, what is the most important characteristic of libraries?

    (A) There were over a thousand free libraries by 1919.
    (B) They provide needed information for knowledgeable citizens.
    (C) They are always funded by taxes.
    (D) They lend materials without restriction.

**Questions 39–40 are based on the following passage.**

There are three European professional cycling stage races in the Grand Tour: Giro d'Italia, Tour de France, and Vuelta a España. The oldest and most enjoyable is the Tour de France, first held in 1903 and usually taking place in July. Originally launched to promote a sports newspaper, it is now the most famous bicycle race in the world. The Giro d'Italia and Vuelta a España are held to be almost as prestigious by professional cyclists and the sport's fans, and together the three races make up the Grand Tour of professional race cycling. The Giro d'Italia was originally mounted a few years after the first Tour de France to promote the newspaper *Gazzetta dello Sport*, but the Vuelta a España first ran in 1935. Originally run in April, not long before the Giro d'Italia, the Vuelta a España now takes place in the fall.

39. In which sentence does the author make a value judgment?

(A) The first sentence
(B) The second sentence
(C) The fourth sentence
(D) The author makes no value judgments.

40. Which is the current annual sequence for the races that make up the Grand Tour?

(A) Tour de France, Giro d'Italia, Vuelta a España
(B) Giro d'Italia, Tour de France, Vuelta a España
(C) Vuelta a España, Giro d'Italia, Tour de France
(D) Vuelta a España, Tour de France, Giro d'Italia

Marcus should have been happy on his wedding day, but he looked dolefully toward the chapel door for his bride-to-be.

41. Which of the following is the meaning of "dolefully" as used in the sentence?

(A) Eagerly
(B) Joyously
(C) Sadly
(D) Warily

**Questions 42–43 are based on the following story.**

# Jovian Mining

"What's the old man like?" Buck asked, as Cole fiddled with the old radio.

"Like all the other damn fools who come out two billion miles to scratch rock, as if there weren't enough already on the inner planets. He's got a rich platinum property. Sells 90 percent of his output to buy his power, and the other 11 percent for his clothes and food."

"He must be an efficient miner, to maintain 101 percent production like that."

"No, but his bank account is. He's figured out that's the most economic level of production. If he produces less, he won't be able to pay for his heating power, and if he produces more, his operation will burn up his bank account too fast."

"I take it he's not after money—just the fun," suggested Buck.

"Oh, no. He's after money," replied Cole gravely. "You ask him—he's going to make his eternal fortune yet by striking a real bed of jovium, and then he'll retire."

"Oh, one of that kind."

"They all are," Cole laughed. "Eternal hope, and the rest of it."

*Source:* Excerpted from *The Ultimate Weapon*, by John W. Campbell, 1936. This work is in the public domain.

42. What is the main idea that emerges in Buck and Cole's conversation?

(A) Miners are practical in the everyday details of their work but have wildly optimistic dreams of making their fortune.
(B) Only the desperate and foolish become miners, especially on the outer planets.
(C) The misunderstood miner is a romantic frontiersman, only interested in the adventure.
(D) Hard and steady work will eventually pay off.

43. It can be inferred from the passage that

(A) most miners eventually lose all their money.
(B) Buck and Cole look down on the miners.
(C) jovium is both rarer and more valuable than platinum.
(D) Buck and Cole have been working together for years.

A wise man once said that you can lead a child to school but you can't make him learn. It's long been established that a person's grit—that is, their perseverance, their confidence, and their endurance—is the greatest predictor of their future success. Yet parents spend a fortune on expensive prep schools and colleges they can hardly afford for kids who refuse to break a sweat. They would be better off sending their kids to military boot camp first and college second. It would be cheaper, and all those push-ups might actually help a kid lift those oh-so-heavy textbook covers.

44. Based on this passage, what underlying belief does the author have?

    (A) Military training helps build "grit."
    (B) Being accepted to college is a good indicator that a student is a diligent, self-reliant learner.
    (C) Students with "grit" don't need to do as much reading in college courses as their classmates with less character.
    (D) Parents who spend a lot of money on their children's education make the children lazy.

### Questions 45–46 are based on the following postcard.

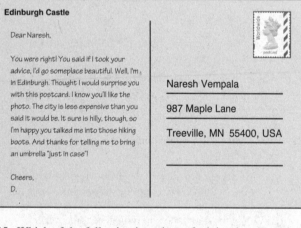

Edinburgh Castle

Dear Naresh,

You were right! You said if I took your advice, I'd go someplace beautiful. Well, I'm in Edinburgh. Thought I would surprise you with this postcard. I know you'll like the photo. The city is less expensive than you said it would be. It sure is hilly, though, so I'm happy you talked me into those hiking boots. And thanks for telling me to bring an umbrella "just in case"!

Cheers,
D.

Naresh Vempala

987 Maple Lane

Treeville, MN 55400, USA

45. Which of the following is a piece of advice that the author did NOT get from Naresh?

    (A) Bring an umbrella.
    (B) Wear hiking boots.
    (C) Visit Edinburgh.
    (D) Buy a photo postcard of Edinburgh Castle.

46. Which of the following questions would the postcard writer have logically asked in order to reach a conclusion based on Naresh's advice?

    (A) Is Edinburgh a beautiful city?
    (B) Is Edinburgh Castle an impressive structure?
    (C) Will Naresh enjoy receiving a postcard?
    (D) Are there less expensive places to visit than Edinburgh?

The night before a workday, I set my alarm for 8:00 AM after I make sure my watch battery is charged. In the morning, when my alarm rings, I hit the snooze button to get 10 extra minutes of blissful sleep. After the alarm rings for the second time, I make a mental checklist of things I have to do at work and any plans I've made for after work. Then it's time to start my day.

47. What does the author of the passage state is the first step in preparing for the workday?

    (A) "I set my alarm for 8:00 AM."
    (B) "I hit the snooze button."
    (C) "I make a mental checklist of things I have to do at work."
    (D) "I make sure my watch battery is charged."

### Questions 48–49 are based on the following passage.

The media are really out of control. When the press gets a story, it seems that within minutes it has produced flashy moving graphics and sound effects to entice viewers and garner ratings. Real facts and unbiased coverage of an issue are totally abandoned in exchange for an overly sentimental or one-sided story that too often distorts the truth. Unless viewers learn to recognize real reporting from the junk on nearly every television channel these days, they will be badly misinformed about current events.

48. In this passage, the author refers to graphics and sound effects in order to

    (A) give examples of features that make news reports more interesting and relevant.
    (B) define through specific examples what he means by "junk."
    (C) draw a distinction between biased and neutral reporting.
    (D) illustrate ways in which the media depart from unbiased news reporting.

49. The author's primary purpose in writing this passage is to

    (A) criticize indiscriminate television viewers.
    (B) support the use of graphics and sound effects to add interest to a news report.
    (C) distinguish between biased and neutral news reporting.
    (D) condemn the media for distorting news reports.

**Questions 50–51 are based on the following passage.**

The first passage below is a newspaper article about recent legislation. The second is a letter to the editor of that newspaper in response to the legislation.

## New Tractor License Requirements

State senators narrowly passed a bill last week that will require minors to have their tractor license (available at the age of 14 1/2 in this state) when working the land with heavy equipment, even on their own family's farms. Prior to this bill's passing, a license was only required when operating a tractor on public rural roads, necessary only when crossing from one field to another. The bill's sponsors argued that while state laws permit children to work in a family business when they would be too young to work under other circumstances, it's necessary to take special steps to protect minors from potentially dangerous work. The bill, which was passed as a Child Labor Law amendment and not part of the Highway Traffic Act, will prevent children too young to hold a tractor license from operating heavy equipment, though not from working on their family farm.

## Thanks for "Taking Care" of Us

I was so pleased to read about how the state senators, desperate for something to do with their time, decided to start adding more restrictions on how struggling farmers can run their business. There have been farmers here longer than there have been state senators, and I should know: my family homesteaded in this county almost two hundred years ago, and we've always taken good care of our kids. But please, by all means, tell us how to raise our children and put food on *your* table, all while ignoring the economic realities of this industry. One season after another, we keep getting asked to do more with less, and we'll keep doing it. Until one day we can't. But I'm sure the state senate will find a way to bail us out. They're so good at dealing with nonexistent problems, they've probably gotten all the practice they need to deal with the real ones they've created.

50. What is the main point of disagreement between the farmer who wrote the response to the news story and the state officials who sponsored and approved the bill?

(A) The state senators want to restrict all children under the age of 14 1/2 from working, while the farmer claims that family-owned businesses need this labor.

(B) The farmer disagrees with the state senators' assumptions about safety issues in child farm labor.

(C) The state senators and the farmer disagree about whether children's safety or farming families' economic security should be a higher priority.

(D) The state senators argue that there is high risk of injury to children from farmwork, while the farmer claims the danger lies only in operating heavy equipment.

51. The farmer who wrote the response to the news article apparently believes that

(A) this bill will make operating farms more difficult for families by preventing them from hiring neighborhood children for lower wages.

(B) the state is actively trying to destroy the agriculture industry.

(C) minor injuries are all part of a day's work and this is a lesson children should learn.

(D) the state overestimates the danger to children of operating tractors.

There are five species of frigate birds, a family of seabirds found across tropical and subtropical oceans. Three of the species are widespread, _____ two are endangered with restricted breeding habitats.

52. Which of the following words best completes the blank?

(A) while
(B) therefore
(C) consequently
(D) because

Fortunately, the election campaign has seen a shift from pejorative vilification to constructive debate in the last few weeks.

53. Which of the following words has a positive connotation as used here?

(A) shift
(B) pejorative
(C) vilification
(D) constructive

IF YOU FINISH BEFORE TIME IS CALLED, YOU MAY CHECK YOUR WORK ON THIS SECTION ONLY. DO NOT TURN TO ANY OTHER SECTION IN THE TEST.

**STOP**

# Mathematics

**Directions** You have 54 minutes to answer 36 questions. Do not work on any other section of the test during this time. You may use a four-function calculator for this section of the test only.

1. What is the decimal equivalent of 4.5%?

   (A) 0.0045
   (B) 0.045
   (C) 0.45
   (D) 4.5

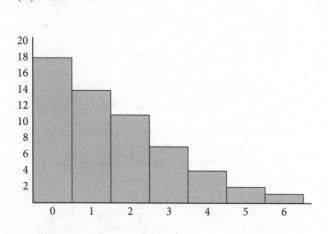

2. Which of the following correctly describes the distribution portrayed by the above graph?

   (A) Skewed right
   (B) Skewed left
   (C) Normal
   (D) Symmetrical

3. $4y + 36 = 128$

   Solve for $y$ in the equation above. Which of the following is correct?

   (A) 23
   (B) 41
   (C) 92
   (D) 164

4. A restaurant worker is cutting oranges. He cuts each orange into six slices and can cut up one orange every 15 seconds. If he maintains this rate, how many slices will he create in 15 minutes?

   (A) 60
   (B) 90
   (C) 225
   (D) 360

5. A study conducted early in the 20th century found that the more telephones that were present in a household, the higher the incidence of cancer. Which of the following must be true about the relationship between telephones and cancer based on the results of the study?

   (A) There was a positive covariance between the number of telephones and the incidence of cancer.
   (B) There was a negative covariance between the number of telephones and the incidence of cancer.
   (C) There was no cause and effect relationship between telephones and cancer.
   (D) Talking on the telephone causes cancer.

6. There are marbles of four different colors in a bag. The ratio of red to white to blue marbles is 3:4:5. There are half as many green marbles as there are blue marbles. What is the least possible number of marbles in the bag?

   (A) 12
   (B) 24
   (C) 29
   (D) 58

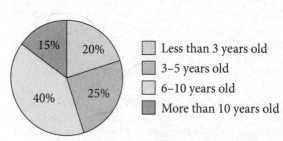

**Age of Apple Trees**

7. A fruit orchard has 300 apple trees. The chart above shows the distribution of ages of the apple trees. How many apple trees are 5 years old or younger?

   (A) 45
   (B) 75
   (C) 135
   (D) 165

8. The children at a nursery school are painting eggs for a holiday party. They paint a total of 30 eggs. They paint 5 of the eggs blue, 5 of the eggs yellow, 5 of the eggs pink, and the remaining eggs green. What fraction of the eggs are painted green?

   (A) $\dfrac{1}{15}$

   (B) $\dfrac{1}{6}$

   (C) $\dfrac{5}{15}$

   (D) $\dfrac{1}{2}$

9. What is the value of $27 \times 47 \times 31 \times 61$?

   (A) 2,399,679
   (B) 2,401,775
   (C) 2,403,094
   (D) 2,405,353

10. $1\dfrac{7}{8} \times 3\dfrac{1}{5}$

    Simplify the expression above.

    (A) $\dfrac{21}{40}$

    (B) $\dfrac{4}{5}$

    (C) $3\dfrac{7}{40}$

    (D) 6

11. A physical therapist is using a wide elastic band to help a patient strengthen his knee after surgery. At the patient's current stage of therapy, he should not exert more than 20 kilograms weight of force. The band being used for this therapy exerts a force of 40 grams of weight for every millimeter it is extended. The relationship between force applied and the distance the band is extended is linear. What is the maximum distance the therapist should allow the patient to extend the band?

    (A) 5 millimeters
    (B) 5 centimeters
    (C) 5 decimeters
    (D) 80 centimeters

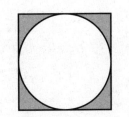

12. A circle is inscribed in a square as shown in the figure above. If the side length of the square is 6 inches, what is the area of the shaded region, in square inches?

    (A) $36 - 9\pi$
    (B) $36 - 6\pi$
    (C) $36 + 6\pi$
    (D) $36 - 3\pi$

13. $4,\ 3.35,\ \dfrac{11}{3},\ \dfrac{13}{4},\ \dfrac{7}{2}$

    Order the numbers above from least to greatest.

    (A) $\dfrac{7}{2}, \dfrac{11}{3}, \dfrac{13}{4}, 3.35, 4$

    (B) $\dfrac{13}{4}, 3.35, \dfrac{7}{2}, \dfrac{11}{3}, 4$

    (C) $4, 3.35, \dfrac{13}{4}, \dfrac{11}{3}, \dfrac{7}{2}$

    (D) $4, \dfrac{11}{3}, \dfrac{7}{2}, 3.35, \dfrac{13}{4}$

14. A nurse in a postsurgical ward records the blood pressure of a certain client no fewer than 2 times per hour and no more than 6 times per hour. Which expression describes the number of times, $n$, that the nurse will record the client's blood pressure in an 8-hour shift?

    (A) $8 \le n \le 48$
    (B) $16 \le n \le 48$
    (C) $16 \ge n \ge 48$
    (D) $16 \le n \le 64$

15. A personal trainer produces her own brand of sports drink to distribute to her clients. She produces the drink by diluting a commercial nutrient mix into a 15 percent concentrated solution. The commercial nutrient mix is sold by the bottle, in bottles containing 10 ounces each. How many bottles of the nutrient mix will the trainer need to buy to produce 240 ounces of her sports drink?

    (A) 3
    (B) 4
    (C) 24
    (D) 36

16. $\dfrac{7}{8}+\dfrac{5}{6}+\dfrac{3}{4}$    $\dfrac{15}{18}$

    Simplify the expression above.

    (A) $\dfrac{5}{8}$

    (B) $\dfrac{5}{6}$

    (C) $2\dfrac{5}{12}$

    (D) $2\dfrac{11}{24}$

17. If the ratio of $a$ to $b$ is 4 to 3 and the ratio of $b$ to $c$ is 1 to 5, what is the ratio of $a$ to $c$?

    (A) $\dfrac{4}{15}$

    (B) $\dfrac{1}{3}$

    (C) $\dfrac{2}{5}$

    (D) $\dfrac{4}{5}$

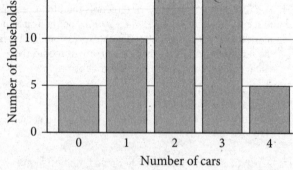

Number of cars

18. The bar graph above shows the number of cars owned per household for 50 households. According to the graph, how many households own at least three cars?

    (A) 4
    (B) 5
    (C) 15
    (D) 20

19. $917 \div 31 \times 4$

    What is the value of the expression above, rounded to the nearest whole number?

    (A) 70
    (B) 94
    (C) 118
    (D) 152

20. A fuel tank initially contains 180 L of fuel. After 360 L are added, the tank is $\dfrac{5}{8}$ full. What is the total capacity of the tank?

    (A) 576 L
    (B) 864 L
    (C) 1000 L
    (D) 1244 L

21. How many milligrams are in 2 kilograms?

    (A) 2,000,000
    (B) 200,000
    (C) 20,000
    (D) 2,000

22. In the following equations, the variable $p$ is independent and $q$ is dependent. In which equation is the relationship between $p$ and $q$ positively covariant?

    (A) $q = p^2 + 4$
    (B) $q = p + 4 - p$
    (C) $q = p + 4$
    (D) $q = 4 - p$

23. Which of the following expressions is equal to
    $$6a + \dfrac{4(a-8)}{2} + a + 1 ?$$

    (A) $6a + 33$
    (B) $9a - 15$
    (C) $9a - 31$
    (D) $11a + 17$

24. A bicyclist regularly travels the same route during training for a race. There are three segments on this route: an uphill segment, a level segment, and a downhill segment. On the uphill segment, the bicyclist travels at 15 mph and covers the distance in 20 minutes. On the level segment, she travels at 20 mph and covers the distance in 1 hour. On the downhill segment, she travels at 30 mph. If the entire trip takes her 2 hours to complete, what is the distance of all three segments combined?

    (A) 32.5 miles
    (B) 45 miles
    (C) 65 miles
    (D) 95 miles

25. Janice received a large bonus, so she treated her friends to lunch at a local restaurant. The total price for the food and beverages was $110.50 before sales tax was added. Later, when Janice was reviewing her monthly charge card statement, she noticed that the total amount she had paid, including the tip and 6% sales tax, was an even $140. Rounded to the nearest tenth, what percentage of the price plus tax was the tip that Janice left for the server?

    (A) 15.0%
    (B) 19.5%
    (C) 20.7%
    (D) 26.7%

26. $2\times(8\times10-5)+5$

    What is the value of the expression above?

    (A) 85
    (B) 155
    (C) 160
    (D) 165

27. A gardener plants a 60-square-foot vegetable garden with carrot seeds and lettuce seeds. In each square foot of the garden, he plants either 6 carrot seeds or 2 lettuce seeds. If he plants two-thirds of the area of the garden with carrot seeds, and the remaining area with lettuce seeds, what is the ratio of lettuce seeds to carrot seeds?

    (A) 6:1
    (B) 1:2
    (C) 1:3
    (D) 1:6

28. April purchased a bottle of spring water on her way to work. After her morning break, she noticed that she had consumed $\frac{2}{7}$ of her water. After her afternoon break, $\frac{1}{3}$ of the water remained. Approximately what was the percentage change in the amount of water left in April's bottle between the two times that she noted the level of the bottle's contents?

    (A) 53%
    (B) 27%
    (C) −53%
    (D) −71%

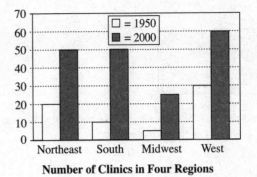

**Number of Clinics in Four Regions**

29. The bar graph above shows the number of clinics in different regions in the years 1950 and 2000. What was the average of the number of clinics in the South and West in 1950?

    (A) 10
    (B) 20
    (C) 40
    (D) 55

30. At a pharmacy, the ratio of containers of a brand-name prescription medicine to the generic version of that medicine is 7:2. If the pharmacy adds 6 more containers of the generic version to its inventory, the ratio becomes 11:4. What was the original total number of containers of the two medicines in stock?

    (A) 11
    (B) 22
    (C) 77
    (D) 99

31. $3+5\times(8+4)\div3-7$

    What is the value of the expression above?

    (A) 14
    (B) 16
    (C) 25
    (D) 30

32. $3m-15=\dfrac{m}{2}+110$

    Solve for $m$ in the equation above. Which of the following is correct?

    (A) 25
    (B) 38
    (C) 50
    (D) 125

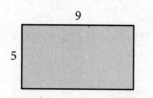

33. What is the area, in square units, of a square that has the same perimeter as the rectangle above?

 (A) 25
 (B) 36
 (C) 49
 (D) 64

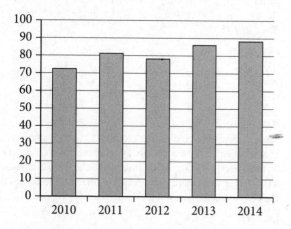

34. The graph above shows a farm's production of sorghum by year. The acreage devoted to sorghum was cut significantly in 2015, and, as a result, that year's sorghum crop was half that of 2012's production. How much sorghum was produced in 2015?

 (A) 36,000 bushels
 (B) 39,000 bushels
 (C) 40,000 bushels
 (D) 42,000 bushels

35. Approximately how many ounces are in four kilograms? (Note: 1 kilogram ≈ 2.2 pounds and 1 pound = 16 ounces.)

 (A) 140.8
 (B) 35.2
 (C) 29.1
 (D) 7.3

36. Jan is a pet sitter who wants to build a kennel and a dog run in her yard. The kennel will be a square enclosure 9 feet on a side, and the dog run will be a rectangular enclosure 6 feet wide by 20 feet long. If she wants to completely fence each enclosure, what is the total length of fencing Jan will need?

 (A) 38 feet
 (B) 62 feet
 (C) 64 feet
 (D) 88 feet

IF YOU FINISH BEFORE TIME IS CALLED, YOU MAY CHECK YOUR WORK ON THIS SECTION ONLY. DO NOT TURN TO ANY OTHER SECTION IN THE TEST. YOU MAY NOW TAKE A 10-MINUTE BREAK.    **STOP**

3/9

# Science

**Directions** You have 63 minutes to answer 53 questions. Do not work on any other section of the test during this time.

1. Which of the following are parts of a neuron?

   (A) Brain, spinal column, and nerve cells
   (B) Autonomic and somatic
   (C) Dendrites, axon, and soma
   (D) Sympathetic and parasympathetic

2. Which of the following organelles is NOT involved in protein translation or processing?

   (A) Ribosome
   (B) Rough ER
   (C) Mitochondrion
   (D) Golgi apparatus

3. Which of the following is primarily absorbed in the ileum?

   (A) Vitamin K
   (B) Carbohydrates
   (C) Water
   (D) Vitamin $B_{12}$

4. Which of the following correctly includes all the layers of the skin, from the deepest layer outward?

   (A) hypodermis, dermis, epidermis
   (B) subcutaneous, sebaceous, dermis
   (C) sebaceous, epidermis, dermis
   (D) dermis, hypodermis, epidermis

5. Which of the following is NOT a possible pairing of period numbers and orbital names?

   (A) 2 and $d$
   (B) 3 and $d$
   (C) 2 and $s$
   (D) 2 and $p$

6. Which of the following is NOT a possible consequence of hypertension?

   (A) Vascular scarring from increased plaque buildup
   (B) Hemoglobin not properly binding to oxygen
   (C) Stroke or aneurysm resulting from blood clots
   (D) Heart or kidney failure from poor vascularization

7. Which of the following is NOT a function of the kidney?

   (A) Filtering blood
   (B) Maintaining blood pressure
   (C) Activating vitamin D
   (D) Storing urea

8. How many milligrams are in 10 grams?

   (A) 100 mg
   (B) 1000 mg
   (C) 10,000 mg
   (D) 100,000 mg

9. In which of the following would blood pressure be the highest?

   (A) Aorta
   (B) Capillaries
   (C) Pulmonary arteries
   (D) Vena cava

**Questions 10–12 are based on the following diagram.**

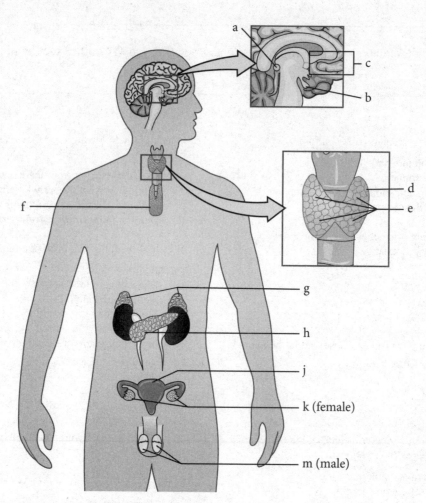

Each letter in the diagram corresponds to a specific anatomical body part. Use the letters above to answer the following questions.

10. Which of the following secretes the hormone that regulates sleep cycle?

    (A) a
    (B) d
    (C) f
    (D) g

11. Which of the following is stimulated to release hormones by an electrical signal?

    (A) b
    (B) c
    (C) e
    (D) k

12. In which of the following would progesterone be produced in response to a surge of luteinizing hormone (LH)?

    (A) b
    (B) j
    (C) k
    (D) m

13. Which of the following is NOT a function of surfactant in the lungs?

    (A) Prevent alveolar collapse
    (B) Increase gas exchange
    (C) Decrease gas exchange
    (D) Decrease surface tension

14. Which of the following correctly describes the sequence of chemical digestion in the stomach?

    (A) Glucagon stimulates the release of gastric juice.
    (B) Gherlin stimulates the release of HCl and pepsin.
    (C) Gastrin stimulates the release of HCl and pepsinogen.
    (D) Goblet cells stimulate the release of pepsin and pepsinogen.

15. Which of the following are responsible for transmitting a motor impulse across the neuromuscular junction?

    (A) Neurotransmitters
    (B) Nodes of Ranvier
    (C) Calcium ions
    (D) Action potentials

16. When the body temperature becomes abnormally high, which of the following homeostatic processes occurs?

    (A) Sweat gland activity and blood flow to the subcutaneous layer of the skin increase, and hair follicles relax.
    (B) Sweat gland activity and blood flow to the subcutaneous layer of the skin increase, and hair follicles contract.
    (C) Sweat gland activity increases, blood flow to the subcutaneous layer of the skin decreases, and hair follicles relax.
    (D) Sweat gland activity decreases, blood flow to the subcutaneous layer of the skin increases, and hair follicles relax.

17. Which of the following is an enzyme that regulates arterial blood pressure?

    (A) Epinephrine
    (B) Renin
    (C) Glucagon
    (D) Nephron

18. Which of the following physical properties changes when volume changes but mass is held constant?

    (A) Electronegativity
    (B) Density
    (C) Atomic radius
    (D) First ionization energy

19. Which of the following could result when the body is exposed to a live pathogen?

    (A) Active immunity
    (B) Passive immunity
    (C) Antigen resistance
    (D) Autoimmune disease

20. A person complains of sciatica, pain that shoots from the lower back through the hips and legs. What is the most likely cause?

    (A) Herniated lumbar disc
    (B) Fractured coccyx
    (C) Bruised calf muscle
    (D) Myocardial infarction

21. A recent editorial critical of a political candidate alleged, among other things, that she is more popular with less educated voters than with those with more education. The candidate believes that she is equally popular among voters across all levels of education. Her campaign manager wants to conduct a poll to ascertain which belief is correct. What would be an appropriate null hypothesis to test with the poll?

    (A) The candidate is more popular among voters with less education than voters with more education.
    (B) Other candidates are more popular among voters with more education.
    (C) There is no correlation between the candidate's popularity and voters' income levels.
    (D) There is no correlation between the candidate's popularity and voters' education.

22. Which of the following is NOT found in smooth muscle?

    (A) Actin
    (B) Myosin
    (C) Sarcomere
    (D) Gap junction

**Questions 23–25 are based on the following information.**

For most substances, the solid phase is the densest, with molecules tightly packed in an orderly pattern. Water is the only substance that is denser as a liquid than as a solid and, as a result, has special properties. The phase diagram of water is shown below.

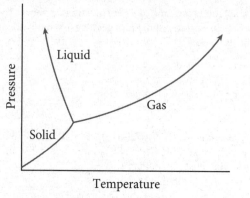

**Phase Diagram of Water**

A scientist set out to determine how the presence of contaminants in water changed its freezing point. The scientist added increasing concentrations of sodium chloride to water and measured the freezing point of each solution. The results are summarized in the following table.

| Solution Composition | Freezing Point (°C) |
|---|---|
| Pure Water | 0 |
| 1M | −2 |
| 2M | −4 |
| 3M | −6 |

**Experimental Results**

23. What would eventually happen to solid ice when the pressure is significantly increased at constant temperature?

 (A) It would become a denser form of ice.
 (B) It would melt to form the less dense liquid state.
 (C) It would melt to form the denser liquid state.
 (D) There would be no change.

24. Which of the following is a valid conclusion that can be made from the freezing point data?

 (A) Salt increases the freezing point of water, enabling it to melt at higher temperatures.
 (B) Salt decreases the freezing point of water, enabling it to melt at higher temperatures.
 (C) Salt decreases the freezing point of water, enabling it to melt at lower temperatures.
 (D) Salt increases the freezing point of water, enabling it to melt at lower temperatures.

25. Which of the following is NOT an endothermic process?

 (A) Melting
 (B) Sublimation
 (C) Vaporization
 (D) Deposition

26. In its final stage, the HIV virus disrupts the immune system by which of the following methods?

 (A) Destroying lymphocytic cells that contain an antigen signature
 (B) Favoring the production of memory cells over immunoglobulins
 (C) Overproducing IgE and triggering a histamine reaction
 (D) Preventing the activation of cytotoxic T cells

27. Which of the following correctly describes the role of the integumentary system?

 (A) Maintains adequate blood volume
 (B) Protects the body against dehydration
 (C) Secretes hormones into the bloodstream
 (D) Expels excess fluid from the body

28. The price of a call option at any point in time depends upon, among other factors, the number of days remaining until the option expires and the price of the underlying stock upon which the option is based. Some representative values are shown in the following table.

| Days Remaining | Stock Price | Call Price |
| --- | --- | --- |
| 30 | $20.00 | $1.00 |
| 60 | $20.00 | $1.75 |
| 90 | $20.00 | $2.00 |
| 30 | $40.00 | $2.00 |
| 60 | $40.00 | $3.50 |
| 90 | $40.00 | $4.00 |
| 30 | $60.00 | $3.00 |
| 60 | $60.00 | $5.25 |
| 90 | $60.00 | $6.00 |

Which of the following is true based on the relationships that can be determined from the data in the table?

(A) Call prices are unrelated to either stock prices or days remaining.
(B) Call prices are positively, linearly related to both stock prices and days remaining.
(C) Call prices are positively, linearly related to stock prices and positively, but not linearly, related to days remaining.
(D) Call prices are positively, but not linearly, related to stock prices and positively, linearly related to days remaining.

29. Which of the following correctly identifies the location of the sternum on the body?

(A) Superior and ventral
(B) Superior and dorsal
(C) Inferior and ventral
(D) Inferior and dorsal

30. Under normal circumstances, which of the following is normally found in urine?

(A) Glucose
(B) Urea
(C) Blood cells
(D) Amino acids

31. Which of the following statements is true of ventricular systole?

(A) The ventricles relax and are passively filled with blood.
(B) The ventricles are forcibly filled with blood from the atria.
(C) The semilunar valves open under increased pressure.
(D) The atrioventricular (AV) valves open under increased pressure

32. A researcher found that 17 percent of people suffering from chronic pain described themselves as very unhappy with their lives and 30 percent said they were somewhat unhappy. When he studied a group of people with the same demographic characteristics who were not experiencing chronic pain, only 6 percent said they were very unhappy with their lives and 17 percent were somewhat unhappy. Based on the results of his study, the researcher concluded that unhappiness is a major cause of chronic pain. Which of the following errors did the researcher make in reaching his conclusion?

(A) He equated correlation with causation.
(B) The study was biased.
(C) He only performed one study.
(D) He did not have a null hypothesis.

33. Which of the following nervous systems work in tandem to maintain homeostasis of the body?

(A) Central and peripheral
(B) Autonomic and sympathetic
(C) Somatic and autonomic
(D) Sympathetic and parasympathetic

34. Which of the following involves chemical digestion?

(A) Salivating
(B) Swallowing
(C) Chewing
(D) Belching

35. Which of the following is NOT composed of macromolecules?

(A) Carbohydrate
(B) Gastric acid
(C) Nucleic acid
(D) Lipid

36. Homeostatic control of blood glucose by insulin and glucagon is achieved by which of the following?

    (A)  A decrease in blood glucose stimulates glucagon; an increase in blood glucose stimulates insulin.
    (B)  An increase in insulin lowers blood glucose; an increase in blood glucose stimulates glucagon.
    (C)  A increase in blood glucose stimulates glucagon; a decrease in blood glucose stimulates insulin.
    (D)  An increase in glucagon lowers blood glucose; a decrease in insulin lowers blood glucose.

37. Balance the chemical equation

    ____ $Hg(OH)_2$ + ____ $H_3PO_4$ → $Hg_3(PO_4)_2$ + ____ $H_2O$

    by identifying the coefficients that correctly fill in the blanks.

    (A)  2, 3, 6
    (B)  3, 2, 6
    (C)  3, 2, 8
    (D)  6, 4, 12

38. Which of the following is a short bone?

    (A)  Phalange
    (B)  Tarsal
    (C)  Scapula
    (D)  Radius

39. Which hormone is responsible for triggering ovulation?

    (A)  Luteinizing hormone
    (B)  Estrogen
    (C)  Corpus luteum
    (D)  Progesterone

40. Which of the following would decrease the rate of diffusion of oxygen from the lungs into the bloodstream?

    (A)  Decreasing the concentration of oxygen in the blood
    (B)  Increasing the surface area of the alveoli
    (C)  Increasing the concentration of carbon dioxide in the blood
    (D)  Increasing the concentration of oxygen in the blood

41. The prescribed dose of a certain medication is 1 deciliter. The amount administered must be accurate to within ±1 percent. The amount being administered should be measured in what unit to the nearest whole number to ensure that the needed accuracy is attained?

    (A)  Decaliters
    (B)  Deciliters
    (C)  Milliliters
    (D)  Microliters

42. Which of the following produces bile?

    (A)  Gall bladder
    (B)  Bile duct
    (C)  Duodenum
    (D)  Liver

43. Which of the following correctly pairs the reproductive structure with its function?

    (A)  Fallopian tubes, site of fertilization
    (B)  Prostate gland, produces sperm
    (C)  Uterus, site of fertilization
    (D)  Testes, produces nourishing fluid for sperm

44. White fur is a recessive trait in a certain species of mammal. A black-furred parent and a white-furred parent produce an offspring that has white fur. Which of the following deductions is supported by the information given?

    (A)  The parents' next offspring will be black.
    (B)  The white-furred parent has a recessive black fur allele.
    (C)  The black-furred parent has a recessive white fur allele.
    (D)  The offspring has one black fur allele and one white fur allele.

45. Which of the following blood vessels contain valves to prevent blood from flowing backward?

    (A)  Arteries
    (B)  Capillaries
    (C)  Ventricles
    (D)  Veins

46. Ohm's law states that $V = IR$, where $V$ is voltage, $I$ is current flow, and $R$ is total resistance. A science class performs an experiment to determine how placing two different resistors, with resistance $r_1$ and $r_2$, in parallel affects the total resistance of a circuit. The experiment uses a constant voltage; as the different resistors are placed in parallel in the circuit, the current flow is measured. From these values of $V$ and $I$, $R$ can be calculated using the proven logic of Ohm's law. Which of the following equations is a hypothesis that can be evaluated with this experiment?

(A) $V = IR$

(B) $R = \dfrac{r_1 r_2}{r_1 + r_2}$

(C) $R = \dfrac{V}{I}$

(D) $r_1 = \dfrac{R \times r_2}{r_2 + R}$

47. Which of the following statements correctly describes the contraction of muscles and change in pressure inside the lungs during inhalation?

(A) The diaphragm and intercostal muscles contract, decreasing pressure in the lungs.
(B) The diaphragm and intercostal muscles contract, increasing pressure in the lungs.
(C) The diaphragm and intercostal muscles relax, increasing pressure in the lungs
(D) The diaphragm and intercostal muscles relax, decreasing pressure in the lungs.

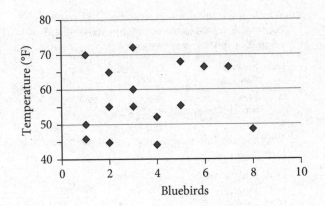

48. A birder records the number of bluebirds he spotted on any given day and the high temperature recorded that day, as shown on the scatterplot above. Which of the following best describes the relationship between the temperature and the number of bluebirds observed based on the data shown?

(A) The number of bluebirds observed correlates positively with temperature.
(B) The number of bluebirds observed correlates negatively with temperature.
(C) There is no apparent correlation between temperature and the number of bluebirds observed.
(D) Temperature is inversely correlated with the number of bluebirds observed.

49. Which of the following cells would NOT be involved in the immune response to a pathogen encountered for the first time?

(A) Macrophages
(B) NK lympocytes
(C) Plasma cells
(D) Dendritic cells

50. Which of the following organs does NOT release a hormone involved in the absorption and/or distribution of nutrients from the digestive tract?

    (A) Stomach
    (B) Pancreas
    (C) Liver
    (D) Small intestine

51. Which of the following is a part of the adaptive immune system?

    (A) Phagocytes
    (B) Inflammation
    (C) Earwax
    (D) T cells

52. Which if the following would lead to a decrease in respiration rate following the onset of hyperventilation?

    (A) Decrease in blood pH
    (B) Increase in blood pH
    (C) Increase in blood carbon dioxide levels
    (D) Increase in blood oxygen levels

53. Which of the following bone cells is responsible for breaking down bone?

    (A) Osteoclasts
    (B) Osteocytes
    (C) Osteoblasts
    (D) Osteons

**IF YOU FINISH BEFORE TIME IS CALLED, YOU MAY CHECK YOUR WORK ON THIS SECTION ONLY. DO NOT TURN TO ANY OTHER SECTION IN THE TEST.**  **STOP**

# English and Language Usage

5/8

> **Directions** You have 28 minutes to answer 28 questions. Do not work on any other section of the test during this time.

1. The art teacher reminded her student to purchase his art supplies _____ a paint brush, palette, easel, and canvas.

   Which of the following punctuation marks correctly completes the sentence?

   (A) .
   (B) :
   (C) ;
   (D) ,

2. David decided to contact the appliance repair company regarding his broken washing machine; although he wanted the machine fixed immediately, he thought it best to request a ballpark figure for the repair fee first.

   Which of the following phrases in the sentence above is informal?

   (A) decided to contact
   (B) fixed immediately
   (C) thought it best
   (D) ballpark figure

3. The famous producers _____ planning to release an exciting new film this upcoming fall.

   Which of the following correctly completes the sentence above?

   (A) are
   (B) is
   (C) will
   (D) be

4. Stella was delighted to see that the children enjoyed there gifts.

   Which of the following corrects an error in the sentence above?

   (A) Change "see" to "sea."
   (B) Change "children" to "childrens."
   (C) Change "enjoyed" to "enjoied."
   (D) Change "there" to "their."

5. At the end of the short-term drug trials, the subjects who had received the medication showed no discernible differences in health outcomes when compared to the subjects who had received the placebo.

   In which of the following would the above sentence most likely appear?

   (A) Letter to the editor
   (B) Short story
   (C) Scientific report
   (D) Advertisement

6. _____ she had left the water running, the sink overflowed onto the floor and into the hallway.

   Which word correctly completes the sentence?

   (A) However
   (B) Because
   (C) Even though
   (D) Unless

7. The researcher <u>disclaimed</u> any knowledge of improper use of funds by his team.

   Which of the following is the meaning of the underlined word in the sentence above?

   (A) Admitted
   (B) Proclaimed
   (C) Blamed
   (D) Denied

8. Which of the following sentences would most likely appear in a novel?

   (A) Walter stepped out of the office building and walked toward his car, careful not to slip on the thin layer of ice that covered the parking lot.
   (B) The suspect was captured close to his home yesterday evening after a neighbor contacted police.
   (C) Our profit margin will continue to increase, provided we implement the customer service initiatives suggested by our relationship management team.
   (D) The leafcutter ant is an unusual species in that it grows its own food to feed its young.

 27

4/7

9. Marcus attempted to <u>disentangle</u> the fawn caught in the snare.

   Which of the following is the meaning of the underlined word in the sentence above?

   (A) Free
   (B) Hunt
   (C) Observe
   (D) Trap

10. The girls' volleyball team will win _____ championship game because each player will play _____ best.

    Which of the following pairs of words correctly completes the sentence above?

    (A) its ; her
    (B) it's ; her
    (C) its ; their
    (D) it's ; its

11. Which of the following examples is a complex sentence?

    (A) A member of the city council has proposed a new ordinance.
    (B) Under the new law, parking on city streets would be free on weeknights, and the mayor would have the authority to suspend parking fees on major holidays.
    (C) Although free parking might draw more patrons to the downtown stores, the city cannot afford to lose any parking revenue.
    (D) The council should vote against the proposed ordinance at this time.

12. Which of the following sentences is an example of incorrect subject-verb agreement?

    (A) Jolie and Daniel went to the movies after dinner.
    (B) The boy with the extra sandwiches is going to share with the girl who forgot her lunch.
    (C) Everyone who lost points on the test have to stay after class.
    (D) The cheerleaders holding the banner are leading the crowd in a cheer.

13. **Types of Research Methodologies**

    1. Quantitative Methods
       a. Description
       b. Application

    2. Qualitative Methods
       a. Description
       b. Application

    If the outline above is used to write a paper, which of the following statements is most likely to appear in that paper?

    (A) Researchers must choose between two types of research methodology.
    (B) Application is a type of description.
    (C) Types of research include quantitative and qualitative methodologies.
    (D) Quantitative methods are preferable to qualitative methods.

14. Which of the following words is spelled incorrectly?

    (A) Reliable
    (B) Enjoyable
    (C) Complyant
    (D) Denial

15. Jarvis dropped the laptop. The laptop was expensive. Then the whole group turned around. Everyone in the cafeteria stared at him.

    Which of the following best states the information above in a single sentence?

    (A) The expensive laptop was dropped by Jarvis and the whole group of people sitting in the cafeteria turned around and stared.
    (B) After Jarvis dropped the expensive laptop, everyone in the cafeteria turned around and stared at him.
    (C) The laptop, which was expensive, was dropped by Jarvis, and the whole group, who sat in the cafeteria, turned around, staring.
    (D) When Jarvis dropped the laptop, then the whole group in the cafeteria turned around and stared at him because it was expensive.

16. Instead of attending the cookout, Ria took a nap because the hot summer weather made her feel lethargic.

   As used in the sentence above, "lethargic" most likely means

   (A) unfriendly.
   (B) bored.
   (C) thirsty.
   (D) weary.

17. Jessica's abrupt departure left her colleagues in a <u>precarious</u> situation, with no one knowing how to answer the clients' many questions.

   As used in the sentence above, "precarious" most likely means

   (A) irresponsible.
   (B) offensive.
   (C) uncertain.
   (D) unforeseen.

18. In my opinion, the children at this school have too much freedom, and not nearly enough discipline; for example, they can interrupt the teacher, leave the classroom during lessons, and fail to turn in assignments without facing any repercussions.

   Which of the following punctuation marks is used incorrectly in the sentence?

   (A) The comma after "opinion"
   (B) The comma after "freedom"
   (C) The semicolon after "discipline"
   (D) The comma after "teacher"

19. Dana did not get dehydrated on her long run because she _____ plenty of water before she began.

   Which verb or verb phrase correctly completes the sentence?

   (A) drank
   (B) had drank
   (C) drunk
   (D) had drunk

20. The phlebotomist was unable to find suitable _____ in the dehydrated patient's arm.

   Which of the following correctly completes the sentence above?

   (A) vanes
   (B) vains
   (C) veins
   (D) vein's

21. A clinical trial recently examined the effectiveness of a new beta blocker. The trial tracked patients using the new drug for a period of 18 months and found no serious side effects. All side effects noted were similar in frequency to side effects reported by the control group taking a placebo. Now the trial should be expanded to include more patients and compare this drug's efficacy to that of existing beta blockers available by prescription. Additionally, the trial should explore the use of this beta blocker in comparison with other drugs commonly prescribed for hypertension.

   Which of the following sentences would be an appropriate concluding sentence for the paragraph above?

   (A) More than 500 patients participated in the clinical study.
   (B) The new beta blocker outperformed the placebo on all measures.
   (C) Finally, if the expanded trial succeeds, the FDA should consider approving the new drug.
   (D) Existing beta blockers do not show similar results in patients over age 35.

22. This summer, my friends are visiting _____ relatives in Europe, and _____ staying for three weeks.

   Which of the following pairs of words correctly completes the sentence above?

   (A) their ; they're
   (B) their ; there
   (C) there ; they're
   (D) they're ; their

23. Which of the following is the best definition of "prescience"?

   (A) Classes taken before a science class
   (B) Knowledge of an event before it happens
   (C) A written order for medicine
   (D) The study of the earth

24. Because Rafael usually enjoys trying new foods, his refusal to visit the restaurant to sample its innovative dishes had his mother scratching her head.

    Which of the following phrases from the sentence is informal?

    (A) trying new foods
    (B) visit the restaurant
    (C) innovative dishes
    (D) scratching her head

25. Gregory trusted Kiera and accepted her offer without reservation.

    As used in the sentence above, "reservation" most likely means

    (A) assignment.
    (B) reliability.
    (C) derivation.
    (D) uncertainty.

26. Which of the following sentences correctly punctuates the dialogue?

    (A) When she found her brother outside, Julie exclaimed, "Michael, there you are! A short while ago, mother said, 'Children, come inside.'"
    (B) When she found her brother outside, Julie exclaimed "Michael, there you are! A short while ago, mother said 'Children, come inside.'"
    (C) When she found her brother outside, Julie exclaimed, "Michael there you are! A short while ago, mother said Children, come inside."
    (D) When she found her brother outside, Julie exclaimed "Michael, there you are! A short while ago, mother said, "Children, come inside.""

27. Lack of sleep is more than just an annoyance. A recent study of high school juniors showed that, on average, students who consistently earn low grades go to bed 40 minutes later and get up 25 minutes earlier than students with high grades. _____, another study shows that when a person sleeps less than 6 hours per night, he or she has difficulty remembering information.

    Which of the following words best completes the sentence above?

    (A) Similarly
    (B) However
    (C) Therefore
    (D) In conclusion

28. The rusty old boat with the torn sails is in danger of sinking during the storm.

    Which of the following is the complete subject of the sentence?

    (A) boat
    (B) The rusty old boat
    (C) The rusty old boat with the torn sails
    (D) The rusty old boat with the torn sails is in danger

**IF YOU FINISH BEFORE TIME IS CALLED, YOU MAY CHECK YOUR WORK ON THIS SECTION ONLY. DO NOT TURN TO ANY OTHER SECTION IN THE TEST.** **STOP**

# Diagnostic Test Answers and Explanations

# Reading

## Questions 1–2: Passage Map

Topic: Detective stories
Scope: Relation to public interest in science
Purpose: To explain how rationalism influenced stories
¶ 1: Detective stories written when science very popular
¶ 2: Perception and nature of science different than today
Author: Fictional detectives showed spirit of science

1. **(B) they wrote about heroes whose rational approach mirrored that of real-life scientists.** This question asks for a detail stated in the passage. The first paragraph states that both writers admired scientists and gave their fictional detective characters scientific attitudes and abilities.

2. **(D) out of place.** This is an uncommon word. One clue is the prefix *mal*, which means "bad"; the only answer choice with a negative connotation is **(D)**. If you are not familiar with the prefix, the word's meaning can still be determined from context. Doyle was described as a lover of science, and from context, "rationalist" has a similar meaning. How does ghost hunting fit with scientific thought? Supernatural beliefs tend to involve a different kind of thinking and aren't usually studied scientifically. Also, the next sentence says "these apparent quirks aside," suggesting that this interest seems odd for a man who loves science. So "malapropos" probably means "strange" or "inappropriate." Choice **(D)** is the correct match. Choice (C) might be tempting, because context suggests a possible relationship between "quirky" and "malapropos." However, the tone of the preceding sentence is not positive or admiring, so it doesn't make sense to say that "malapropos" describes a behavior that is endearing.

3. **(B) Courts should stop awarding such excessive settlements.** Sorensen does not make a suggestion in the passage, so to answer this question, you must make an inference. The passage states that Sorensen believes high settlements are a travesty and burden the courts. The rest of the passage explains that these awards set a precedent and provide an incentive for more of these lawsuits. You can infer that Sorensen feels the that the high awards are what lead to a greater workload for the courts. Therefore, predict that he would suggest not awarding such high settlements. Choice **(B)** is a match for that prediction. Choice (A) might seem like a valid inference, since having fewer lawsuits would logically place less of a burden on the courts, but Sorensen's

focus is on the amount of settlements, not on the number of cases brought. Make sure to base your answers to inference questions on the information in the stimulus.

4. **(C) wipe off and replace the drain plug.** According to the passage, "[w]hen the oil is drained fully," you should next wipe off the drain plug and the plug opening and replace the plug. Choice **(C)** is a match for this step in the sequence.

## Questions 5–10: Passage Map

Topic: Happiness
Scope: Where it comes from
Purpose: To explain and endorse Haidt's happiness hypothesis
¶ 1: Two theories of happiness: within/without
¶ 2: Haidt: happiness comes from between
Author: Agrees with Haidt

5. **(D) happiness requires a combination of the right internal attitude as well as external life circumstances.** To answer this question about the passage's main idea, use your summary of topic, scope, and purpose. The author endorses Haidt's idea that happiness comes from "between," requiring both internal and external factors. This matches choice **(D)**. The author describes Buddhism and utilitarianism, but the purpose is not to critique them, even though Haidt's hypothesis is presented as correct. Nor is the wisdom of ancient proverbs the main idea, although the passage acknowledges they contain some wisdom that science has confirmed. The statement in answer choice (C) can be inferred from the happiness hypothesis, but this is one aspect of that idea and not the overall focus of the passage.

6. **(A) Utilitarianism** This detail question can be researched in the first paragraph, which discusses several belief systems. Utilitarianism's stance on happiness is briefly defined as the view that "life circumstances happen to satisfy our desires." This is an example of a view that happiness comes from "without," that is, from outside factors rather than from one's own attitude and perception. The question stem's reference to "the state of the world" is another way of saying "without," so utilitarianism, choice **(A),** is the correct belief system.

7. **(D) To provide an example of a belief system in which happiness is held to be influenced by external factors** The question asks why the author described utilitarianism in a particular location, so focus on the structure of the passage. The first sentence poses a rhetorical question about where happiness comes from, within or without. This is followed up with examples of belief systems that hold these contrasting views. Utilitarianism is given as the single example of happiness coming from without (based on life circumstances), and it is not mentioned again. Choice **(D)** is therefore the correct answer. Note that this answer choice uses the term "influenced by external factors" instead of "from without." Look for the correct idea in the answer choice; it may be expressed in different words than in the passage.

8. **(A) To argue that both internal attitude and life circumstances play a role in a person's happiness** To answer this question, you need to determine the author's point of view and purpose in writing. The author goes beyond just explaining the topic, personally showing support for Haidt's happiness hypothesis by saying Haidt "shows" and "establishes" his idea. The author not only describes Haidt's belief in the "between" theory of happiness but argues that Haidt's hypothesis is supported by evidence. Thus, the author's purpose is to argue that Haidt's idea about happiness is correct. While choice (C) also says the author is making an argument, it does not correctly describe the author's point.

9. **(B) It would challenge the claim that happiness comes from "without."** This question requires you to analyze the effect that new evidence would have on the argument made in the passage. A glance at the answer choices shows that you need to consider how the three points of view described in the passage—happiness comes from within, without, or between—are either supported or undermined by the information given in the question stem. The study says there is a correlation between few material goods and happiness, suggesting that happiness comes more from within than from without. Thus, predict that this evidence would support the within viewpoint and challenge the without and between views. Choice **(B)** is a match for the prediction that the evidence would challenge the without perspective.

10. **(B) Because there is more than one way to be happy, even someone in difficult circumstances can find joy with the right outlook.** The question asks you to infer which of the answer choices is contrary to the author's point of view. The most specific prediction you can make is that the author agrees with Haidt's "between" hypothesis, so any answer choice that contradicts this hypothesis, including any statement that is based primarily on the "within" or "without" hypotheses, will be correct. Choice **(B)** is based on the "within" hypothesis, saying that external circumstances do

not determine happiness, so the passage author would disagree with this statement. Choices (A) and (C) both state the importance of external and internal factors, and neither choice states that one factor is irrelevant, so they do not contradict the "between" hypothesis. Likewise, choice (D) does not contradict the "between" hypothesis, since it only states that internal factors are related to happiness, not that internal factors are exclusively important.

11. **(A)**

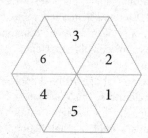

The question presents a hexagon composed of numbered triangles and asks you to follow a series of three instructions. Follow the instructions step-by-step.

1. Switch the positions of numbers 1 and 6.

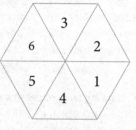

2. Switch the positions of numbers 2 and 5.

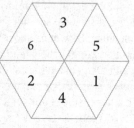

3. Switch the positions of numbers 4 and 5.

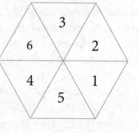

12. **(B) Appreciative** The author notes that some people have negative feelings toward snakes but uses the key phrase "on the contrary" to introduce some positive attributes snakes possess. Thus, predict a positive word and choose "Appreciative." The author is not disgusted, (A); that would be more appropriate to describe those he disagrees with. Considering the author's appreciation for snakes, it would be incorrect to say he was (C), uninterested, in them. There is no reason to believe that the author is fearful, (D).

13. **(A) January.** The letter writer notes that she lives in the Rocky Mountains and there is currently snow on the ground. Because this is a response to a birthday card, you can conclude that the writer's birthday has occurred recently, and because she lives in the Rocky Mountains, she is in the Northern Hemisphere. Therefore, her birthday occurs during the winter. Of the choices, only January is a winter month.

14. **(B) Contact the Student Association and name some movies by Akira Kurosawa the Association should show.** The question requires you to read the three stimuli and draw a conclusion based on the information you are provided. Jack will not state a preference for Hollywood Horror because *Throne of Blood* is not a horror movie but rather an adaptation of *Macbeth*, a famous quasi-historical tragedy about a Scottish king. He is unlikely to choose English Spy Movies because there is no evidence he is interested in the course on Fleming and le Carré. However, because you know that he is writing a paper on Akira Kurosawa for the Shakespeare Adaptation course, you can infer that he will ask the Student Association to show some movies by Kurosawa so he can bring his experience of watching them to his class.

## Questions 15–16: Passage Map

Topic: Toby's transition from childhood
Scope: Baseball as a marker of transition; Toby's last game
Purpose: To tell a story about an important life milestone
¶ 1: Importance of baseball to Toby and his father; Toby soon moving on to adulthood
¶ 2: Anticipation of a good game with dad watching

15. **(A) To tell a story about a significant life milestone** This is a fictional narrative. The author might share his personal beliefs through his characters, but the main goal here is to introduce those characters and tell a story about them.

16. **(D) eager.** Although uneasiness and sadness would be possible answers given the circumstances, the tone of the story and description of the boy's actions does not suggest either of these emotions. The boy is clearly looking forward to the game and is happy that it won't be cancelled due to poor weather.

## Questions 17–18: Passage Map

Passage 1: Homework = not fun but useful
Passage 2: Homework = too much time/stressful, probably not useful

17. **(C) They disagree over whether the benefit of completing homework is worth the effort.** It is clear that the first writer is in favor of assigning a lot of homework while the second one is not. The question is why they disagree. Both authors note that completing a large amount of homework is difficult. The first author suggests that this builds character and sets students up for later success. In contrast, the second author suggests that doing a lot of homework is frustrating, interferes with family time, and will not be very useful to the child's future life. So the points of disagreement are whether homework is as beneficial as is claimed and whether any benefits gained are worth the cost. Choice **(C)** is a match for one of these predictions.

18. **(B) A survey of students in kindergarten through grade 12 found that most considered their academic load to be minimal and unchallenging.** There is one thing both authors agree on: homework is difficult. They disagree about whether this is a good thing: one states that homework's difficulty supports a child's development, and the other says it stresses the child out and undermines family time. If the idea that homework is difficult is undermined, then both arguments are weakened. Therefore, choice **(B)** is correct. Choice (A) weakens the first author's argument only, (C) weakens the second author's argument, and (D) is irrelevant to both arguments.

19. **(A) provide a supporting detail for the main idea.** The first sentence introduces the main idea, that "[t]he English language is an amalgam of several other languages, but relies most heavily on Latin." To support this, the author provides an example of an English word that is derived from a Latin prefix and root. Choice **(A)** describes this use of the word "ambidextrous" and is thus correct. Choice (B) is incorrect because the topic is the English language, not this particular word. (C) is incorrect because the paragraph states that we don't translate the word literally from the Latin but instead give it a somewhat different meaning in English. Choice (D) is incorrect because although the root and prefix of "ambidextrous" are Latin, it is an English word.

20. **(A) She is explaining the basis for a marketing decision.** Asafa is laying out the reasons a decision was made by noting the relevance of social media to a marketing campaign. She is not ignoring Janelle as in choice (B); she directly states that the memo answers Janelle's question, and she thanks Janelle for her input. Although the memo begins with the word "Sorry," this relates to a delay in responding, not to any outcome, so choice (C) is incorrect. Finally, Asafa is not suggesting that Janelle use social media, (D).

## Questions 21–23: Passage Map

Topic: Astronomy
Scope: Brightness/visibility of objects
Purpose: Explain how improved perception of objects advances astronomy
¶ 1: Moons of Jupiter visible with telescope, proved solar system model; recent technology advanced understanding more
¶ 2: Brightness related to size, distance
Chart: Shows object brightness, higher number means fainter

21. **(D) astronomy has advanced based on our ability to perceive different celestial objects.** This is a main idea question, and the main idea of this passage appears in the first few sentences and is captured in the passage map. Choice **(D)** correctly identifies the main idea, that being able to see relatively faint objects with technology has been key to increasing astronomical knowledge.

22. **(C) the more powerful the telescope, the fainter the objects it can be used to discover.** This inference question does not point to any particular part of the passage, so consult your map and make a mental checklist of the author's key ideas. The correct answer will logically follow from one or more of these. Then check each answer choice against your understanding of the passage. It is noted in the passage that Galileo discovered Jupiter's moons when the telescope became available, and Jupiter's moons are fainter than Earth's own moon (because a higher number means an object is harder to see). These pieces of information strongly imply that telescopes make fainter objects easier to see. The passage also states that the more powerful Hubble telescope allows greater detail to be seen, further supporting the idea that stronger telescopes allow people to see more. None of the other answer choices are supported by the passage.

23. **(A)** $-26.7$ The passage states that brighter objects have a lower apparent magnitude. The brightest object on the table is Earth's moon (Luna), which has a negative value. Because the sun is obviously brighter than the moon, it must have a lower apparent magnitude, that is, less than $-12.6$. Only one value in the answer choices is less than $-12.6$—that's $-26.7$, choice **(A)**.

24. **(C) Some foods taste better when cooked in salted water.** In the last sentence, Chef Marion names pasta as an example of a food that tastes better when cooked in salted water. A statement about which food tastes better reflects the chef's opinion; someone else might think food cooked in unsalted water tastes better. Choice (B) is a scientific fact, not an opinion. Although (A) might be true, Chef Marion does not express an opinion about the healthfulness of foods. You might be tempted by (D), thinking that cooking in hotter water equates to cooking more quickly, but the passage does not support

this idea; it could be that the higher temperature cooks pasta through more thoroughly in the same time, for example.

25. **(A) painting small areas with blue and other colors** Careful reading of both the stimulus and question are vital to getting a correct answer. The question asks for a step that is *not* part of painting a room. There are an infinite number of activities that aren't part of painting a room! Because you can't predict which one will be in the answer choices, check each choice against the passage and eliminate those that are mentioned. The only one not mentioned is choice **(A)**: patches of the wall should be painted different shades of one color (blue is the example used in the passage), not blue and other colors.

## Questions 26–27: Passage Map

Topic: Charles Frederick Worth
Scope: Importance as designer, businessperson
Purpose: Argue that he had lasting impact on fashion industry

26. **(C) Its quality of construction and luxuriousness of materials** Worth is described as the "inventor of haute couture," and this is described as establishing new standards for the construction and luxury of clothing. Choice (B) is a detail about the particular customers Worth served, not the clothing he designed. Choice (A) relates to a quality that would not be expected of haute couture; this contrast is signaled by the key word "[d]espite." Nothing in the passage connects choice (D) with haute couture; this is a description of the way the designer ran his business, not his clothing.

27. **(B) Many fashion designers today seek to be well-known among people who cannot afford their clothes.** The author's conclusion, signaled by the key word "[t]hus," is that today's fashion industry has been shaped in part by Worth's passion for self-promotion, which was so great that even women who could not afford his clothes knew who he was. To strengthen the argument, therefore, look for an answer choice that provides further evidence that modern fashion designers are famous beyond their customer base. Choice **(B)** matches this prediction. Choice (A) only reinforces that Worth was important to the history of fashion, not that he had an impact on the contemporary fashion world. Choice (C) is about the lasting impact of his clothing designs, but the author's argument is about the lasting impact of his business model. Whether Worth made money, choice (D), is beside the point, because the author's conclusion is about "superstar" designers—that is, very famous designers, not necessarily rich ones.

28. **(A) Jason had been late to work earlier in the week.** This is an inference question that asks what was *not* implied by the passage. Check each answer choice against what is implied in the story. Because Jason is explaining why he was late,

you can infer that everything he mentions about traffic and detours slowed him down. Thus, he drove down Maple and was affected by the lane closure, as in choice (B). He drives a large truck and couldn't take the faster detour, (D), and due to driving the large truck, he couldn't park in the smaller spaces, (C). Not implied is the idea that he had been late earlier in the week. The passage begins, "What a week it had been!" but that exclamation could refer to any kind of difficulties, not necessarily other days when Jason was late to work.

29. **(D) Problem and solution** The passage states that King George V wanted to recognize the contributions of noncombatants in World War I but was unable to do so and goes on to explain that the MBE was established to solve this deficiency. The passage, therefore, notes a problem and identifies a solution as in choice **(D)**. Choice (A) might have been tempting because the passage discusses a king, the kind of prominent person about whom biographies are often written. However, the focus of the passage is on why the MBE was created and what purpose it serves today; King George V is a supporting detail in that story.

30. **(A) A pooling of hospitals' and clinics' procurement of surgical tools, such as laser scalpels, so these instruments are purchased at lower cost** This inference question requires you to use information from the text and the chart. The author of the passage states that the best opportunities for cost savings lie in the categories that are the biggest percentage of healthcare costs. The pie chart shows that these involve hospitals, choices (B) and (D); physicians and clinics, choice (B); and prescription drugs, choice (C). The passage explains that *nondurable* medical supplies are disposable items, so you can infer that *durable* medical equipment is multiuse items, like surgical tools. At 1%, durable medical equipment is a much smaller category than those involved in the other answer choices, and therefore choice **(A)** is the strategy the author would least likely adopt to achieve cost savings.

31. **(B) It assumes that one daycare worker will be required for each parent who wants to return to work.** The question asks you to identify a problem in the way the letter writer supports her conclusion with evidence. The author's argument is that parents returning to work will not gain financially, because the amount they spend on daycare will almost equal their own daily earnings. However, the argument assumes that each parent will be fully responsible for the wage of a single daycare worker. Common sense suggests that each daycare worker will be responsible for more children than those dropped off by a given parent. For example, if 2 daycare workers are responsible for 20 children of 15 parents, then those parents share the cost of those workers. This is the major flaw in the argument. Choice (A) might be tempting; most parents will need the

daycare worker to take care of the children while the parent is driving to and from work, so the hours that daycare is needed would be more than the hours the parent works. However, this actually strengthens the argument that daycare costs would be too high. Choice (C) is part of the mayor's argument, not the letter writer's. Choice (D) does not describe a flaw in the argument; having a personal opinion on a subject does not invalidate an argument as long as the conclusion proceeds logically from the evidence.

32. **(B) Pleasant** The figure of speech "sunny disposition" is an appropriate way to describe a pleasant person, someone who is always smiling, for example. The other choices all have negative connotations.

33. **(A) Challenging** Martina's choice of words ("waste valuable time") in her response to Thomas reveals that she is challenging his suggestion. Although her first comment is phrased as a question, she is speaking rhetorically and is not really interested in answer, so choice (D), "puzzled," is incorrect. There is nothing "encouraging," (B), or "understanding," (C), in her tone. Indeed, with the words "Everyone knows," Martina is quite dismissive toward Thomas.

### Questions 34–38: Passage Map

Topic: Public libraries in America
Scope: Carnegie's support
Purpose: Explain why he supported, positive impact

34. **(C) Public libraries, which are important resources for educating people in a democracy, benefited greatly from Andrew Carnegie's library funding.** To answer this main idea question, it is important to consider the entire passage. Consult your map, where you have jotted notes about the topic, scope, and purpose. Overall, the passage is about Andrew Carnegie's support for public libraries, which are described as being important to "to inform a literate and thoughtful citizenry." The answer that reflects both of these ideas is **(C)**, which summarizes the entire passage. Choice (A) is only about Carnegie, choice (B) is the opposite of the facts in the passage, and choice (D) is only partially correct. Carnegie did believe in free libraries, but nothing in the passage indicates that he believed libraries are the foundation of a thriving democracy.

35. **(A) to serve as an example of Carnegie's support for libraries.** Throughout the passage, the author highlights Carnegie's funding of libraries and his desire to make these sources of knowledge available to all people. The author uses the Washington library as a concrete example of the results of Carnegie's support; the dedication inscribed on the library

provides evidence as to why Carnegie put his money toward public libraries. Choice **(A)** is a match for this prediction. Choices (B) and (D) are out of scope; neither beautification of cities nor access to public buildings in general is mentioned in the passage. Choice (C) reflects the author's viewpoint and does not relate to the use of the Washington library as an example.

36. **(B) Immigrates from Scotland; becomes wealthy; builds the Allegheny library** Research the passage for the progression of events in Carnegie's life. Carnegie is first mentioned at the end of the third sentence. That sentence describes him as a "steel tycoon," and the next sentence describes him as a "self-educated Scottish immigrant." From this, you can infer that he was poor in Scotland, immigrated, and became very wealthy. A few sentences later, the keyword "first" introduces the first library Carnegie build, in Allegheny. This sequence of events matches choice **(B)**. Choice (A) is not only out of order but also out of scope; there is no indication that Carnegie returned to Scotland. Choices (C) and (D) are also out of order.

37. **(D) The very wealthy can afford to downplay the importance of money.** Remember that the correct answer to an inference question, though not stated in the passage, must be true given the information that is stated. The author's parenthetical comment relates to the fact that Carnegie had become a very wealthy man by being a "ruthless businessman" and keeping the wages of his workers down, yet said he prioritized knowledge over money. The author is commenting on the fact that someone with no need to focus on financial security has the luxury of valuing knowledge, and the author extends this insight to wealthy people in general. Thus, the correct answer is choice **(D)**. Choice (A) reflects Carnegie's expressed viewpoint but not the author's. Choices (B) and (C) misrepresent the author's point; the author does not judge Carnegie's stated belief in the importance of knowledge.

38. **(B) They provide needed information for knowledgeable citizens.** In the first sentence, the author states that libraries were prized. She goes on to write that "they were deemed important sources of knowledge to inform a literate and thoughtful citizenry." Though choice **(B)** states this in different words, it is a match for what the author writes in the passage. Choice (A) is stated in the passage but is a relatively minor detail. Choice (D) is also true according to the passage, but this is a description of how libraries work, not why they are fundamentally important. Choice (C) is contradicted by the passage; the author states that libraries are often funded by taxes, but as Carnegie's library building efforts make clear, this was not always the case. Be careful of answer choices with the extreme word "always," because they are only correct if the author uses equally extreme language.

## Questions 39–40: Passage Map

Topic: Pro cycling "Grand Tour"
Scope: The three races
Purpose: Inform reader of some history

39. **(B) The second sentence** In the second sentence, the author expresses the opinion that the Tour de France is the "most enjoyable" of the Grand Tour races. The first sentence states a fact, and the fourth sentence reflects a value judgment ("most prestigious") made by other people, not the author.

40. **(B) Giro d'Italia, Tour de France, Vuelta a España** Correctly answering this detail question requires careful reading of the passage. You are told that the Tour de France is usually held in July. You are also told that the Vuelta a España was "originally run in April, not long before the Giro d'Italia," which means the latter race is held shortly after April. Now, you are told, the Vuelta a España takes place in the fall. So, the current running order of the Grand Tour is the Giro d'Italia (sometime shortly after April), the Tour de France (usually in July), and the Vuelta a España (sometime in the fall). Note that choice (A) is the order in which the races were first run, but this is not what the question is asking for.

41. **(C) Sadly** This is the meaning of "dolefully." If you weren't sure of the word's meaning, the sentence provides clues. The contrasting word "but" means Marcus was feeling the opposite of "happy." Therefore, you can infer that "dolefully" is similar in meaning to "sadly." Choice (D), "warily," also has a negative connotation, but it means "being worried about potential danger," and there is no reason to think Marcus was afraid of his future wife, only that he was not happy for some reason.

## Questions 42–43: Passage Map

Topic: Mining in space
Scope: The "old man's" foolish optimism
Purpose: To tell a story, describing a setting and lifestyle
In these ¶s, two men discuss a miner who is losing money while hoping to strike it rich; Buck and Cole poke fun at the "old man's" dreams.

42. **(A) Miners are practical in the everyday details of their work but have wildly optimistic dreams of making their fortune.** This question asks for the overall theme of the two characters' dialogue, in which the character of a miner, the "old man," is made clear through the viewpoint of Buck and Cole. The correct answer will express their characterization of the miner. The miner spends 101% of his output, that is, 1% more than he makes; thus, he is slowly losing money. It's then explained that he is operating at maximum efficiency in the

sense of making his losses as small as possible. When Buck asks about the miner's motives, Cole clarifies that he wants to get rich and retire. So his goal is to make his money last as long as possible in hopes of striking it rich, a goal the two characters view with skepticism. Finally, Cole says "all" miners have this dream. Thus, the miner is both shrewd in managing his operation and foolish in envisioning his future. Choice **(A)** expresses the overall gist of the passage. The other choices are either contradicted by the passage or express only part of its meaning.

43. **(C) jovium is both rarer and more valuable than platinum.** Because this is an inference question, the correct answer choice will be something that follows from statements in the passage, and the other answer choices will be either untrue or not necessarily true. The passage states that the miner has a "rich" platinum mine but is losing money, meaning there is a lot of the metal but it is not worth enough to cover the cost of mining it. The fact that the miner hasn't found jovium yet indicates that it is rarer than platinum, and the fact that he expects to retire if he does find jovium means it is more valuable. Beyond what you know from the passage itself, it is common knowledge that rare things tend to be more valuable than common things, so when you infer one, you can reasonably infer the other. None of the other statements can be inferred from the passage. Choice (A) is extreme; there isn't enough information here to know what eventually happens to most miners. Choice (B) is not supported: Buck and Cole poke fun at the miners, but they do not express a negative opinion or view themselves as better than the miners. Choice (D): While Buck and Cole appear to be friendly, they may have been friends for years without working together, or they may have become friendly quickly.

44. **(A) Military training helps build "grit."** The author is arguing that children without grit get less from their education, and that expensive schools are therefore a waste. He argues that these children should go to boot camp instead of prep school. The assumption is that boot camp will help them build character, or "grit." Choice (B) is the opposite of what the author believes, as is (C), because the point of grit is to do more work and learn more. Choice (D) might be tempting, but the author only suggests that lazy children are sent to expensive schools, not that sending the kids to those schools actually makes them lazy.

45. **(D) Buy a photo postcard of Edinburgh Castle.** The writer states that Naresh advised a trip to Edinburgh, (C); talked the writer into buying hiking boots, (B); and told him to bring an umbrella, (A). On the other hand, he writes that he is surprising Naresh with this postcard, so **(D)** is the correct choice.

46. **(A) Is Edinburgh a beautiful city?** Naresh advised the writer to "go someplace beautiful." Using Naresh's opinion as evidence, the writer concluded that he should go to Edinburgh. To move from this evidence to this conclusion, the writer must have determined that Edinburgh is beautiful by asking the question in choice **(A)**. The postcard writer decided to visit Edinburgh despite being told by Naresh that it was expensive, so evaluating whether Edinburgh was more or less expensive than other places was not essential to reaching the decision to go there. Choice (D) is incorrect.

47. **(D) "I make sure my watch battery is charged."** The author states that she sets her alarm before a workday only after she ensures her watch battery is charged. The other two steps take place when she wakes the next day.

**Questions 48–49: Passage Map**

Topic: News reporting
Scope: Inaccuracy, bias
Purpose: To criticize

48. **(D) illustrate ways in which the media depart from unbiased news reporting.** Throughout, the author contrasts an ideal of unbiased news coverage with the biased reporting that actually occurs. Graphics and sound effects are mentioned in the second sentence, where according to the author they are used to "entice viewers and garner ratings." The next sentence continues: "Real facts . . . are totally abandoned." Thus, graphics and sound effects are examples of what the media does to make a story interesting, which, in turn, leads to inaccuracy and bias. Choice **(D)** is a match for this prediction. Choice (A) is true in that the graphics and sound effects are designed to make the story interesting, but relevance is not mentioned in the passage. Furthermore, the author presents these examples to say something negative about the news media, not something positive. The author considers biased news "junk," not the graphics and sound effects that are features of that news, as in choice (B). Similarly, the author does distinguish two kinds of reporting, but not solely on the basis of graphics and sound effects, (C); the distinction lies in accuracy and bias.

49. **(D) condemn the media for distorting news reports.** From the very first sentence, the author severely criticizes the news media for abandoning "[r]eal facts and unbiased coverage of an issue . . . in exchange for an overly sentimental or one-sided story that too often distorts the truth." Choice **(D)**, which uses the strong word "condemn," meaning to express strong disapproval, reflects this purpose. Choice (A) might be tempting, but the author isn't criticizing viewers; instead, she is warning them of the dangers of distorted news reports. (B) is

the opposite of the author's point. The author does distinguish between biased and neutral reporting, but simply explaining the difference is not her primary purpose, (C).

### Questions 50–51: Passage Map

Topic: Minors workings on family farms
Scope: License requirements to operate heavy equipment
Purpose: The first passage explains the goal of the bill. The second passage argues against it.
Passage 1: News article; kids age 14 1/2 up need license to operate tractors
Passage 2: Law will hurt farming families; parents know better than government how to run business, raise kids

50. **(B) The farmer disagrees with the state senators' assumptions about safety issues in child farm labor.** The argument of the state officials, as described in the news article, is that restricting minors' access to farm equipment will make those children safer. The farmer argues that this law will make farmers' lives more difficult and that the officials know little about how to keep children safe on farms. The key disagreement, then, is about whether the senators understand the safety concerns at issue, answer choice **(B)**. Choice (A) is out of scope because the debate is about children on farms operating heavy equipment, not children doing any kind of work. Choice (C) is incorrect as neither party compares safety and economic security. Choice (D) is incorrect: the senate has passed a law restricting the operation of heavy equipment, not farmwork in general, and the farmer claims "we've always taken good care of our kids," meaning that farmwork poses little risk.

51. **(D) the state overestimates the danger to children of operating tractors.** The word "apparently" indicates that this is an inference question, so the correct answer choice will include an idea believed by the second author but not explicitly stated. The crux of the second author's argument is that this bill makes farm families' lives more difficult without improving safety, because farmers know better than legislators how to raise their children safely, choice **(D)**. He does not imply that safety is not important, choice (C), nor does he imply that the state is intentionally trying to hurt the agriculture industry, (B). Indeed, he implies they are hurting the industry due to ignorance. There's no reference to hiring children to work on land not owned by their family, so choice (A) is irrelevant.

52. **(A) while** The author states that three species of frigate birds are widespread but two are endangered with restricted breeding habitats, so look for a word that signals contrast. Choice **(A)**, "while," matches the prediction.

53. **(D) constructive** This word means "helping to improve." Choice (A), "shift," is neutral, simply meaning "a change." The words "pejorative" ("belittling") and "vilification" ("harsh criticism") have negative meanings. If you weren't sure of the words' meanings, you could use context clues to find the answer. The word "Fortunately" indicates that the campaign has changed in a positive manner. Thus, it has changed "from [a bad thing] to [a good thing]," and the latter phrase will contain the word with a positive connotation.

# Mathematics

1. **(B) 0.045** This question asks you to convert a percent to a decimal. You may have memorized the very useful shortcut "Move the decimal two places to the left and drop the % sign." This will efficiently produce the correct answer to this straightforward question. However, be sure to understand the process as well. Convert the percentage to a fraction by placing the expression over 100 and then change the fraction to a decimal by using place value: $4.5\% = \dfrac{4.5}{100} = \dfrac{4.5(10)}{100(10)} = \dfrac{45}{1000} = 0.045$.

2. **(A) Skewed right** The question presents a bar graph and asks for a description of the distribution indicated by the shape of the graph. *Skew* describes the direction of the "tail" of a graph (i.e., the part of the graph with fewer data values). Because this graph's tail is to the right, the graph indicates a distribution that is skewed right.

3. **(A) 23** The question provides an equation with a variable on one side and a value on the other, and it requires you to isolate the variable. Use inverse operations to isolate $y$. First, subtract 36 from both sides to yield $4y = 92$. Next, divide both sides by 4 to yield $y = 23$.

4. **(D) 360** The question provides the rate at which the worker slices oranges and the number of slices per orange, and it asks for the number of slices the worker will produce in 15 minutes. First, calculate how many oranges the worker can cut up in one minute: $\dfrac{60 \text{ seconds per minute}}{15 \text{ seconds per orange}} = 4$ oranges per minute. Next, calculate how many oranges he can cut up in 15 minutes: 4 oranges per minute $\times$ 15 minutes = 60 oranges in 15 minutes. Finally, calculate the number of slices: 60 oranges $\times$ 6 slices = 360 slices.

5. **(A) There was a positive covariance between the number of telephones and the incidence of cancer.** You are provided survey data: the more telephones in a household, the more likely it was that a member of the household had cancer. Then

the question asks which of the answer choices best describes the relationship between those two variables. Based on the limited information given, all you can conclude is that there is a positive relationship between telephones and cancer. This positive relationship is a covariance between the two measurements, so choice (A) is correct. Choice (B) is the opposite. Choice (D) says that there is a cause-and-effect relationship (that talking on the phone causes cancer), and choice (C) says that there is no cause and effect involved. A common error in logic is to assume that a correlation between two things means that a cause-and-effect relationship exists. There is not enough information here to know whether there is or is not a causal relationship between telephones and cancer, so both (C) and (D) are incorrect.

6. **(C) 29** The question provides the part-to-part ratio of three of the four colors of marbles in a bag (red, white, and blue). It also states that there are half as many green marbles as there are blue marbles. You need to find the minimum total number of marbles that satisfies these facts. Because the number of green marbles is half that of blue marbles, restate the part-to-part ratio by adding green at the end. The number in the ratio representing blue is 5, so the number representing green is half that, or $2\frac{1}{2}$. Thus, the ratio becomes $3:4:5:2\frac{1}{2}$. However, there won't be half a marble, so double all the values to get 6:8:10:5. While the total number of marbles could be the sum of the values in the part-to-part ratio multiplied by any number, the question asks for the *least* possible number, so just add $6 + 8 + 10 + 5$ to get 29, choice **(C)**.

7. **(C) 135** The pie chart provides the percentages of apple trees of different ages, and the question tells you the total number of trees. You need to find the number of trees 5 years old or younger. Find the segments of the chart that include ages of 5 years or younger. The chart indicates that 20% of the trees are less than 3 years old and 25% are from 3 to 5 years old, so add these two percentages: $20\% + 25\% = 45\%$. Now calculate 45% of the total number of trees: $0.45 \times 300 = 135$.

8. **(D)** $\frac{1}{2}$ The question provides the total number of eggs and the number of eggs painted each color other than green, and it asks for the fraction of eggs that are painted green. Begin by determining the number of eggs that are painted a color other than green: 5 blue + 5 yellow + 5 pink = 15 eggs that are not green. Subtract this number from the total number of eggs to calculate the number that are green: 30 total eggs −15 eggs that are not green = 15 green eggs. Thus, the fraction of green eggs to total eggs is $\frac{15}{30}$. Because this fraction does not appear among the answer choices, simplify: $\frac{15}{30} = \frac{1}{2}$.

9. **(A) 2,399,679** The question asks for the product of four 2-digit numbers. The answer choices are closely spaced, so estimating will not suffice. Rather than accessing the calculator, however, look at the last digits of the four numbers. The last digit of the product of $27 \times 47 \times 31 \times 61$ is the same as the last digit of $7 \times 7 \times 1 \times 1 = 49$—the last digit is 9. The only answer choice that ends in 9 is **(A)**. This shortcut doesn't always work because there could be more than one answer choice that ends in the target number. However, it is so fast and simple that it is always worth a try, especially in a case like this where every answer choice ends with a different digit.

10. **(D) 6** You are asked to multiply two mixed numbers. Change each number to an improper fraction: $1\frac{7}{8} \times 3\frac{1}{5} = \frac{15}{8} \times \frac{16}{5}$. Simplify before multiplying if possible by dividing out common factors from the numerator and denominator: $\frac{15 \times 16}{8 \times 5} = \frac{3 \times 2}{1 \times 1}$. Now multiply the numerators and then the denominators: $\frac{6}{1} = 6$. Alternatively, you could round the first fraction up to 2 and the second fraction down to 3. Then $2 \times 3 = 6$, and even if this were not the exact answer, only choice **(D)** is close.

11. **(C) 5 decimeters** A wide elastic band requires 40 g weight of force to stretch it 1 mm. The force-to-distance relationship is linear, so each additional millimeter of stretch will add 40 grams of resistance. The maximum force permitted is 20 kg. The question asks how far the band can stretch to produce that much force. The information in the question is in different metric units, and the answer choices are presented in various metric units as well, so conversion of units will be part of solving this question. Begin by converting 20 kg to 20,000 g. Then, to determine the distance that would create that much force, divide 20,000 g by 40 g/mm to get 500 mm. Choice (A), 5 mm, is clearly incorrect. None of the other answer choices are stated in mm. Since there are 10 mm per cm, 500 mm = 50 cm, so (B) is incorrect as well. There are 10 cm per decimeter, so 50 cm = 5 decimeters and choice **(C)** is correct.

12. **(A) 36 − 9π** The question provides a circle inscribed in a square, and it asks you to find the area of that region of the square not bounded by the circle. Find the area of each shape and then subtract the area of the circle from the area of the square. The area of a square is side length squared: $6^2 =$ 36 square inches. Because the side length of the square is 6 inches, this must also be the diameter of the circle. The area formula for a circle is $\pi r^2$. Because the diameter is 6 inches, the radius is 3 inches, so the area of the circle is $\pi 3^2 = 9\pi$ square inches. Thus, the area of the shaded region is $36 - 9\pi$ square inches.

13. **(B)** $\frac{13}{4}$, **3.35**, $\frac{7}{2}$, $\frac{11}{3}$, **4** You are asked to order the numbers from least to greatest. Given the mix of fractions and decimals, it may be easiest to convert the fractions to decimals: $\frac{11}{3} = 3.6\overline{6}$, $\frac{13}{4} = 3.25$, $\frac{7}{2} = 3.5$. Now compare the numbers: $\frac{13}{4} < 3.35 < \frac{7}{2} < \frac{11}{3} < 4$.

14. **(B) 16 ≤ *n* ≤ 48** The question provides the minimum and maximum number of times the nurse will record the client's blood pressure each hour and the duration of the shift in hours, and it asks for the expression that reflects the number of times the blood pressure will be recorded. To calculate the range of the possible number of times *n* the nurse will record blood pressure over the entire shift, multiply the minimum number of times per hour and the maximum number of times per hour by the number of hours in the shift: minimum: 2 times per hour × 8 hours = 16 times; maximum: 6 times per hour × 8 hours = 48 times. Thus, *n* is greater than or equal to 16, and less than or equal to 48.

15. **(B) 4** The question provides the sports drink's concentration level, the amount of nutrient mix in each bottle, and the total amount of sports drink the trainer will produce. You need to determine how many total bottles of nutrient mix the trainer will need. Determine the quantity of the nutrient mix needed by multiplying the amount of sports drink by the concentrate level: 15% of 240 ounces = 0.15 × 240 ounces = 36 ounces of nutrient mix. Next, determine how many bottles of nutrient mix the trainer will need to purchase by dividing the total amount of mix needed by the amount of mix per bottle: 36 ounces of nutrient mix ÷ 10 ounces per bottle = 3.6 bottles. Because the trainer has to purchase the nutrient mix by the bottle, she'll need to buy 4 bottles.

16. **(D)** $2\frac{11}{24}$ To add fractions with different denominators, you first need a to find common denominator. The least common denominator (LCD) of these fractions is 24. Using 24 as the denominator, rewrite each fraction: $\frac{7}{8} + \frac{5}{6} + \frac{3}{4} = \frac{7 \times 3}{8 \times 3} + \frac{5 \times 4}{6 \times 4} + \frac{3 \times 6}{4 \times 6} = \frac{21}{24} + \frac{20}{24} + \frac{18}{24}$. Add the numerators of the fractions: $\frac{21 + 20 + 18}{24} = \frac{59}{24}$. Simplify the fraction: $2\frac{11}{24}$.

17. **(A)** $\frac{4}{15}$ The question provides values for the ratios of *a* to *b* and *b* to *c* and asks for the ratio of *a* to *c*. To work with these ratios, translate them into their fractional representations: $\frac{a}{b} = \frac{4}{3}$ and $\frac{b}{c} = \frac{1}{5}$. The ratio $\frac{a}{c}$ can be calculated by multiplying the two known ratios: $\frac{a}{b} \times \frac{b}{c} = \frac{a}{c}$. Substitute the known values for those ratios to get $\frac{4}{3} \times \frac{1}{5} = \frac{4}{15}$, which is choice **(A)**.

18. **(D) 20** The graph shows the number of households that own zero, one, two, three, or four cars. The question asks you to determine how many households own three or more cars. The graph indicates that 15 households own three cars and 5 households own four cars. Add these together: 15 households + 5 households = 20 households.

19. **(C) 118** The question asks for the value of an expression "to the nearest whole number," which, along with the wide spacing of the answer choices, is a clue that estimating would be a good approach. Round 31 down to 30 and roll 917 down to 900. Now simply solve 900 ÷ 30 × 4 = 30 × 4 = 120. The only answer choice close to that estimate is **(C)**. Although you have access to a calculator on the TEAS, in this case, estimating is probably just as quick and avoids the risk of data entry errors.

20. **(B) 864 L** The question states that a tank contains 180 L + 360 L = 540 L and that it is $\frac{5}{8}$ full. You must find the total capacity of the tank. Set up the proportion $\frac{540}{C} = \frac{5}{8}$. Cross multiply to get $8 \times 540 = 5C$. Simplify the calculations by first dividing both sides by 5: $8 \times 108 = C$; $864 = C$. Answer choice **(B)** is correct.

21. **(A) 2,000,000** The question provides an amount in kilograms and asks for a conversion from kilograms to milligrams. Use dimensional analysis (the fact that multiplying or dividing a value by 1 does not change the value) to convert from kilograms to milligrams: 2 kilograms × $\frac{1,000 \text{ grams}}{1 \text{ kilogram}}$ × $\frac{1,000 \text{ milligrams}}{1 \text{ gram}}$ = 2,000,000 milligrams.

22. **(C)** *q* = *p* + 4 The question asks you to determine which of the equations in the answer choices results in a positive covariance between the two variables. Choice (A) may be tempting, but because *q* is a function of *p* squared, *p* can become a smaller and smaller negative number yet *q* will continue to get larger. Eliminate (A). The equation in (B) simplifies to *q* = 4, so there is no relationship with *p*. In **(C)**, as *p* increases, so does *q*, so the two variables are positively covariant. In choice (D), as *p* increases, *q* decreases, so the two are negatively covariant.

**K**

23. **(B) $9a - 15$** The question presents an algebraic expression containing a single variable and asks you to find the equivalent expression among the answer choices. Simplify and combine like terms to isolate the variable $a$. First, simplify the fraction by dividing the numerator by 2 to yield $2(a - 8)$. Next, distribute the 2 to get $2a - 16$. Now combine like terms: $6a + 2a + a = 9a$ and $-16 + 1 = -15$. Finally, add the resulting terms: $9a + (-15) = 9a - 15$. Note that another way to solve would be to substitute a number for $a$. If $a = 2$, then the expression equals $(6)(2) + \dfrac{4(2-8)}{2} + 2 + 1 = 3$. Plugging in 2 for $a$ in each of the answer choices produces 3 only in choice **(B)**.

24. **(B) 45 miles** The question provides the number of segments of a trip, the bicyclist's speed for each segment of the trip, and the time it takes to cover the first two segments, as well as the time for the entire trip. You are asked to determine the entire distance. Use the formula rate $\times$ time = distance. First, calculate the distance of the uphill segment: 20 minutes $\times$ 15 mph $= \dfrac{1}{3}$ hour $\times$ 15 mph = 5 miles. Next, the level segment: 1 hour $\times$ 20 mph = 20 miles. To find the distance of the downhill segment, first calculate the time it takes to travel this segment by subtracting the time of the other two segments from the entire trip length: 2 hours $-$ 1 hour 20 minutes = 40 minutes. Next, calculate the distance: 40 minutes $\times$ 30 mph $= \dfrac{2}{3}$ hour $\times$ 30 mph = 20 miles. Finally, add all three distances: 5 miles + 20 miles + 20 miles = 45 miles.

25. **(B) 19.5%** The question provides a price before sales tax, the sales tax rate, and the total amount including a tip. You are asked what percentage of the price plus tax was the tip. A key element of this question is the amount of the meal plus tax. Apply the 6% tax rate to the base amount: $\dfrac{6}{100} \times 110.50 = 0.06 \times 110.50 = \$6.63$. Add this tax to the amount for food and beverages: $\$110.50 + \$6.63 = \$117.13$. Because the total charge was \$140, the amount of the gratuity must have been $\$140 - \$117.13 = \$22.87$. Calculate the percent tip relative to the bill with tax added: $\dfrac{t}{100} = \dfrac{22.87}{117.13}$. Cross multiply to get $117.13t = 2287$. Divide both sides of the equation by 117.13 to get $t = 19.5\%$, which is choice **(B)**. Choice (C) is the tip amount as a percentage of the bill *before* tax, and choice (D) ignores tax altogether.

26. **(B) 155** You are asked the value of an expression with multiple operations. The order of operations is important. Use PEMDAS. Start inside the parentheses, doing multiplication/division first and then addition/

subtraction: $2 \times (80 - 5) + 5 = 2 \times (75) + 5$. Next, multiply: $2 \times 75 + 5 = 150 + 5$. Last, add: $150 + 5 = 155$.

27. **(D) 1:6** The question provides the total area of the garden, the number of carrot seeds planted per square foot, the number of lettuce seeds planted per square foot, and the fraction of the garden's area planted with carrot seeds. You need to solve for the ratio of lettuce seeds to carrot seeds. Begin by calculating the number of square feet planted in carrots: $\dfrac{2}{3} \times 60$ square feet = 40 square feet. Multiply this by the number of carrot seeds per square foot: 40 square feet $\times$ 6 carrot seeds = 240 carrot seeds total. Next, calculate the remaining square footage: 60 total square feet $-$ 40 square feet planted with carrot seeds = 20 square feet planted with lettuce seeds. Multiply this number by the number of lettuce seeds per square foot: 20 square feet $\times$ 2 lettuce seeds = 40 lettuce seeds total. Finally, set up the ratio of lettuce seeds to carrot seeds and simplify: 40:240 = 1:6. Make sure you have the ratio of lettuce to carrot seeds and not the other way around.

28. **(C) $-53\%$** The question provides the fractional contents of a bottle of water at two different times and asks for the percentage change of the contents between those times. Note that the first measurement is that $\dfrac{2}{7}$ of the water had been *consumed*, which means that $\dfrac{5}{7}$ remained. The percentage change is the second observed amount less the first amount divided by the first amount and converted to percent, or $\dfrac{\frac{1}{3} - \frac{5}{7}}{\frac{5}{7}} \times 100\%$.

Multiply every term by 21 to eliminate the fractions:

$$\frac{21\left(\frac{1}{3}\right) - 21\left(\frac{5}{7}\right)}{21\left(\frac{5}{7}\right)} \times 100\% = \frac{7 - 15}{15} \times 100\%.$$

This equals $-53\%$ to the nearest percent, so choice **(C)** is correct. Note that because water is consumed and no water is added $\left(\frac{1}{3} < \frac{5}{7}\right)$, the percentage change must be negative. Thus, you could eliminate choices (A) and (B) on that basis alone.

29. **(B) 20** The graph shows the number of clinics in four regions for the years 1950 and 2000. The question asks for the average of the number of clinics in two of the regions in 1950. Find the number in each region in 1950 (the white bars), then calculate their average. In the South, the number of clinics in 1950 was 10; in the West, the number of clinics in

1950 was 30. Apply the average formula: sum of terms divided by number of terms: $\dfrac{10+30}{2}=\dfrac{40}{2}=20$.

30. **(D) 99** The question states that the ratio of two quantities is 7:2 and that if the amount of the first item were increased by 6, the new ratio would be 11:4. You need to solve for the original total number of the two items. The ratio 7:2 gives the relative amounts of brand-name and generic medicine, but the actual amounts could be any multiple of the ratio, so express this as $\dfrac{7x}{2x}$. When 6 more containers of the generic medicine are added, the quantity of that item is $2x + 6$. The ratio of the new amounts is 11:4, so set up the proportion $\dfrac{7x}{2x+6}=\dfrac{11}{4}$. Cross multiply to get $28x = 22x + 66$, so $6x = 66$ and $x = 11$. This is not the answer to the question; it is the multiplier for the initial ratio. The total number of items before the extra 6 were added was $7x + 2x = 9x$. Because $x = 11$, there were 99 containers.

31. **(B) 16** You are asked for the value of an expression with multiple operations. The order of operations is important. Use PEMDAS. Start inside the parentheses:

$3+5\times(8+4)\div3-7=3+5\times(12)\div3-7$. Next, multiply and divide, from left to right:

$3+5\times12\div3-7=3+60\div3-7=3+20-7$. Finally, add and subtract, from left to right: $3+20-7=23-7=16$.

32. **(C) 50** The question provides an equation with the same variable on each side, and it asks you to solve for the variable. Use inverse operations to isolate $m$. First, add 15 to both sides to yield $3m=\dfrac{m}{2}+125$. Next, subtract $\dfrac{m}{2}$ from both sides to yield $3m-\dfrac{m}{2}=125$. To make calculations easier, multiply each term by 2 to eliminate the fraction: $(2)3m-(2)\dfrac{m}{2}=(2)125$; $6m-m = 250$. Simplify on the left to yield $5m = 250$. Now divide both sides by 5 to yield $m = 50$.

33. **(C) 49** The question provides a diagram of a rectangle with its dimensions, and it asks you to determine the area of a square that has the same perimeter as the rectangle. Begin by determining the perimeter of the rectangle. Perimeter of a rectangle is two times length plus two times width: $(2 \times 9) + (2 \times 5) = 18 + 10 = 28$. Because this is the perimeter of the rectangle, it is also the perimeter of the square. The area of a square is side times side, so you'll need to determine the side length of the square to calculate its area. The perimeter of a square is four times its side length. Therefore, you can find side length by

dividing perimeter by four: $28 \div 4 = 7$. Now multiply this length times itself to find the area of the square: $7 \times 7 = 49$.

34. **(B) 39,000 bushels** The graph displays yearly production of sorghum, and you are asked for the production in 2015. No value is shown for 2015, but the question states that 2015 production was half that of 2012. First, estimate the 2012 production from the graph; it was approximately 80,000 bushels. Half that would be 40,000 bushels. However, a closer look at the column for 2012 production shows that it is a couple thousand *less* than 80,000 bushels. This makes choice **(B)**, 39,000 bushels, correct. Choice (A), 36,000, is half the production of 2010, and choice (D) is half that of 2013.

35. **(A) 140.8** The question provides an amount in kilograms and asks for a conversion to an amount in ounces. Use dimensional analysis (the fact that multiplying or dividing a value by 1 does not change the value) to convert kilograms to ounces:

$$4 \text{ kilograms} \times \frac{2.2 \text{ pounds}}{1 \text{ kilogram}} \times \frac{16 \text{ ounces}}{1 \text{ pound}} = 140.8.$$

Alternatively, you could efficiently use estimation. Because there are a little more than 2 pounds per kilogram, 4 kilograms are about 8 pounds. Then 8 pounds times 16 ounces in every pound is 128 ounces. Because you rounded the number of pounds per kilogram down, the answer is actually somewhat more than 128 ounces. Only choice **(A)** is anywhere close.

36. **(D) 88 feet** The question provides the shapes and dimensions of two enclosures and asks for the total length of fencing needed to enclose each completely. To calculate the total length of fencing needed, calculate the perimeter of each of the enclosures separately and then combine the two values. The perimeter of a square is four times the side length, so the kennel's perimeter is $4 \times 9$ feet = 36 feet. The perimeter of a rectangle is two times length plus two times width, so the dog run is $(2 \times 20 \text{ feet}) + (2 \times 6 \text{ feet}) = 52$ feet. Add the two perimeters: 36 feet + 52 feet = 88 feet.

# Science

1. **(C) Dendrites, axon, and soma** The question asks about parts of the neuron. Recall that soma, nucleus, axon, and dendrites are parts of a neuron. The correct answer will contain some or all of these terms and not any others. Choice **(C)** is a match. Choice (A) describes parts of the nervous system, whereas choices (B) and (D) are divisions of the nervous system.

2. **(C) Mitochondrion** This question is asking you for an organelle that is *not* involved in protein production. Recall that mitochondria are responsible for energy production and are not

involved in protein production. The ribosome and the rough ER, choices (A) and (B) respectively, are responsible for protein translation. The Golgi apparatus, (D), is involved in protein modification.

3. **(D) Vitamin B$_{12}$** This question is asking about absorption specific to the ileum, the third part of the small intestine, so eliminate any substance that is absorbed elsewhere in the digestive tract. Vitamin K, (A), is absorbed throughout the intestinal tract, not primarily in the ileum. Carbohydrates, (B), are primarily absorbed in the jejunum, another part of the small intestine. Water, (C), is absorbed in the stomach and large intestine.

4. **(A) hypodermis, dermis, epidermis** This question is asking about the layers of the skin. Recall that the skin has three layers: hypodermis, dermis, and epidermis. The dermis is the middle layer that contains the sebaceous glands (which appear in choices (B) and (C)). The lower layer is the hypodermis, and the surface layer is the epidermis. This matches answer choice **(A)**.

5. **(A) 2 and *d*** This question is asking for a pairing that is *not* possible. Recall that the period number will limit the possible orbitals. In period 2, the only possible orbital names are *s* and *p*, so choices (C) and (D) can be eliminated because they are possible. By the same logic, you can choose choice **(A)**, because orbital *d* cannot appear with period 2. In period number 3, the possible orbital names are *s*, *p*, and *d*, so (B) is a possible pairing and can be eliminated.

6. **(B) Hemoglobin not properly binding to oxygen** This question is asking which factor is *not* a secondary effect of hypertension. Recall that *hypertension* is a term for chronic high blood pressure. Thus, you can eliminate all answer choices that could result from increased pressure in the blood vessels. Minor tearing to the blood vessels can result from the increased pressure, which in turn would cause scar tissue to accumulate, as in choice (A). Vascular scarring can act like a net to catch other particles in the circulatory system, including platelets and cholesterol, causing clots to form. These can both decrease blood flow to vital organs by restricting blood flow, as in choice (D), or can break off and result in a stroke, (C). Choice **(B)** is correct. Poor oxygenation resulting from hypertension is caused by blocked blood vessels, not improper hemoglobin binding.

7. **(D) Storing urea** This question is asking for a role the kidneys do *not* perform, so three of the answer choices will correctly state the kidneys' function. Recall that the kidneys filter blood to remove waste products, choice (A), and they reabsorb water to stabilize blood pressure, (B). The kidneys also convert vitamin D to its active form, as in choice (C). While the kidneys filter urea from the blood, urea (in the form of urine) is stored in the bladder prior to excretion. The correct answer is choice **(D)**.

8. **(C) 10,000 mg** This question is asking for a unit conversion. Recall that 1 gram is equal to 1000 milligrams, so 10 grams must be equal to $10 \times 1000 = 10,000$ milligrams.

9. **(A) Aorta** This question is asking about the variance of blood pressure over different parts of the circulatory system. Recall that blood pressure is highest as it leaves the heart, so predict that the correct answer will be a large artery. This matches choice **(A)**. Though blood is also being pumped directly from the right ventricle to pulmonary arteries, choice (C), the left ventricle is pumping blood through the aorta to the entire body and thus pumps with more force. Blood pressure is lowest in the capillaries, choice (B), and the vena cava, (D), is part of the venous system.

10. **(A) a** The question is asking you to match an endocrine process to the proper endocrine gland. Recall that melatonin is the hormone that regulates sleep, and it is secreted by the pineal gland. The pineal gland is indicated by letter *a* on the diagram. Letter *d* refers to the thyroid gland, which regulates metabolism; *f* to the thymus, which produces T cells; and *g* to the adrenal glands, which regulate blood pressure as well as release estrogen, androgens, epinephrine, and cortisol, among other secretions.

11. **(B) c** Given the glands and organs represented in the diagram, this question is asking about communication within the endocrine system. Recall that most endocrine organs receive and relay chemical signals in the form of hormones. The exception to this is *c*, which refers to the hypothalamus. The hypothalamus receives electrical impulses from the brain. The label *b* refers to the pituitary gland, which is stimulated by one of several hypothalamic hormones; *e* refers to the parathyroid glands, which are stimulated chemically by calcium; and *k* refers to the ovaries, which are stimulated by LH or FSH.

12. **(C) k** This question is asking about the relationship between luteinizing hormone (LH) and progesterone. Recall that LH is released from the pituitary gland, labeled *b* on the diagram. In males, it stimulates the production of testosterone in the testes, labeled *m*. In females, it stimulates ovulation. After ovulation, the follicle develops into the corpus luteum, which secretes progesterone. This occurs in the ovaries, labeled *k*. The label *j* refers to the uterus.

13. **(C) Decrease gas exchange** This question is asking for a function that surfactant does *not* perform. Recall that surfactant decreases surface tension to prevent lung collapse and serves as a medium for gas exchange. Thus, answer choices (A), (B), and (D) can be eliminated. Surfactant does not decrease gas exchange, so choice **(C)** is correct.

14. **(C) Gastrin stimulates the release of HCl and pepsinogen.** This question is asking about chemical digestion in the stomach. Recall that the stomach secretes two main hormones (gastrin and ghrelin) and three main enzymes (gastric lipase, pepsinogen, and HCl). Gastrin stimulates the release of HCl and pepsinogen, which is converted to pepsin in the presence of acid. This matches choice **(C)**. Gherlin, choice (B), stimulates the appetite, not the exocrine cells of the stomach. Goblet cells, (D), are present in the stomach, but they release mucus. Glucagon, (A), is secreted by the pancreas.

15. **(A) Neurotransmitters** The question is asking what occurs at the synapse between a motor neuron and muscle fiber. Recall that neurotransmitters, such as acetylcholine, are released from the motor neuron and transmit the motor impulse to the muscles. Choice **(A)** is correct. After the neurotransmitters bind to the muscle fibers, calcium ions, (C), are released. The nodes of Ranvier, (B), are gaps in the axon's myelin sheath, and action potentials, (D), propel the motor impulse along the neuron.

16. **(A) Sweat gland activity and blood flow to the subcutaneous layer of the skin increase, and hair follicles relax.** This question is asking about thermoregulation. Recall that one of the primary roles of the integumentary system is to maintain internal body temperature. Sweat glands lower the body temperature via evaporative cooling. Blood vessels dilate to increase heat loss by convection and conduction. Hair follicles relax, causing hairs to lie flat on the skin's surface to prevent heat from becoming trapped against the skin. This response to increased body temperature matches answer choice **(A)**.

17. **(B) Renin** This question is asking about the enzymatic regulation of blood pressure in arteries. Recall that blood pressure can be controlled by vasodilation or vasoconstriction of the blood vessels and by changes to the volume of water that is excreted or reabsorbed by the kidneys, so predict that the correct answer affects one of these processes. Choice **(B)** matches your prediction. Renin is a renal enzyme that activates hormones responsible for regulating blood pressure and fluid balance. Epinephrine, choice (A), is a hormone that causes vasodilation or constriction; however, the question specifically asks for an enzyme. The nephron, (D), is the functional unit of the kidney. Glucagon, (C), is a pancreatic hormone.

18. **(B) Density** The question asks what property is affected when mass is held constant but volume is changed. Recall that density is defined as mass over volume, so if mass is held constant and volume is changed, the density will also change. It gets larger when the volume is decreased and smaller when the volume is increased.

19. **(A) Active immunity** This question is asking about the body's response to a live pathogen. Recall that pathogens trigger the immune system to create antibodies as well as memory B cells and T cells. These memory cells will respond to that specific pathogen if it is detected again in the future, there by establishing active immunity, choice **(A)**. Passive immunity, (B), is produced from exposure to antibodies, not the pathogen. By definition, an antigen, (C), is any substance that triggers an immune response. Autoimmune diseases, (D), occur when an immune response is triggered against the body's own cells.

20. **(A) Herniated lumbar disc** This question tests your ability to infer a logical cause-and-effect relationship. The term "sciatica" refers to the sciatic nerve, which is the largest single nerve in the human body and branches from the lower spine into the buttocks and legs. If you did not recall the anatomy of the sciatic nerve, because the symptom is pain "that shoots from the lower back through the hips and legs," you could infer the problem likely relates to a spinal nerve. The most likely cause of the symptoms would be a problem in the upper lumbar or lower thoracic discs, so choice **(A)** is correct. The coccyx (tailbone) is at the lowest end of the spine and is not the site of any spinal nerves, so damage there is not likely to cause the noted symptoms; eliminate (B). A bruised calf muscle would cause pain in the lower leg only, so (C) is incorrect. A myocardial infarction (commonly called a "heart attack," as the root *cardia* suggests) would not produce pain in the lower body, so eliminate (D).

21. **(D) There is no correlation between the candidate's popularity and voters' education.** The campaign manager wants to find out whether the candidate is equally popular among voters at all educational levels or whether she is more popular among voters with less education. The question asks for an appropriate null hypothesis for the manager's study. A null hypothesis states that there is no relationship between variables. In this case, the variables under study are the candidate's popularity and voter education level. Choice **(D)** correctly states that there is no relationship between these two variables. Choice (A) states a possible research, or experimental, hypothesis—that there is a relationship between the variables. Choice (B) makes a statement about other candidates, which is not the topic of the proposed poll. While there may be a direct relationship between voter income and education, the poll will examine the relationship between education and attitude toward this candidate, so choice (C) is incorrect.

22. **(C) Sarcomere** This question is asking about the anatomy of smooth muscle. Recall that smooth muscle is unstriated muscle that does not have individual neuromuscular junctions. Actin and myosin, choices (A) and (B) respectively, are

present in smooth muscle tissue, but they are *not* arranged into sarcomeres; this is why smooth muscle does not appear striated. The same logic confirms choice **(C)** as correct. Gap junctions, (D), occur in both smooth and cardiac muscle tissue, where they allow cells to contract in tandem.

23. **(C) It would melt to form the denser liquid state.** This question requires usage of the figure provided. According to the phase diagram, water is liquid at high pressures since the solid liquid line has a negative slope. Thus, if pressure were increased but temperature remained the same, solid ice would melt to liquid water since the liquid form is denser. Solids are not compressible, so the water will not change volume to become more dense—eliminate (A). Choice (B) is opposite to the correct answer because the liquid state is more dense.

24. **(C) Salt decreases the freezing point of water, enabling it to melt at lower temperatures.** Based on the information in the table, as more salt is added, the freezing point of water decreases. A lower freezing point means that the ice will melt at a lower temperature. Choices (A) and (D) can be eliminated since the addition of salt decreases, not increases, the freezing point. Choice (B) can also be eliminated since a decrease in freezing point would cause ice to melt at lower, not higher, temperatures.

25. **(D) Deposition** This question is asking for the process that does not require an input of heat. Recall that heat must be added to go from a solid to a liquid to a gas. Deposition, going from gas straight to a solid, will release heat. Melting, (A), going from solid to liquid; sublimation, (B), going from solid to gas; and vaporization, (C), going from liquid to gas, all require heat input.

26. **(D) Preventing the activation of cytotoxic T cells** This question is asking about the final stage of HIV infection, otherwise known as acquired immune deficiency syndrome (AIDS). Recall that the HIV virus replicates inside, and thus destroys, helper T cells, so you can predict the answer will relate to the role of these cells. This matches choice **(D)**. Helper T cells produce cytokines that activate the cytotoxic T cells. Choice (C) describes the cause of allergies, and (B) describes the changes that occur as antigen levels subside in a functioning immune system. The adaptive immune system responds to antigen signatures, as in choice (A).

27. **(B) Protects the body against dehydration** This question is asking about the role of the integumentary system. Recall that the integumentary system consists of the skin, hair, nails, and sweat glands. Predict that the integumentary system acts as a barrier against the outside world. Choice **(B)** matches this prediction, as the skin is a waterproof barrier that prevents

excessive fluid loss. While some fluid is lost through the sweat glands, it is the genitourinary system (choices (A) and (D)) that controls blood volume by regulating fluid loss. Choice (C) describes a role of the endocrine system.

28. **(C) Call prices are positively, linearly related to stock prices and positively, but not linearly, related to days remaining.** Note that you do not need to know anything about investing in the stock market to answer this question. Focus on what is being tested, which is the relationship between a dependent variable and two independent variables. Everything needed to determine the correct answer is contained within the question and table.

The question states that call prices are a dependent variable and the price of the underlying stock and the days remaining until expiration are independent variables. The accompanying chart displays some values of these three variables. The question asks you to determine which of the answer choices correctly describes the relationships among the variables. To determine the relationship of a dependent variable to a particular independent variable when there are multiple independent variables, hold the other independent variables constant. There are three table rows with 30 days remaining. The stock prices for those entries are $20, $40, and $60 and the call prices are $1, $2, and $3. So, if the days remaining are held constant at 30, the option price is $\frac{1}{20}$ of the stock price, and the relationship between these two variable is positive and linear. Eliminate choices (A) and (D). Similarly, for a stock price of $20, as the days remaining go from 30 to 60 to 90, the call prices are $1.00, $1.75, and $2.00. When the stock price increases from $30 to $60, the call price increases $0.75, but when the stock goes up another $30 to $90, the call price increases $1.25. Therefore, call prices are positively, but not linearly, related to days remaining, and choice **(C)** is correct.

29. **(A) Superior and ventral** This question is asking where the sternum is located in relation to the coronal and transverse planes. Recall that the sternum is located in the top half of the body in the front, so it is on the superior side of the transverse plane and on the ventral side of the coronal plane.

30. **(B) Urea** This question is asking about the normal components of urine. Recall that the body excretes wastes that have been filtered from the blood through the urine, so predict that the answer is a waste product. This matches choice **(B)**. Urea is a metabolic byproduct that is removed from the blood by the kidneys. Glucose, (A), in the urine can be an indication of diabetes. The presence of blood cells, (C), or protein (amino acids), (D), in the urine could indicate kidney damage.

**31. (C) The semilunar valves open under increased pressure.** This question is asking about ventricular systole. Recall that systole indicates a contraction of the heart muscle, so predict that the answer will refer to what occurs as the ventricles contract. This matches answer choice **(C)**: as the ventricles contract, the increased pressure forces open the semilunar valves, allowing blood to be ejected from the heart into the arteries. Atrial systole forces open the AV valves, as in choice (D), and ejects blood into the ventricle, (B). The ventricle is relaxed, (A), during ventricular diastole.

**32. (A) He equated correlation with causation.** The question describes a study that found a group of people who experience chronic pain were less happy than a comparable group that were not experiencing chronic pain. The researcher concluded that unhappiness "is a major cause of chronic pain." The question asks for the flaw in the researcher's reasoning. Although the numerical results do suggest a positive correlation between chronic pain and unhappiness, nothing in the study indicates whether sadness caused pain, pain caused sadness, or some third variable caused both. Choice **(A)** is correct. The fact that the two groups in the study had "the same demographic characteristics" discredits choice (B). If a study is properly performed, one study can test (but not prove) a hypothesis, so eliminate (C). Choice (D) is intriguing because no mention is made of the researcher's initial hypothesis, null or otherwise. Nevertheless, the presence or absence of the null hypothesis was not the reason for the researcher's unsupported conclusion.

**33. (D) Sympathetic and parasympathetic** This question is asking about homeostatic regulation. Recall that *homeostasis* refers to maintaining a stable internal environment. Predict that homeostasis is regulated by the two divisions of the autonomic nervous system that work in opposition to one another: sympathetic and parasympathetic. This matches answer choice **(D)**. The sympathetic division causes "fight or flight" responses, and the parasympathetic returns the body to its resting state.

**34. (A) Salivating** This question is asking for an activity that is part of chemical digestion. Recall that chemical digestion is the process by which food is broken down at the molecular level by acids, bases, or enzymes, so predict that the answer will involve a chemical agent. Choice **(A)** matches this prediction. Saliva contains two enzymes that break down carbohydrates and lipids. Choices (B) and (C), swallowing and chewing respectively, are examples of mechanical digestion. Belching could occur when stomach gasses build up as the result of digestion, but it is not a digestive process.

**35. (B) Gastric acid** The question asks you to identify which of the answer choices is *not* made up of macromolecules. Recall that the four most common macromolecules in biology are carbohydrates, lipids, proteins, and nucleic acids, so the correct answer will be a substance that is not one of these. Gastric acid is composed of three simple compounds, HCl, KCl, and NaCl, none of which are macromolecules, so choice **(B)** is correct. The other choices are all macromolecular substances.

**36. (A) A decrease in blood glucose stimulates glucagon; an increase in blood glucose stimulates insulin.** This question is asking about the regulation of blood glucose levels. Recall that blood glucose is regulated by two opposing hormones—glucose and insulin—operating as a negative feedback loop, and that insulin stimulates the cells to uptake glucose. Glucagon acts in an antagonistic fashion, meaning it acts to oppose insulin. Choice **(A)** matches this prediction. Glucagon is secreted when blood glucose is low; it causes glucose to be released from the cells, raising blood sugar levels. When blood sugar levels are high, insulin is secreted to lower the levels. Choice (B) is partly true; an increase in insulin lowers blood glucose. However, it is a *decrease* in blood glucose that stimulates glucagon. Choices (C) and (D) describe the opposite of what occurs.

**37. (B) 3, 2, 6** The question shows a chemical equation with the numbers of both reactants and one product missing. Your task is to find the coefficients that are needed to balance the equation. Since the coefficient of $Hg_3(PO_4)_2$ is known to be 1 because there is no blank preceding it, that is a good place to start. In order to get 3 atoms of Hg as a product of the reaction, there must be the same number in the reactants. The only source of this component is $Hg(OH)_2$, so the first missing number is 3. Similarly, 2 atoms of P are required because the subscript 2 applies to everything inside the parentheses, so the second blank is 2. Next look at H. There are $3 \times 2 = 6$ H in the first reactant and another 6 in the second reactant for a total of 12 H. Thus, 6 $H_2O$ will balance the equation, and choice **(B)** is correct. Verify this answer by checking the number of O. There are $3 \times 2 = 6$ plus $2 \times 4 = 8$ for a total of 14 O on the input side, and $4 \times 2 = 8$ plus $6 \times 1 = 6$ for a total of 14 on the output side—the O balances.

**38. (B) Tarsal** This question is asking you to correctly identify a short bone. Recall that short bones are wider than they are long. The tarsals of the foot are short bones. The phalanges of the fingers and toes, choice (A), are long bones; the scapula of the shoulder, (C), is a flat bone; and the radius of the forearm, (D), is a long bone.

**39. (A) Luteinizing hormone** This question is asking you to identify the hormone that induces ovulation. Recall that a spike in luteinizing hormone at day 14 in the menstrual cycle will trigger ovulation. Estrogen, choice (B), triggers the thickening of the endometrium, and progesterone, (D), maintains it. The corpus luteum, (C), is not a hormone. Instead, it is the remaining tissue after the follicle ruptures.

40. **(D) Increasing the concentration of oxygen in the blood** Recall that the rate of diffusion is proportional to the concentration gradient and to the surface area. To decrease the rate, either the concentration gradient or surface area must be smaller. The air always contains more oxygen than the blood, but by increasing the concentration of oxygen in the blood, the difference in concentration between the air and the blood becomes smaller, thus decreasing the rate of diffusion.

41. **(C) Milliliters** The question mentions a dosage amount in deciliters and asks what unit should be used to ensure that the dosage is accurate to within $\pm 1\%$ when measured to the nearest whole number. A deciliter is 0.1 L, and 1% converts to 0.01, so the required degree of accuracy is 0.1 L $\times$ 0.01 = 0.001 L, which is one-thousandth of a liter. The prefix for thousandth is *milli*, so choice **(C)** is correct.

42. **(D) Liver** This question is asking about bile production. Recall and predict that bile is produced in the liver, choice **(D)**. Bile is stored in the gall bladder, (A). It passes through the bile duct, (B), and is secreted into the duodenum (C).

43. **(A) Fallopian tubes, site of fertilization** This question is asking which reproductive structure is correctly paired with its function. Recall that follicles mature in the ovaries and fertilization of the ovum occurs in the fallopian tubes. Sperm are produced in the testes, and the prostate and seminal vesicles produce the nourishing and lubricating fluids for the sperm.

44. **(C) The black-furred parent has a recessive white fur allele.** The question states that white fur is a recessive trait and that a black-furred parent and a white-furred parent have a white-furred offspring. You must select the answer that is a valid deduction. Because white fur is a recessive trait, any white-furred member of the species must have two white fur alleles; this applies to both the white-furred parent and the offspring. Thus, the offspring must have acquired a white fur allele from the black parent. The black-furred parent must, therefore, have the recessive white fur gene, making choice **(C)** correct. The traits of one offspring have no bearing on the traits of subsequent offspring, so eliminate choice (A). The question states that the white fur allele is the recessive one, so (B) is incorrect. As already predicted, a white-furred animal of this species must have two white fur alleles; (D) is incorrect.

45. **(D) Veins** This question is asking about the anatomical presence of valves in blood vessels. Recall that valves prevent the backflow of blood. Because the blood pressure is lower as

blood is returned to the heart, you could predict that valves will be present in the blood vessels of the venous system. Choice **(D)** matches your prediction.

46. **(B)** $R = \dfrac{r_1 r_2}{r_1 + r_2}$ A class conducts an experiment to determine how placing different resistors in parallel affects the total resistance of a circuit. Voltage ($V$), which is held constant, is set by the researchers. The researchers also choose the resistors, $r_1$ and $r_2$. As the students place different resistors in parallel, they measure current flow ($I$). Then Ohm's law, $V = IR$, allows total resistance, $R$, to be calculated. The question asks for an equation that represents a hypothesis the class could be testing. Recall that a hypothesis is about the effects of independent variables on a dependent variable.

Choice (A) restates Ohm's law, which is a given, so it is not the hypothesis. Choice (C) merely rearranges Ohm's law. Eliminate these choices. Choice (D) calculates $r_1$ in terms of the other resistor and total resistance. But $r_1$ is known and controlled by the experimenters; after all, they choose each resistor to place in the circuit. This is not a dependent variable in this experiment. Choice **(B)** predicts that the resistance calculated using Ohm's law will be the product of the two resistors divided by their sum, and this is a hypothesis about the response of a dependent variable to manipulation of independent variables that can be tested by this experiment.

47. **(A) The diaphragm and intercostal muscles contract, decreasing pressure in the lungs.** The question pertains to muscle contraction and air pressure in the lungs. During inhalation, the diaphragm and intercostal muscles simultaneously contract, increasing the volume of the lungs, causing the pressure to drop. Air will subsequently flow into the lungs.

48. **(C) There is no apparent correlation between temperature and the number of bluebirds observed.** The scatterplot shows the data gathered by a bird-watcher, and you must identify the relationship between those two variables. Examine the pattern of the data points. There were three days when six or more birds were seen, and the temperatures on those days varied widely. Similarly, the recorded temperatures ranged from just over 40°F to 70°F on the days when only one bird was spotted. Thus, there is no discernible relationship between bluebirds and temperature; choice **(C)** is correct.

49. **(C) Plasma cells** This question is asking about the immune response to a new pathogen. Recall that a new pathogen would trigger the innate immune system. Therefore, predict that the answer will be a component of the adaptive immune system or not be a part of the immune system at all. Choice **(C)** is a match. Plasma cells are differentiated B cells that produce antibodies after being exposed to a known

antigen. Macrophages, (A); NK lympocytes, (B); and dendritic cells, (D), are all leukocytes of the innate immune system.

50. **(C) Liver** Because this question is asking about which organ does *not* secrete a hormone involved in nutrient absorption/distribution, you can predict that three of the answer choices will secrete hormones involved in digestion. Gastrin, a hormone that stimulates the release of HCl, is secreted by the stomach and the duodenum (part of the small intestine), as in choices (A) and (D), respectively. Secretin, a hormone that stimulates the release of pancreatic enzymes, is secreted from the pancreas, (B), as well as from the duodenum, (D). Other hormones with roles in digestion include insulin and glucagon (both from the pancreas) and cholecystokinin (CCK, from the small intestine). The liver, choice (C), creates bile, a key digestive enzyme but *not* a digestive hormone.

51. **(D) T cells** This question is asking about one part of the immune system. Recall that the adaptive immune system responds to specific antigens. This is in contrast to the innate immune system, which has a nonspecific response. T-cells are activated by the presence of specific antigens, so choice (D) is correct. Phagocytes, (A), ingest a variety of detritus in the blood, including dead cells and pathogens. Inflammation and earwax, choices (C) and (D) respectively, are part of the innate immune system.

52. **(B) Increase in blood pH** This question is asking what happens during hyperventilation that would lead to a decrease in respiration rate. The medulla oblongata in the brain stem changes respiration rate in response to changes in blood pH. Hyperventilation would lead to a large drop in blood $CO_2$ levels, causing the concentration of $H^+$ and $HCO_3^-$ to drop, resulting in an increase in blood pH. In response, the medulla oblongata would decrease the respiration rate.

53. **(A) Osteoclasts** The question asks what type of cells break down bone. Recall that osteoclasts break down or cleave bone. Osteoblasts, choice (C), help to build bone, and an osteocyte, (B), is the most common cell in mature bone. Osteons, (D), are not cells but are cylindrical structures within compact bone.

# English and Language Usage

1. **(B) :** This sentence begins with an independent clause (if a period followed "supplies," the sentence would express a complete thought. However, the missing punctuation mark introduces a list of items that could not stand alone as another sentence. The colon in choice (B) is the correct punctuation mark to introduce a list after an independent clause.

2. **(D) ballpark figure** The question indicates that the sentence has informal usage in it, so read looking for figures of speech that would not be appropriate for formal academic writing. The phrase "ballpark figure" in choice (D) is an informal expression that means "rough estimate." The other phrases in the answer choices are examples of formal or standard uses of the English language.

3. **(A) are** The subject of the sentence is the plural noun "producers." The missing word is part of the verb, which must agree in number with the subject. Choice (B) is incorrect because it is singular. Choice (C), "will," might be tempting because the new film will be released in the future. However, "will planning" is not the correct form of the future tense for an ongoing action; "will be planning" would be needed. Choice (A) correctly uses the plural "are," and it places the planning for the future release of the film in the present, a logical order of events.

4. **(D) Change "there" to "their."** In this sentence, the correct homophone is the plural possessive pronoun *their*.

5. **(C) Scientific report** Different publications require different writing styles for the intended audience to understand and appreciate the information. The tone, subject matter, and word choice of a piece of writing can indicate the type of publication in which it did or should appear. The sentence in this question, about a scientific study, is written in a formal tone using scientific wording such as "subjects" (instead of *people*). This type of text would most likely appear in a scientific report, choice **(C)**.

6. **(B) Because** The missing word introduces a subordinate or dependent clause and must express the cause-and-effect relationship between the act of leaving the water on and the overflowing of the sink. Only choice (B) properly expresses the relationship between the dependent clause and the independent clause.

7. **(D) Denied** The prefix *dis-* suggests reversal or removal, which indicates the meaning will be close to the opposite of *claim*. To "unclaim" knowledge is to *deny* knowledge, and choice (D), "Denied," is a match. If the researcher had "proclaimed" his knowledge of wrongdoing, he would have announced it.

8. **(A) Walter stepped out of the office building and walked toward his car, careful not to slip on the thin layer of ice that covered the parking lot.** A novel is a written narrative that tells the story of fictional characters and events. The style is typically descriptive, and the tone can vary depending on the subject matter. Choice (A) is the sentence most likely to be found in a novel because it narrates the actions of a specific character

and has a descriptive style. Choice (B) refers to recent events related to a crime and would likely be found in a news report. The tone of choice (C) is very formal and contains jargon that would likely be found in a business memo. Choice (D) is also formal, but the factual content indicates that it belongs in a scientific article.

9. **(A) Free** The prefixes *dis-* and *en-* are attached to the root word *tangle*. *En + tangle* means "tangled together." *Dis + en + tangle* means the opposite: "not tangled together." Choice **(A)**, "Free," matches this prediction. Context clues are helpful as well: the words "caught" and "snare" indicate being trapped, so you can infer that Marcus is attempting to "free" the fawn.

10. **(A) its ; her** A glance at the answer choices indicates that this question deals with pronoun rules. The first blank requires a singular, neuter pronoun to refer to its antecedent, "team." The second blank needs a singular, female, possessive pronoun because it is referring to each individual player on the girls' team.

11. **(C) Although free parking might draw more patrons to the downtown stores, the city cannot afford to lose any parking revenue.** A complex sentence is composed of an independent clause and a least one dependent clause. Choices (A) and (D) are simple sentences because they each only contain one independent clause. Choice (B) is comprised of two independent clauses joined by "and," so it is a compound sentence. In choice **(C)**, the first clause is dependent, since it does not express a complete thought by itself, while the second clause could stand alone as a complete sentence, making it independent.

12. **(C) Everyone who lost points on the test have to stay after class.** Analyze each sentence for subject–verb agreement; a singular subject requires a singular verb, and a plural subject requires a plural verb. You are looking for the *incorrect* example. In choice (A), the past tense verb "went" can be paired with either a singular or a plural subject, so this sentence is correct as written. The subject of the sentence in choice (B) is "boy," which correctly agrees with the singular verb "is going." In choice (D), the plural subject "cheerleaders" agrees with the plural verb "are leading." The subject of the sentence in choice **(C)** is the singular pronoun "everyone," which does not agree in number with the plural verb "have."

13. **(C) Types of research include quantitative and qualitative methodologies.** The title of this sample outline indicates that it presents ways to conduct research. The items are listed in a logical fashion, using heading levels to indicate relationships. The outline indicates that both quantitative and

qualitative methods are available to researchers, not that they need to choose one or the other, as in choice (A). Application and description are separate categories, so eliminate (B). Quantitative methods are listed first, but this does not imply that they are preferable to qualitative methods; eliminate (D).

14. **(C) Complyant** Each of these words involves a spelling rule that frequently causes trouble. The root word of choice (B), *enjoy*, correctly follows the rule for adding a suffix to a word that ends in *-oy*. Choices (A), (C), and (D) have root words that end in *y* preceded by a consonant (*rely, comply, deny*). Only **(C)** fails to follow the rule for adding a suffix beginning with a vowel, which is to change the *y* to *i*.

15. **(B) After Jarvis dropped the expensive laptop, everyone in the cafeteria turned around and stared at him.** The correct answer needs to convey the same meaning as the original sentences. Choice **(B)** conveys the information clearly and fluently, in the correct sequence. Choice (A) uses passive voice and lacks a comma after "Jarvis," which is needed because this answer choice is a compound sentence. Choice (C) also uses passive voice, and by placing the ideas in short modifying clauses, it produces a choppy effect. Choice (D) changes the meaning by using "because" to introduce a cause-and-effect relationship between the cost of the laptop and people turning to look; they may well have turned around because they heard the loud noise of some object falling without knowing what it was, let alone whether it was expensive.

16. **(D) weary.** If you are not certain of the meaning of "lethargic," use context clues to predict the correct answer. The phrase "took a nap" suggests that Ria was tired, so you can infer that feeling "lethargic" means being "tired." Choice **(D)**, "weary," is a match. If you read the word "weary" back into the sentence in place of "lethargic," it makes sense.

17. **(C) uncertain.** The context clues suggest that a precarious situation is one in which it is difficult to know how to behave or proceed. "Uncertain" is a match for this prediction.

18. **(B) The comma after "freedom"** This question asks about punctuation, and the sentence contains a number of commas and one semicolon. The semicolon is used correctly to join two independent clauses that express closely related thoughts. The comma in choice **(B)** incorrectly separates the two terms of the compound direct object—"freedom" and "discipline."

19. **(D) had drunk** This question is testing two important concepts—verb tense and irregular verb forms. To determine the tense of the missing verb, analyze the context clues and decide the logical order of the events described in the sentence. In this sentence, Dana did something with water prior

to running. When an action is completed prior to another past action, past perfect tense is correct. Eliminate choices (A) and (C). The verb *to drink* is an irregular verb that changes its spelling to "drank" in past tense and "drunk" in the past perfect tense. Choice **(D)** uses the proper tense and correct spelling of the verb *to drink* for this sentence.

20. **(C) veins** The context clues suggest the correct word relates to a blood vessel; of the homophones *vanes*, *vain*, and *vein*, only choice **(C)** is a type of blood vessel. With an apostrophe, the word "vein's" is singular and possessive; a correct construction with this word would be "The vein's lining may become irritated."

21. **(C) Finally, if the expanded trial succeeds, the FDA should consider approving the new drug.** This question tests your understanding of paragraph structure. The paragraph gives details of a drug trial that has taken place and of a proposed trial of the drug. The concluding sentence will provide a logical next step in the sequence of events or outcome of the series of trials. Choice **(C)** begins with the key word "finally," indicating that it is a concluding statement, and this sentence recommends a future action based on what has come before. The other choices offer supporting details about the clinical study and the drug.

22. **(A) their ; they're** The answer choices in this sentence are all homophones, meaning they sound alike but have different spellings, definitions, and even parts of speech. The context clues in the sentence help clarify which word is needed in each blank. The first blank requires a possessive adjective, narrowing the choices down to (A) and (B). The second blank must include a subject and helping verb, so the contraction *they're*, short for "they are," in choice **(A)** is correct.

23. **(B) Knowledge of an event before it happens** The root and affixes suggest "prescience" most nearly means "knowing" (*sci*), "before" (*pre-*), and "the state of something" (*-ence*). Thus, predict this word means "knowing something beforehand." This matches choice **(B)** very well.

24. **(D) scratching her head** This question asks about informal usage, so read the sentence looking for language that would not be appropriate for formal academic writing. The phrase

"scratching her head" is an informal, figurative expression that is used to describe confusion in response to a unexpected situation.

25. **(D) uncertainty.** "Trusted" provides a context clue; because he trusts her, Gregory is likely to be certain or confident in Kiera's sincerity. Therefore, the phrase "without reservation" most likely means "without condition" or "with certainty." To act "with certainty" means to act "without uncertainty," making choice **(D)** the correct answer. A reservation can be a thing that is set aside, or assigned, for some use (e.g., "We have a table reserved for dinner"), but that meaning does not fit the context here, making (A) incorrect.

26. **(A) When she found her brother outside, Julie exclaimed, "Michael, there you are! A short while ago, mother said, 'Children, come inside.'"** Recall that in direct dialogue, the quoted text is separated from the speaker by a comma. The sentence in choice **(A)** correctly introduces Julie's quote and the quote inside her quote with a comma. The quotation of the mother's words is properly offset with a pair of single quotation marks.

27. **(A) Similarly** The blank in the sentence must be filled by a transition word that links a sentence about one study to a sentence about another study. Both studies support the idea that lack of sleep affects people's cognitive skills. The word "Similarly" reflects this relationship between the sentences. All the other answer choices would signal contrasting ideas.

28. **(C) The rusty old boat with the torn sails** The complete subject of a sentence includes the simple subject and all words and phrases in the sentence that describe it. In this sentence, "boat" is the simple subject. The article "The," the adjectives "rusty" and "old," and the prepositional phrase "with the torn sails" all serve to describe the boat.

# Kaplan Study Planner for the TEAS

The tables below correspond to the content areas of the test. For each test content area—*Reading, Mathematics, Science, and English language and usage*—circle the question numbers that you answered correctly in the second column. Write the number of questions you answered correctly in the third column. For purposes of this diagnostic test, count all of the questions toward your score.

To calculate the percentage correct for each content area, enter the number of questions you got right in the numerator (top part) of the fraction. Then do the calculations: divide the number you got right by the number of questions in the content area and multiply that result by 100. Follow the same procedure for calculating your overall percentage; here you are dividing by the number of questions on the test, which is 170.

If you do not have time to review all of the lessons in this book, target the areas where you have the most opportunity to improve your score. Note that if a school you are applying to considers scores in each content area, then you will want to focus most on the content areas in which you missed the greatest *percentage* of correct answers. However, if a school considers the composite (overall) score, then focusing on the areas in which you missed the greatest *number* of questions can raise your composite score the most.

## Reading, 53 questions

| Lesson | Pretest Question Numbers | # Correct |
|---|---|---|
| **Chapter 1: Main Ideas and Supporting Details** | | |
| Lesson 1: Strategic Reading | 5, 19, 21, 34, 42, 48 | 4 out of 6 |
| Lesson 2: Reading for Details | 1, 6, 26, 38, 40, 45 | 6 out of 6 |
| Lesson 3: Making Inferences | 3, 10, 13, 22, 28, 37, 44, 51 | 6 out of 8 |
| Lesson 4: Understanding Sequences of Events | 4, 11, 25, 36, 47 | 5 out of 5 |
| **Chapter 2: Passage Structure and Word Choices** | | |
| Lesson 1: Understanding the Author's Purpose and Point of View | 8, 12, 15, 20, 24, 33, 39, 49 | 8 out of 8 |
| Lesson 2: Using Text Structure and Features | 7, 29, 35, 52 | 3 out of 4 |
| Lesson 3: Determining Word Meaning | 2, 32, 41, 53 | 3 out of 4 |
| **Chapter 3: Integrating Ideas to Draw Conclusions** | | |
| Lesson 1: Comparing and Contrasting Multiple Sources | 14, 17, 50 | 1 out of 3 |
| Lesson 2: Making Inferences About Fiction | 16, 43 | 1 out of 2 |
| Lesson 3: Evaluating an Argument | 9, 18, 27, 31, 46 | 2 out of 5 |
| Lesson 4: Integrating Data From Different Formats | 23, 30 | 1 out of 2 |
| **Total *Reading*** | | 40 out of 53 |

$$100 \times \frac{\phantom{xx}}{53} = \underline{\phantom{xx}}\%$$

# Mathematics, 36 questions

| Lesson | Pretest Question Numbers | # Correct |
|---|---|---|
| **Chapter 1: Arithmetic and Algebra** | | |
| Lesson 1: Arithmetic | 1, 10, 13, 16, 26, 31 | ____ out of 6 |
| Lesson 2: Algebra | 3, 23, 32 | ____ out of 3 |
| Lesson 3: Solving Word Problems | 4, 8, 14, 15, 24, 36 | ____ out of 6 |
| Lesson 4: Ratios, Percentages, and Proportions | 6, 11, 17, 20, 25, 27, 28, 30 | ____ out of 8 |
| Lesson 5: Estimating and Rounding | 9, 19, 34 | ____ out of 3 |
| **Chapter 2: Statistics, Geometry, and Measurements** | | |
| Lesson 1: Tables, Charts, and Graphs | 7, 18 | ____ out of 2 |
| Lesson 2: Statistics | 2, 29 | ____ out of 2 |
| Lesson 3: Covariance and Causality | 5, 22 | ____ out of 2 |
| Lesson 4: Geometry | 12, 33 | ____ out of 2 |
| Lesson 5: Converting Measurements | 21, 35 | ____ out of 2 |
| **Total *Mathematics*** | | ____ out of 36 |

$$100 \times \frac{\phantom{x}}{36} = \underline{\phantom{xx}}\%$$

# Science, 53 questions

| Lesson | Pretest Question Numbers | # Correct |
|---|---|---|
| **Chapter 1: Human Anatomy and Physiology** | | |
| Lesson 1: Human Anatomy and Physiology: An Overview | 2, 29 | ____ out of 2 |
| Lesson 2: The Skeletal System | 38, 53 | ____ out of 2 |
| Lesson 3: The Neuromuscular System | 1, 15, 22, 33 | ____ out of 4 |
| Lesson 4: The Cardiovascular System | 6, 9, 31, 45 | ____ out of 4 |
| Lesson 5: The Respiratory System | 13, 40, 47, 52 | ____ out of 4 |
| Lesson 6: The Gastrointestinal System | 3, 14, 34, 42, 50 | ____ out of 5 |
| Lesson 7: The Genitourinary System | 7, 17, 30 | ____ out of 3 |
| Lesson 8: The Endocrine System | 10, 11, 12, 36 | ____ out of 4 |
| Lesson 9: The Reproductive System | 39, 43 | ____ out of 2 |
| Lesson 10: The Immune System | 19, 26, 49, 51 | ____ out of 4 |
| Lesson 11: The Integumentary System | 4, 16, 27 | ____ out of 3 |
| **Chapter 2: Biology and Chemistry** | | |
| Lesson 1: Macromolecules: Carbohydrates, Proteins, and Lipids | 35 | ____ out of 1 |
| Lesson 2: Heredity | 44 | ____ out of 1 |
| Lesson 3: Atoms and the Periodic Table | 5 | ____ out of 1 |
| Lesson 4: Properties of Substances | 18 | ____ out of 1 |
| Lesson 5: States of Matter | 23, 24, 25 | ____ out of 3 |
| Lesson 6: Chemical Reactions | 37 | ____ out of 1 |
| **Chapter 3: Scientific Procedures and Reasoning** | | |
| Lesson 1: Scientific Measurements and Relationships | 8, 20, 41 | ____ out of 3 |
| Lesson 2: Designing and Evaluating an Experiment | 21, 28, 32, 46, 48 | ____ out of 5 |
| **Total *Science*** | | ____ out of 53 |

$$100 \times \frac{\phantom{xx}}{53} = \underline{\phantom{xx}} \%$$

# English and language usage, 28 questions

| Lesson | Pretest Question Numbers | # Correct |
|---|---|---|
| **Chapter 1: Spelling, Punctuation, and Sentence Structure** | | |
| Lesson 1: Spelling | 4, 10, 14, 20, 22 | ___ out of 5 |
| Lesson 2: Punctuation | 1, 18, 26 | ___ out of 3 |
| Lesson 3: Sentence Structure | 6, 11, 28 | ___ out of 3 |
| **Chapter 2: Grammar, Style, and the Writing Process** | | |
| Lesson 1: Grammar | 3, 12, 19 | ___ out of 3 |
| Lesson 2: Formal and Informal Style | 2, 5, 8, 24 | ___ out of 4 |
| Lesson 3: The Writing Process | 13, 15, 21, 27 | ___ out of 4 |
| **Chapter 3: Vocabulary** | | |
| Lesson 1: Using the Correct Word | 7, 9, 16, 17, 23, 25 | ___ out of 6 |
| **Total *English and language usage*** | | ___ out of 28 $100 \times \dfrac{\quad}{28} = \_\_ \%$ |

| Total | |
|---|---|
| | ___ out of 170 $100 \times \dfrac{\quad}{170} = \_\_ \%$ |

# Reading

Understanding written material will be critical to your success in a nursing or health science program and to your ability to care for clients as a health care professional. Whether reading a textbook, a patient's chart, a healthcare facility's policies, or research study results, you will need to be able to grasp an author's main idea and purpose in writing, evaluate trends or patterns in words and data, focus on important details, draw appropriate conclusions on the basis of what you've read, and apply information and conclusions to your work. The TEAS *Reading* content area tests your ability to perform these tasks.

**Questions by Content Area**

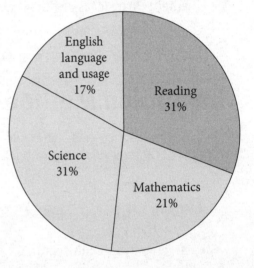

## The TEAS Reading Content Area

Of the 170 items on the TEAS, 53 will be in the *Reading* content area, and you will have 64 minutes to answer them.

While you have on average just over a minute per question, most questions will require reading a short passage or a figure or table first. As a rule of thumb, if you invest about 45 seconds in reading a paragraph of text, a table, or a figure and take about 30 seconds to answer each question, you will stay on pace to complete the *Reading* section.

> *Example:* A three-paragraph text passage has four questions associated with it.
>
> 45 seconds × 3 paragraphs = 2 minutes 15 seconds
>
> 30 seconds × 4 questions = 2 minutes
>
> Reading the passage and answering four questions takes 4 minutes 15 seconds.

Of course, some passages, tables, and figures are very short and will take much less than 45 seconds to read, while others are longer and will require more time to map. Some questions will not refer to any information beyond what's in the question itself. The key is to work at a steady pace. Reading in a hurry because you are worried about time will lead to choosing wrong answers.

Of the 53 *Reading* questions, 47 will be scored and 6 will be unscored. You won't know which questions are unscored, so do your best on every question.

The 47 scored *Reading* questions come from three sub-content areas:

| Sub-content Areas | # of Questions |
|---|---|
| Key ideas and details | 22 |
| Craft and structure | 14 |
| Integration of knowledge and ideas | 11 |

To help you prepare for these questions, this part of your book is divided into three chapters:

- Chapter 1: Main Ideas and Supporting Details
- Chapter 2: Passage Structure and Word Choices
- Chapter 3: Integrating Ideas to Draw Conclusions

# The Kaplan Method for Reading

Reading on the TEAS requires a **strategic** approach. Following the Kaplan Method for Reading helps you get the correct answer efficiently, without wasting time.

## KAPLAN METHOD FOR READING

**Step 1:** Read the stimulus strategically.*

**Step 2:** Analyze the question.

**Step 3:** Research.

**Step 4:** Predict the answer.

**Step 5:** Evaluate the answer choices.

* If there is only one question on a stimulus, switch the order of steps 1 and 2. If there is no stimulus, begin with Step 2.

## Step 1: Read the stimulus strategically.

The *stimulus* is the passage, figure, or chart on which the questions are based. Reading *strategically* means paying special attention to the **topic** and **scope** of the stimulus. The topic is the subject the author is writing about, and the scope is the specific aspect of that topic in which the author is interested. In a passage, the topic and scope are often found in the first few sentences. In a figure or graph, they are often found in the title, headings, and labels. Also, seek to understand the author's **purpose** in writing. Often, this is to explain a process, describe a topic, or outline information, but sometimes the author is presenting a particular point of view or seeking to persuade the reader.

When the stimulus is a passage of more than a few sentences or a figure or table of any complexity, you should also take notes as you read. Your notes should sum up the important ideas of the stimulus. Write notes in your own words and use abbreviations and symbols. Your notes become a **map** of the stimulus, both summarizing important information and helping you find details to answer questions. Investing time in understanding the stimulus helps you answer the questions more efficiently.

*Note:* Some questions do not refer to a stimulus. When this is the case, proceed directly to step 2. Also, if there is only one question on a stimulus, read the question first (step 2) and then read the stimulus strategically as you research the answer to that question (combining steps 1 and 3).

## Step 2: Analyze the question.

Determine exactly what the question asks you to find. Is it asking for the author's main point or primary purpose in writing? Or is it asking for a detail from the stimulus? Or is it asking you to make an inference based on the stimulus? Or is it asking why the author included some detail or feature? How you research your map and the stimulus and what you will look for in a correct answer depend on the task in the question.

## Step 3: Research.

Research the answer in the stimulus. If you mapped it in step 1, your map will help you find the right place quickly; read your notes and, as needed, the appropriate portion of the stimulus.

If you are reading the stimulus for the first time, because there is only one question on the stimulus, then make sure to read it strategically. Many TEAS questions require you to grasp the big picture of a stimulus, interpret a detail in context, or connect the dots between different details.

## Step 4: Predict the answer.

Before looking at the answer choices, *predict* the correct answer. Having the answer clearly in mind before looking at the choices will help you choose the correct answer and not be misled by choices that "sound right" but aren't actually correct.

Some questions are open-ended and don't allow for a precise prediction. Examples are "Based on the passage, what conclusion can you reasonably draw?" or "Which of the following questions are answered by the passage?" Even in these cases, you can review your map and prepare a mental checklist of the important ideas and information in the stimulus. The correct answer will align with one of those.

## Step 5: Evaluate the answer choices.

Evaluate the answer choices looking for a match for your prediction and eliminating choices that do not match. If the answer you expected is not there, revisit Steps 2–4 to refine your thinking.

# CHAPTER ONE

# MAIN IDEAS AND SUPPORTING DETAILS

## LEARNING OBJECTIVES

- Identify the author's main idea and the details used to support that idea
- Identify the relevant information to answer a question
- Make logical inferences based on information provided
- Use the relationship of events in a sequence to answer a question or achieve a result

Of the 47 scored *Reading* questions, 22 (47%) will be in the sub-content area of *Key ideas and details*. With these questions, the TEAS tests your ability to read for the "big picture" and for important details, as well as to draw inferences from your reading and apply what you learn from text.

This chapter addresses these skills in four lessons:

**Lesson 1:** Strategic Reading

**Lesson 2:** Reading for Details

**Lesson 3:** Making Inferences

**Lesson 4:** Understanding Sequences of Events

**Reading Questions by Sub-content Area**

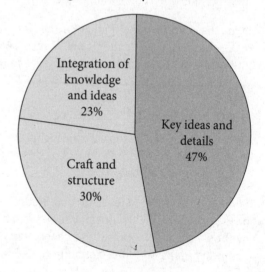

# LESSON 1

# Strategic Reading

## LEARNING OBJECTIVES

- Identify the author's main idea
- Identify supporting details

## Main Idea

Many TEAS questions ask you to identify the main idea, which is the subject the author is writing about or the point he or she is making in the stimulus. You can identify the main idea by asking yourself, "What does the author want me to know?" You should also ask, "Why does the author want me to know it?" Sometimes the writer will be simply describing or explaining a topic, and other times the author will be trying to persuade you of a particular point of view.

The correct answer to a question about the main idea, topic, or author's primary purpose in writing is broad enough to reflect the entire stimulus, but not so broad that it goes beyond the author's point. Eliminate answer choices that are supporting details; these answers are too narrow.

## Supporting Details

Other questions ask about details the author includes to support the main idea. Details are explicitly stated in the stimulus, and important details in passages—the kind of details you are likely to see a question about—are usually indicated by keywords indicating contrast, emphasis, or a sequence. Contrast keywords, which signal a different idea or example, include "however" or "on the other hand." "Especially" or "surprisingly" are examples of emphasis key words, signaling a fact or idea the author thinks is important. Words like "first," "second," and "third" or a series of dates indicate a sequence of events or steps. Details may also be highlighted by structural features of the text, like headings.

Follow along as a TEAS expert answers first a main idea question and then a supporting detail question.

Like most superheroes, the Incredible Hulk possesses supernatural abilities. Among other talents, he has unlimited strength and the ability to leap several miles. Though theoretically capable of great evil, he is on the side of good, an especially important position given the time in which he first appeared in Marvel comics. First created at the height of post–World War II paranoia about nuclear war, the Incredible Hulk stories offer a fascinating look at the dual nature of human beings. On the one hand, he is a mild-mannered, bespectacled scientist. On the other, he is a raging, rampaging beast. More than a statement about the dangers of the Atomic Age, the Hulk is a reflection of the two sides in each of us—the calm, logical human and the raging animal.

| Question | Analysis |
|---|---|
| | **Step 1:** The author begins by describing the Incredible Hulk. This description lays the foundation for the author to argue that the Incredible Hulk symbolizes the dual nature of human beings. |
| The author's primary purpose is | **Step 2:** This is a main idea question. Consider the entire passage to determine the author's purpose. |
| | **Step 3:** The author's main point is summarized in the last sentence. The other sentences in the paragraph are supporting details. |
| | **Step 4:** Predict that the correct answer is about what the Incredible Hulk symbolizes. |
| (A) to explain the confusion people can feel due to their dual nature. | **Step 5:** The author does not discuss any confusion people might feel about their dual nature. |
| (B) to argue that the Incredible Hulk symbolizes more than the particular concerns of his time. | Correct. This matches your prediction. The author's purpose is to argue that the Incredible Hulk symbolized not only post–World War II anxiety about nuclear war but also a more universal concern about human nature. |
| (C) to discuss the cultural and psychological importance of comic books in the post–World War II era. | The passage is not about comic books in general, only about the Incredible Hulk. |
| (D) to critique people's fears about nuclear war in the mid-twentieth century | This suggests that the author has an opinion about people's fears, but the author's opinion is about what the Incredible Hulk symbolized. |

Here is a test expert's approach to a supporting detail question.

| Question | Analysis |
|---|---|
| According to the author, the comic book character of the Incredible Hulk first appeared | **Step 2:** This question asks for a detail—information stated in the passage. |
| | **Step 3:** Your map shows that the relevant detail is in the middle of the paragraph, where the author places the superhero in historical context. The sentence with this detail begins: "First created at the height of post–World War II paranoia . . . ." |

| Question | Analysis |
|---|---|
|  | **Step 4**: Predict an answer that restates this sentence. |
| (A) during a lull between wars. | **Step 5**: The passage does not mention a period between wars. |
| (B) after a nuclear attack. | The author notes anxiety about nuclear war but does not mention an actual nuclear attack. |
| (C) in a period of fear about nuclear war. | Correct. This choice matches your prediction. |
| (D) during a protest about atomic power. | The passage mentions fear of nuclear war but not protests over atomic power. |

Now practice answering a main idea and a supporting detail question yourself. After reading and mapping the passage and answering each question, check your work against the explanations that follow.

In a remote valley of Baja California, Mexico, a small group of Kumeyaay Indians retain their traditional way of life. It was here that Eva Salazar learned the ancient art of basket weaving from her tribal elders. Among the Kumeyaay, women have the crucial responsibility of making baskets, which are important artifacts of everyday life. Kumeyaay baskets, tightly woven with expressive designs, were made mostly for utilitarian purposes—for cooking, storing food products in, gathering ingredients, and even, when turned upside down, wearing as hats. As traditional objects of art, they are also valued for their aesthetic beauty.

Following in her ancestors' footsteps, Eva Salazar uses traditional materials to weave her intricate baskets, primarily the strong, sharp reed known as juncus, as well as yucca, sumac, and other plants. She colors the reeds with black walnut, elderberry, and other natural dyes. Eva specializes in coiled baskets, made by starting the weaving at the bottom center of the basket and adding coils upward, then stitching the coils together. The shapes and decorations echo traditional forms. Her most ambitious work is a basket measuring almost three feet in diameter, which took her two years to weave and represents a masterpiece of Native American art.

Which of the following correctly states the main subject of the passage?

(A) Native American basket weaving
(B) A master basket weaver
(C) Uses of natural plants and dyes
(D) Kumeyaay traditions

## Explanation

### Step 1:

Topic: Kumeyaay Indian basket weaving
Scope: master weaver Eva Salazar
Purpose: inform
¶ 1: Importance and uses of baskets for the Kumeyaay
¶ 2: Eva Salazar—how she makes baskets

**Step 2:** This is a main idea question.

**Step 3:** Look at the topic and scope in your map to determine the main idea.

**Step 4:** Predict that the topic is Eva Salazar and her basket weaving.

**Step 5:** Only one answer choice mentions a specific basket weaver, so **(B)** is correct. Choice (A) is too broad. Choice (C) is a detail mentioned in the passage but not the main idea. Choice (D) goes beyond the point of the passage: the subject is basket weaving only, not all Kumeyaay traditions.

> The passage supports the statement that Salazar has followed in her ancestors' footsteps by stating that she
>
> (A)   mainly makes very large baskets.
> (B)   is also a skilled storyteller of traditional tales.
> (C)   uses natural materials and dyes.
> (D)   teaches basket weaving to college students.

## Explanation

**Step 1:** The passage is the same as for the previous question.

**Step 2:** This question asks for a detail stated in the passage. The detail concerns Salazar's relationship with her ancestors.

**Step 3:** Your map shows you that details about Salazar are mostly in the second paragraph, so start your research there. The first two sentences are details about this master basket weaver "following in her ancestors' footsteps" by using traditional materials and dyes.

**Step 4:** Predict that the answer will have something to do with using traditional materials.

**Step 5:** The correct answer is choice **(C)**. None of the other answer choices matches your prediction.

## KEY IDEAS

- Main idea questions ask about the overall topic or purpose of the passage.
- Supporting detail questions ask about evidence the author uses to develop the topic.
- Approach reading strategically, focusing on the passage's topic and scope and the author's purpose in writing.
- Make a prediction before evaluating the answer choices so you do not waste time thinking about or researching incorrect answers.

# Strategic Reading Practice Questions

**Questions 1–6 refer to the following passage.**

In modern society, a form of folktale called the urban legend has emerged. These stories persist both for their entertainment value and for the transmission of popular values and beliefs. Urban legends are stories many have heard, claimed as true, but never actually verified. If you try to confirm one, it turns out that the people involved can never be found. Researchers of urban legends call the elusive participant in these supposedly "real-life" events a "FOAF": friend of a friend.

One classic urban legend involves alligators in the sewer systems of major metropolitan areas. According to the story, before alligators were a protected species, people vacationing in Florida purchased baby alligators to take home as souvenirs. After the novelty of having a pet alligator wore off, people would flush their souvenirs down the toilet. The baby alligators found a perfect growing environment in city sewer systems, where to this day they thrive on an ample supply of rats.

Urban legends also change with the times. In today's world of medical advances, one legend is that unsuspecting people are kidnapped, anesthetized, and subjected to an operation. They wake up with a kidney removed. Though even minimal research can dispel many legends, some seem plausible enough to be taken as true, at least initially. Occasionally, they have turned up on legitimate news broadcasts; more often, though, they are repeated through emails and social media.

1. The main focus of the passage is
    (A) traditional folktales.
    (B) urban legends.
    (C) friends of friends.
    (D) medical advances.

2. According to the passage, the successful urban legend contains all of the following characteristics EXCEPT
    (A) the topics of urban legends can change with the times.
    (B) messages that conform to popular values.
    (C) the qualities of a folktale.
    (D) a basis in reality.

3. Which of the following claims about urban legends is stated in the passage?
    (A) Their themes change with the times.
    (B) Most urban legends can be verified.
    (C) Urban legends are traditional forms of folklore.
    (D) Urban legends are mostly transmitted by national media.

4. The author of the passage is primarily concerned with
    (A) alligators living in Florida sewers.
    (B) kidney donors.
    (C) a new form of folklore.
    (D) researching urban legends.

5. According to the passage, urban legends are
    (A) restricted to cities.
    (B) easy to trace back to their source.
    (C) never taken seriously.
    (D) aligned with popular beliefs.

6. Which of the following is NOT explicitly stated in the passage?
    (A) Pet alligators were supposedly abandoned in sewers.
    (B) All urban legends instill fear in listeners.
    (C) Social media are frequent transmitters of urban legends.
    (D) Urban legends can be entertaining.

**Review your work using the explanations in Part Six of this book.**

# LESSON 2

# Reading for Details

## LEARNING OBJECTIVES

- Identify the relevant information in text to answer a question
- Identify the relevant information in a graphic to answer a question

## Details in Text

The TEAS tests your ability to glean relevant information from many different types of printed communication, including announcements, academic essays, advertisements, instructions, and memos. The test will include communications you might encounter in school, at work, or at home or around town.

Some TEAS questions require you to find specific information that is stated within a passage or depicted in a graphic. The TEAS will word these questions in a variety of ways:

> What reason does the author give to avoid mixing chemicals X and Y before sterilization?

> According to the passage, which of the following is a kind of ornament commonly found in Gothic cathedrals in England?

> At what time will the Annual General Meeting be held?

The correct answer to a detail question will be information or an idea that can be found in the stimulus. It may state the information using the same words as are in the stimulus, or it may paraphrase the information. Note that sometimes wrong answer choices will be information that is in the stimulus but do not answer the question asked. These choices might be tempting because they look familiar, but by analyzing the question to determine exactly what you are being asked for (step 2 of the Kaplan Method for Reading), you will avoid these traps.

Study how a TEAS expert would answer this detail question, one of several questions about the stimulus.

> To the Editor:
>
> Lately, there has been a good deal of discussion about whether or not a new bridge should be constructed over the Millville River. I firmly believe that this structure should be completed at the earliest opportunity, for some very good reasons. The current bridge is clearly decrepit, and indeed must be closed several months a year for much-needed maintenance. Our city should be embarrassed by the nuisance this inconvenience brings to commuters and tourists.
>
> Some might argue that our city cannot afford the considerable expense required for a bridge so far from the town center, but this concern can easily be dealt with. The state governor has made it clear that she considers infrastructure a matter of primary concern and will lobby the federal government for funding. And, as our city expands with new subdivisions providing housing to accommodate our booming population, the Millville River route will only see more and more traffic in the future.

| Question | Analysis |
|---|---|
| | **Step 1:** Read the passage strategically. The letter has two paragraphs. The first states why the author believes a new bridge is needed. The second paragraph introduces a possible objection to the project—its expense—but dismisses this objection before moving on to a prediction about the city's population. |
| What does the letter writer say about the expense of constructing the new bridge? | **Step 2:** This is a detail question. You are looking for something the author says about the cost of the new bridge. |
| | **Step 3:** According to your passage map, information about cost is in paragraph 2—it's a possible barrier to construction. Research that paragraph. |
| | **Step 4:** The author states that the governor has prioritized the bridge project and will lobby for federal funds to pay for it. Look for an answer choice that says either the bridge will be expensive or that it will funded at least in part with federal dollars. |
| (A) It can be recouped by a newly instituted road tax. | A road tax is never mentioned in the letter. Eliminate. |
| (B) The high cost means the project will not proceed. | This prediction is contrary to the letter writer's opinion, which is that money can be found for the bridge. |
| (C) It can be met with federal funds. | Correct. This matches your prediction. |
| (D) It is the sole responsibility of the state. | Although the governor has said that infrastructure is a primary concern of the state, there is no suggestion that the state must be the sole funder. Indeed, the opposite is the case. |

Now you try one. After answering the question, check your work against the explanation that follows.

## First Annual Memorial Day Concert
*Free to the Public!*

**When:** May 26, noon to sunset

**Where:** Granville Park

**Kickoff:** Welcome speech from special guest Mayor Edugyan

**Performances:** The Campertown College Marching Band, the River Valley Elementary School Children's Choir, and Marco Whicker and the Sunset Singers

According to the poster, who will concert attendees see first on stage?

(A) The Campertown College Marching Band
(B) Marco Whicker and the Sunset Singers
(C) Mayor Edugyan
(D) This question cannot be answered from the information on the poster.

## Explanation

**Step 2:** This is a detail question asking about the program order of a concert. Note the question asks about the first person on stage, not first performer. Look for the part of the poster that indicates the sequence of events.

**Steps 1 and 3:** The announcement is divided into different sections. Look for the parts of the poster that indicate the sequence of events. At the top is the name of the event and the information that it's free. Then a section marked "When" states the date and time of the event. Following that is information about the location and, finally, who will be speaking or performing.

**Step 4:** The "kickoff" is a welcome speech by the mayor, so predict that the mayor appears on stage first.

**Step 5:** Choice **(C)** matches your prediction and is correct; a welcome speech kicking off the event logically precedes the performances. Choice (A) is incorrect: although the marching band is the first performer listed, it will follow Mayor Edugyan's kickoff address. Choice (B) is also incorrect because the mayor's kickoff precedes all the performances. Finally, choice (D) is incorrect because the poster does provide the information you're asked for.

# Details in Graphics

The TEAS also tests your ability to identify relevant information presented in graphical form such as maps, graphs, charts, or illustrations. TEAS questions might require you to read examples of graphical representation, recognize figures and graphics within a piece of text, or determine relationships between visual elements.

Study this example of how an expert would approach a question accompanied by an information-laden graphic:

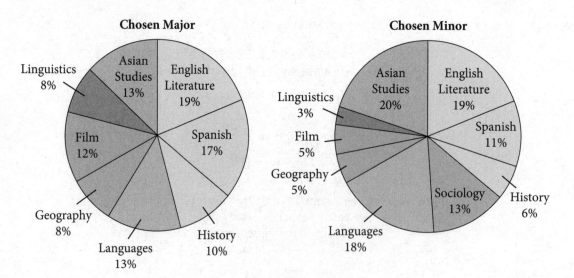

Total students = 500

Brockmeier Liberal Arts College Student Survey Results

| Question | Analysis |
|---|---|
| At Brockmeier College, students do not major and minor in the same field. According to the charts, what percentage of Brockmeier College students choose Film as their major or as a minor field of study? | **Step 2:** The question asks for the total percentage of students who choose Film as a major or minor. |
| | **Steps 1 and 3:** The two charts provide data from a survey of 500 students—specifically percentages of students in each major (left) and minor (right). Because the question asks about majors and minors, look at both pie charts and read the percentages from the Film "slice." |
| | **Step 4:** Because students never major and minor in the same field, the percentages can be added: 12% report Film as their major, while another 5% report it as their minor. Add: $12 + 5 = 17$. |
| (A) 5 | **Step 5:** This is the percentage of Film minors. |
| (B) 12 | This is the percentage of Film majors. |
| (C) 17 | Correct. This matches your prediction. |
| (D) 85 | If you calculated the number of students with Film as a major or minor, then you would get 85. However, the question asks for the percentage, and percentages are directly stated in the charts. |

## KEY IDEAS

- Read each question stem carefully so you know exactly what it is asking.
- When researching the answer to a detail question, don't get distracted by extraneous information.
- Pay attention to headings and labels in graphics so you know the location of key information.

# Reading for Details Practice Questions

**Questions 1–2 refer to this passage.**

Most life is fundamentally dependent on photosynthetic organisms that store radiant energy from the Sun. In almost all the world's ecosystems and food chains, photosynthetic organisms such as plants and algae are eaten by other organisms, which are then consumed by still others. The existence of organisms that are not dependent on the Sun's light has long been established, but until recently they were regarded as anomalies.

Over the last 20 years, however, research in deep-sea areas has revealed the existence of entire ecosystems in which the primary producers are chemosynthetic bacteria that are dependent on energy from within the Earth itself. Indeed, growing evidence suggests that these sub-sea ecosystems model the way in which life first came about on this planet.

1. The passage states that most life depends ultimately on which of the following?

   (A) Photosynthetic plants and algae
   (B) Sub-sea ecosystems
   (C) Chemosynthetic bacteria
   (D) Sunlight

2. According to the passage, which of the following statements is true about both photosynthetic and chemosynthetic organisms?

   (A) Both are at the base of their respective food chains.
   (B) Both are capable of receiving energy from the Earth.
   (C) Sunlight is the basic source of energy for both.
   (D) Chemosynthetic organisms are more abundant than photosynthetic organisms.

**Questions 3–4 refer to the following timeline.**

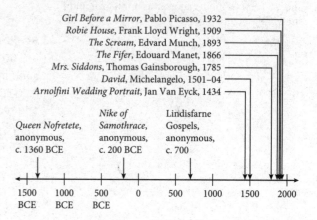

3. How many works of art predate the Common Era?

   (A) 1
   (B) 2
   (C) 3
   (D) 8

4. Which pair of artworks have creation dates that are furthest apart?

   (A) *Nike of Samothrace* and Lindisfarne Gospels
   (B) *Arnolfini Wedding Portrait* and *Mrs. Siddons*
   (C) *The Scream* and *Robie House*
   (D) *Robie House* and *Girl Before a Mirror*

**Questions 5–6 refer to the following map.**

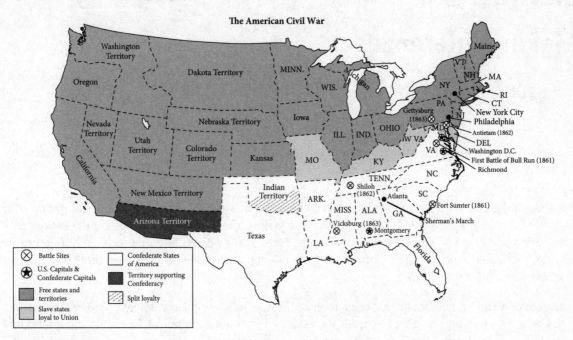

The American Civil War

5. Which battlefield site shown is furthest north?

(A) First Battle of Bull Run
(B) Shiloh
(C) Antietam
(D) Gettysburg

6. Which of the following slave states did NOT join the Confederacy?

(A) Texas
(B) Arizona
(C) West Virginia
(D) Ohio

**Review your work using the explanations in Part Six of this book.**

# LESSON 3

# Making Inferences

## LEARNING OBJECTIVES

- Make logical inferences from statements in a stimulus or question stem
- Apply knowledge of inferences to identify and eliminate false and unsupported conclusions

The TEAS will often ask questions about facts or beliefs that are suggested or implied, but not actually stated outright in the passage. These require you to make correct **inferences** based on the provided information and common knowledge. For example, if you saw a person put on a raincoat before heading outside, you would probably infer that it was either raining or expected to rain, even though no one has said anything about the weather.

There are two main requirements for any inference. First, it has to logically follow from the information that's given. An inference is either logically necessary or very likely to be true based on the information given and common sense. Second, inferences are always unstated. When a fact is stated explicitly, it does not need to be inferred.

Incorrect answer choices to inference questions can be eliminated when they contradict the passage, contradict facts that can be inferred from the passage, are contrary to common sense and general knowledge, or are not implied or suggested by the passage at all.

Follow along as a TEAS expert maps a passage and answers two inference questions.

Dear Applicant,

Thank you for applying to our recent job advertisement. We've been rated one of the best companies to work for as well as one of the top companies in our industry. We believe that success is due to the people who work here. Each of our employees has the right skill set for their role and is the best possible fit for their team. We want to maintain the high-functioning ability of our teams. Therefore, we consider each new team member's application with great care.

You can be confident that your qualifications will be given the same thoughtful consideration we give to those of all prospective new employees. This is often the slowest step of the hiring process, and we would appreciate your not calling us during this period for updates on your application. If you have not heard from us within 15 business days of receiving this letter, then we wish you good luck in your job search and invite you to reach out to us about future opportunities.

| Question | Analysis |
|---|---|
| | **Step 1:** Paragraph 1 establishes that this is a letter acknowledging receipt of a job application. It provides information about the company's goals and how they influence the hiring process. Paragraph 2 explains that the applicant may hear back within 15 business days, but if not, encourages them to apply again. |

| Question | Analysis |
|---|---|
| If the job applicant who received the letter above does not hear anything further after one month, what conclusion should she draw? | **Step 2:** This is an inference question. Consider both paragraphs, but especially the second, as well as the information given in the question. |
| | **Step 3:** Paragraph 2 explains whether and when an applicant can expect to hear back. The response should come, if at all, within 15 days. |
| | **Step 4:** It can be clearly inferred that a person who does not hear from the company within 15 days has not been selected for an interview (if they were, there would be no reason to wish the applicant luck or encourage them to apply for future openings). It can also be inferred that the company does not think the applicants it declines to interview are among the top choices (paragraph 1). Predict that this applicant was not selected to be interviewed. |
| (A) The company misplaced her contact information. | **Step 5:** This choice is contradicted by the fact that the company has already sent her a letter acknowledging her application. |
| (B) The hiring manager did not feel she was likely to be the best fit for the role or team. | Correct. This is a good match for the prediction. |
| (C) The company has not yet determined whom to interview. | The statement in paragraph 2 implies the company does not take more than 15 business days to contact interviewees. Eliminate. |
| (D) The company is leaning toward hiring someone else but is not ready to rule her out. | There is no support for this. It can be inferred from paragraph 2 that anyone not selected for an interview will remain uncontacted without being explicitly told they were rejected, so the lack of contact does not imply a final decision is still pending. |

Here is another inference question on the same passage.

| Question | Analysis |
|---|---|
| Based on the letter, which of the following can be concluded about the company? | **Step 2:** This is an inference question. |
| | **Step 3:** The question stem does not point to a particular part of the passage. Review your passage map so you have the letter writer's important points in mind. |
| | **Step 4:** Predict the correct answer will be supported by information in the passage. |

| Question | Analysis |
|---|---|
| (A) The company expects a large number of applicants for the positions it advertises. | **Step 5:** The first paragraph mentions the job was advertised, so the company has potentially reached a large number of job seekers. This is a generic form letter that doesn't even mention the applicant's name. The letter also implies that applicants should expect to hear back within 15 business days or not at all. It's reasonable to assume from these facts that the company is trying to minimize the amount of time spent communicating with each applicant, which makes sense when there is a large number of applicants. Choice **(A)** is therefore a well-supported conclusion. |
| (B) The company is fairly small. | Nothing in the passage implies this answer choice is true. |
| (C) The company has low standards for its employees. | This is directly contradicted in the first paragraph. |
| (D) The company is brand new. | There is nothing in the passage to support this answer choice. In fact, the statement that the company and its employees are the best implies some history of performance. |

Now practice answering some inference questions on your own. After reading and mapping the passage and answering the question, check your work against the explanation that follows.

Packaging on many popular foods is deceiving to consumers. Too often, the print is small and hard to read. Even if you can read it, it's often confusing or intentionally vague. This is especially true on the nutrition label. Consumer protection advocates say the government ought to do something about the nutrition labels on food because the existing laws don't go far enough.

One recent example of legislation that would have addressed these concerns is a bill, which unfortunately died in committee, that would have forced American distributors to include information related to hormones and antibiotics in meat. There is no ingredient list on a package of ground beef to tell consumers what chemicals they may be ingesting, and perhaps there won't be for some time. But don't consumers have a right to information about what they're putting in their bodies?

The author of the passage would probably support which of the following?

    (A)    A ban on magazine advertisements for cigarettes
    (B)    Unsolicited grocery store flyers
    (C)    Fine print on a contract
    (D)    Allergy information prominently listed on food labels

## Explanation

### Step 1:

Topic: Incorrect/dishonest food package labels
Scope: Why the gov't should do more to protect consumers
Purpose: To argue for more gov't regulation
¶ 1: Why food labels are bad; advocates say gov't should do something
¶ 2: Example of law author supports—info on hormones/antibiotics in meat; law failed
Author: Such laws are needed

**Step 2:** The words "probably support" make this an inference question.

**Step 3:** Your map tells you the author's overall position on the topic and says it's in paragraph 2. For confirmation, you could look at the rhetorical question at the end of the passage.

**Step 4:** Predict that the author would most likely support greater information about food content being made available to consumers.

**Step 5:** Match your prediction with correct answer **(D)**. The author does not take a position on advertisements of unhealthy products, so it cannot be concluded that the author would support choice (A). Choice (B) is unrelated to the main argument of the passage, which is about food labels, while choice (C) is something the the author would likely be against, based on the complaint about hard-to-read ingredient lists.

> Based on the passage, it is reasonable to assume that
>
> (A)  food label laws are primarily an American issue.
> (B)  nutrition is not a top priority for the average consumer.
> (C)  most companies do not voluntarily provide clear and accurate information on food labels.
> (D)  the government has only recently begun to regulate the food industry.

## Explanation

**Step 2:** The words "Based on the passage" and "reasonable to assume that" tell you this is an inference question.

**Step 3:** The question does not focus on a specific part of the passage, so answer choices need to be checked and eliminated one at a time. Review your passage map so you have the letter writer's important points in mind.

**Step 4:** The correct answer choice will be a valid inference from the passage.

**Step 5:** Match your prediction to answer choice **(C)**. It can be inferred from the statement that "existing laws don't go far enough" that a majority of companies in the food industry do not provide more information than legally required. None of the other answer choices are directly contradicted in the passage, but neither are they implied.

## KEY IDEAS

- Recognize key terms that signal inference questions.
- Predict what ideas an author would agree with by using the author's statements to infer a logical conclusion.
- Evaluate answer choices by checking whether they logically follow from the passage; eliminate choices that are not fully supported.

# Making Inferences Practice Questions

**Questions 1–5 refer to the following passage.**

In the dog days of summer, there's a difficult choice to make: tripping over a collection of noisy, bulky fans or running up the electric bill with pricey air-conditioning. But at least it's a choice. In the winter months, high heating bills seem to be simply a fact of life. But there is an alternative: the Arizona Desert product line. It's no longer necessary to choose between economy and comfort. You can have both.

On cold nights, lower your thermostat and plug in the time-tested Arizona Desert electric blanket, which *Consumer Services* magazine calls "the most reliable and best value available by a wide margin." Enjoy your coffee on those chilly mornings in our newest product, the Arizona Desert heated robe. Like our blanket, this robe, the first of its kind, contains our patented heating system with an unobtrusive motor that is as silent as it is invisible. Heating coils warm a fluid, which is then circulated by the motor through tubes sewn into the tough but soft insulating fabric. The temperature can be adjusted to within one degree, and the robe or blanket heats up in minutes.

The tough tubing keeps the heated fluid, with our patented chemical formula, completely sealed. It never needs to be replaced, so you are never exposed to any risk of contact with it. If the tubing cracks or tears, or the motor fails, just bring the product immediately to your nearest supplier and get a replacement—no questions asked. Do not try to repair or replace any parts yourself. Using a mere 100 watts for the blanket and 75 watts for the robe (less than the average toaster uses), these products will run for less than 15 cents per day. This is a heating solution that pays for itself, and then pays you.

1. The above passage is most likely excerpted from

    (A) an advertising brochure.
    (B) a consumer reporting magazine.
    (C) a government report.
    (D) a personal email from a close friend.

2. The final paragraph implies that

    (A) the Arizona Desert products are a viable alternative to a standard toaster.
    (B) consumers who use Arizona Desert products will lower their heating costs.
    (C) toasters contribute a major portion of the average household energy budget.
    (D) cost is not a major factor in determining approaches to heating.

3. From the passage, the reader can determine that

    (A) electric blankets are more expensive to purchase than central heating.
    (B) air conditioners use more energy than fans.
    (C) the Arizona Desert company is a new start-up.
    (D) electric blankets are used primarily by those without central heating.

4. Which of the following would the passage's author likely consider least important to a person thinking of purchasing an electric blanket or robe?

    (A) Energy savings
    (B) Safety
    (C) Comfort
    (D) Country of manufacture

5. The warning label on the blanket would likely NOT include which of the following statements?

    (A) Warning! Chemical fluid—toxic!
    (B) Avoid submerging in water, as electric shock could occur.
    (C) Choking hazard—do not swallow.
    (D) Do not disassemble or modify any part of the heating mechanism.

**Review your work using the explanations in Part Six of this book.**

# LESSON 4

# Understanding Sequences of Events

## LEARNING OBJECTIVES

- Identify key words and phrases that denote order and steps
- Apply an understanding of the relationship of events or steps in a sequence to answer a question
- Follow a set of instructions to achieve a result

## Series of Events or Actions

When the TEAS presents a stimulus that focuses on the order of events or actions, it is vital to identify the words that tell you in what order to perform the steps or how events happened in relation to each other. To tackle such passages, timelines, or other figures, look for certain key words and phrases.

Sequence and timing key words and phrases place steps chronologically. Here are some examples: *first, second, third; before, after, next, finally, later; by the time, when/once* [something has happened]; *in the mid-1990s, after the turn of the century.*

Continuation key words may indicate that one step or event is over and the next is beginning. Examples include *moreover, furthermore, also,* and *in addition.*

Following directions requires you to read carefully, noting what materials are needed and what to do with them. A series of actions may be described out of order, as in this example:

> Until the customer has completed the purchase, be available to answer questions.

Here, being available to answer questions happens first, before the customer finishes the purchase. This order of events is indicated by the key word "Until." When a stimulus involves a number of steps given out of order, jotting them down in order may help you keep them straight.

Here are the directions for making tea. Follow along as a TEAS expert answers a question about the sequence of steps.

| Question | Analysis |
|---|---|
| Before boiling water to make tea, make sure you have tea bags ready. Fill a kettle with water and put it on the stove over medium to high heat. While the water is warming, take out the cups you will use. After the water reaches a boil, turn off the heat and pour some into each cup. Finally, add the tea bags. | **Steps 1 and 3:** The paragraph lists the steps to making tea. The steps are not in first, second, third order. Note the words "while," "after," and "finally." These tell you the correct order.<br><br>Look for "tea bags" to determine where they come in the process. The tea bags appear twice, once at the beginning (when you get them ready) and again at the end (when you add them). It's the latter action that this question mentions, so back up one step from there. |

| Question | Analysis |
|---|---|
| The step prior to placing tea bags in the cups is | **Step 2:** This question asks you to correctly identify a particular step in a process. |
| | **Step 4:** Predict that the step prior to adding tea bags is pouring water into the cups. |
| (A)   taking out the cups. | **Step 5:** This step is done while the water is heating. Eliminate. |
| (B)   getting the tea bags ready. | This is the first step in the process. Eliminate. |
| (C)   pouring water into the cups. | Correct. This matches your prediction; it's the step immediately before adding tea bags. |
| (D)   putting the water on to boil. | This is part of the second step, after getting the tea bags ready; eliminate. |

## Following Instructions

The TEAS may give you a set of instructions and ask you to follow them. Then you must find an answer choice that matches the result. Here's an example of how an expert would tackle this kind of question.

| Question | Analysis |
|---|---|
| Start with the list of letters below. Follow the directions to change the list.<br><br>a d e h n o<br><br>1.   Reorder the list of letters above by placing the vowels in alphabetical order followed by the consonants in reverse alphabetical order.<br>2.   If a letter is a consonant, add the vowel that comes after it in the alphabet directly after it in the list.<br>3.   If a letter is a vowel, add the consonant that comes after it in the alphabet directly after it in the list. | **Steps 1 and 3:** There are six letters, three vowels and three consonants, and the letters are in alphabetical order. The instructions ask you to (1) reorder the letters, (2) add vowels to the list after the consonants, and (3) add consonants to the list after the vowels. |
| After step 3, which letter is in the middle of the list? | **Step 2:** This question asks you to reorder a list of letters by following a set of instructions. |

| Question | Analysis |
|---|---|
| | **Step 4:** Follow the instructions, step-by-step.<br><br>1.  a e o n h d<br>2.  a e o n *o h i d e*<br>3.  a *b e f o* p n *o* p h i *j* d e *f*<br><br>Note that in (2), you insert the vowels after the consonants in the rearranged list, the list that is the output of (1). Then in (3), you insert the consonants in the list that is the output of (2).<br><br>There are now 15 letters in the list. Count in from both ends to find the middle letter. It is the 8th letter, with 7 letters on either side.<br><br>a b e f o p n **o** p h i j d e f |
| (A)  h<br>(B)  n<br>(C)  o<br>(D)  p | **Step 5:** The correct answer is **(C)**. After the list has been rearranged and added to according to the instructions, *o* is in the middle of the list. |

## KEY IDEAS

- When reading a stimulus, note key words and phrases that indicate sequence and time.
- If events or steps are given out of order, construct the proper order mentally or by jotting some notes.
- When following instructions, work step-by-step, making sure to apply the instructions in one step to the result of the previous one.

# Understanding Sequences of Events Practice Questions

**Questions 1–4 are based on the following instructions.**

**Creating an Ikebana Floral Arrangement**

*Materials:*

- Shallow dish
- Floral "frog" (disc with short spikes that hold flowers in place)
- Flowers, stems, and other plant material in at least three different lengths

*Instructions:*

First, fill the dish with 1½ inches of water. Then, place the frog in the dish at the 7:00 position. Put the longest stem at the 11:00 position on the frog. Next, place the second-longest stem on the frog at the 8:00 position, then place the third-longest stem in the 4:00 position.\* Now, continue placing all other plant material in any position that pleases you.

\*Lean the first three stems toward the right.

1. Based on the information in the steps, where is the third-longest stem placed?

   (A) At the 4:00 position
   (B) At the 8:00 position
   (C) At the 11:00 position
   (D) At any pleasing position

2. The first step in making an ikebana arrangement is

   (A) placing the frog.
   (B) using all plant material.
   (C) adding water to the dish.
   (D) placing the longest stem in the frog.

3. Suppose a florist has four items: a bamboo stem of 4 inches, a chrysanthemum of 5½ inches, an iris of 3 inches, and a pine branch of 8 inches. According to the directions, in what order would the florist place the plants in the frog?

   (A) pine, iris, chrysanthemum, bamboo
   (B) iris, bamboo, chrysanthemum, pine
   (C) pine, chrysanthemum, bamboo, iris
   (D) bamboo, pine, chrysanthemum, iris

4. After the third-longest stem, all other stems should be placed

   (A) in any place.
   (B) at the left.
   (C) at the right.
   (D) in the center.

**Questions 5–8 refer to the following passage.**

Construction of the Golden Gate Bridge, connecting San Francisco with Marin County, was started in 1933 and finished in 1937. At the time, it was the longest suspension bridge in the world at 4,200 feet, though it lost this title when the Verrazano-Narrows bridge was built in New York in 1964. On the Golden Gate's first day, May 27, only one person was allowed to walk across the bridge, but the next day 200,000 people walked across it. Currently pedestrians can walk the bridge until 6:00 PM Pacific Standard Time, but skateboards, roller skates, and electric scooters are not allowed at any time. Cars, however, cross at all times, at a rate of approximately 112,000 vehicles per day, having paid a toll only in the southbound direction toward San Francisco.

5. If a person wanted to cross the bridge at 8:00 PM Pacific Standard Time, he or she would need to do so

   (A) on an electric scooter.
   (B) in a car.
   (C) on a skateboard.
   (D) on foot.

6. The Golden Gate Bridge was the longest suspension bridge in the world until

   (A) 1934.
   (B) 1944.
   (C) 1954.
   (D) 1964.

7. On May 28, 1937, how many pedestrians crossed the bridge?

   (A) 1
   (B) 4,200
   (C) 112,000
   (D) 200,000

8. In 1936, the Golden Gate bridge was

    (A) begun.
    (B) finished.
    (C) open.
    (D) under construction.

9. Start with the numbered squares below. Follow the directions to rearrange them.

| 1 | 2 | 3 | 4 | 5 | 6 | 7 | 8 |
|---|---|---|---|---|---|---|---|
| 9 | 10 | 11 | 12 | 13 | 14 | 15 | 16 |

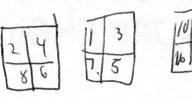

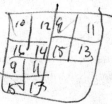

1. Make a larger square out of the first four even-numbered squares, placing the lowest-numbered square in the upper left corner and placing the squares from least to greatest in clockwise fashion.
2. In the same manner as in step 1, make a larger square from the first four odd-numbered squares.
3. In the same manner as in step 1, make a larger square from the remaining even-numbered squares.
4. In the same manner as in step 1, make a larger square from the remaining odd-numbered squares.
5. Using the 4 × 4 squares created in steps 1–4, make a larger square. Place the square containing the single largest number in the upper left and proceed counterclockwise, each time selecting the remaining 4 × 4 square containing the largest number.

Which of the following statements is true regarding the result of steps 1–5 above?

    (A) The square numbered 15 is to the right of the square numbered 6.
    (B) The square numbered 10 is above the square numbered 15.
    (C) The square numbered 2 is to the left of the square numbered 12.
    (D) The square numbered 6 is below the square numbered 15.

**Review your work using the explanations in Part Six of this book.**

# PASSAGE STRUCTURE AND WORD CHOICES

## LEARNING OBJECTIVES

- Determine an author's point of view on a subject and purpose in writing about it
- Analyze how a writer uses rhetorical mode and various features of text to communicate clearly to an audience
- Discover the meanings of words through use of context and references and distinguish among a word's various meanings

Of the 47 scored *Reading* questions, 14 (30%) will be in the sub-content area of *Craft and structure*. The TEAS tests your ability to discern an author's purpose in writing, especially the author's point of view on a topic and potential biases he or she may hold. The TEAS also evaluates your understanding of the different kinds, or modes, of texts, as well as how an author uses features—such as typographical variety, headings, and tables of contents—to help the reader grasp the material. In addition, questions will ask you to analyze how a writer uses style and word choice to convey particular meanings.

This chapter addresses these skills in three lessons:

**Lesson 1:** Understanding the Author's Purpose and Point of View

**Lesson 2:** Using Text Structure and Features

**Lesson 3:** Determining Word Meaning

**Reading Questions by Sub-content Area**

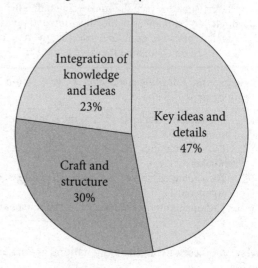

Integration of knowledge and ideas 23%

Key ideas and details 47%

Craft and structure 30%

# LESSON 1

# Understanding the Author's Purpose and Point of View

**LEARNING OBJECTIVES**

- Identify the overall purpose of a stimulus based on tone, structure, and key words
- Analyze key words and passage structure to determine the author's point of view
- Distinguish between facts and opinions in text

All pieces of text are written for a **purpose**. Sometimes, the intention behind a piece of writing is very simple. For example, the warning on a propane tank was written to **inform** users about safe handling procedures. An even simpler example would be the big red EXIT over an emergency door. Sometimes the author of a passage has a more complex purpose in mind: a mass email sent out on behalf of a political party may be intended to **persuade** readers to adopt a particular viewpoint on a social issue, with the hope that readers will then vote a certain way, provide financial support to the party, or even try to convince others of that same perspective.

While an author's **point of view** is most obvious in a persuasive text, even informational texts sometimes reveal an author's attitude toward a subject.

## Determining Purpose and Point of View

Recognizing the author's purpose when reading a stimulus will help you to quickly answer questions about the author's intent and attitude, including any biases the author holds, as well as the intended context and audience of the piece. Questions may ask "With which of the following statements would the author likely agree?" "Which idea would the author most sympathize with?" and "What is the author's opinion on [some issue or topic] likely to be?"

The author's purpose may be to tell a story, provide information, change your mind, or just entertain you. If the **tone** of the writing is factual and straightforward, as in an instruction booklet or a news report, the author is likely seeking to inform or relate events. If the tone of the passage is more emotional (angry, sarcastic, excited, happy, or sad), the author is more likely to be trying to persuade you of something. Keep an eye out for any **key words** that signal authorial opinion—for example, *misguided*, *brilliant*, or *impressive*.

In a persuasive passage, the author will express a clear point of view and ask the reader to accept it. An author may also express a point of view in a passage that is informative. The author's attitude will be reflected by his choice of words, the way he structures the passage (what information is given the most focus), and the sources he draws on, if any. An article that refers to *homeless youth* reveals a different attitude toward the subject than an article that refers to *scruffy young vagabonds*. An essay that cites news reports reflects a less biased approach to the topic than an essay that references "what most people think" or "what's been said on the Internet."

When persuasion is the goal, the author will make an **argument**. That is, the author will promote a point of view, or **conclusion**, and will present **evidence** to support that conclusion. Conclusions are always opinions, while evidence may be either facts or opinions.

Follow along as a TEAS expert maps a passage and answers two questions about the author's purpose and point of view.

Different people have different approaches to choosing a personal computer. Some people pick a new computer at random, falling victim to the latest trend or advertisement. These people often regret their decisions in the long run. On the other hand, people who do thorough research before purchasing a computer are much happier with their decisions over time. When you are shopping for a new computer, conducting research is an important step.

The best source for unbiased information is a respected consumer reporting magazine like *Technology Reports Monthly* or *Desktop Computer Shopper*. These magazines have built a reputation for unbiased, accurate reporting their readers can rely on. Unlike retail salespeople or advertisers, these publications seek to provide consumers with accurate information so they can select the right computer for them.

| Question | Analysis |
|---|---|
|  | **Step 1:** Topic: computers<br>Scope: consumer decisions<br>Purpose: to give advice<br>¶ 1: Research key to choosing right computer<br>¶ 2: Rely on consumer mags—unbiased |
| What is the author's goal in writing this passage? | **Step 2:** This is a question about the author's overall purpose. |
|  | **Step 3:** Look at your passage map. |
|  | **Step 4:** Predict that the author wants to provide advice to consumers about how to make good decisions. |
| (A) To argue that retail salespeople are generally untrustworthy | **Step 5:** Though the author implies that it might be in a retail salesperson's best interest to mislead consumers, this choice is too extreme. Furthermore, it is definitely not the author's primary purpose. |
| (B) To provide advice to nonexperts about how to select the right personal computer | Correct. The author provides information in this passage, but with the ultimate goal of suggesting what consumers *should* do when choosing a computer. |
| (C) To share an opinion about which computer magazines offer the best information on technology | The author only mentions the two trustworthy magazines as examples of where people can find unbiased information. Be careful not to confuse details with the main goal of the passage. |
| (D) To provide information about consumers' retail computer purchases | Though this may be tempting, the author quickly moves on from discussing how many consumers make purchasing decisions to how they *should* make purchasing decisions, first explaining the consequences of poor planning and then advising how to make an informed choice. |

Here is another question based on the same passage.

| Question | Analysis |
|---|---|
| If the author of the passage were planning to purchase a new dishwasher, which of the following sources of information would the author be most likely to trust? | **Step 2:** The question asks you to understand and apply the author's point of view to buying a dishwasher, a topic not discussed in the passage. |
| | **Step 3:** The passage map captures the author's point of view that consumer reporting magazines are unbiased. Researching paragraph 2 finds that these magazines provide reporting "readers can rely on," a strong positive opinion. |
| | **Step 4:** Predict that the author would look for an unbiased source of information, especially a consumer reporting publication or any other unbiased third party with a reputation for honesty. |
| (A) The Acme Appliance Company's dishwasher brochure | **Step 5:** Incorrect. The author would consider advertising copy from a dishwasher manufacturer biased. |
| (B) An entertainment website's list of the most popular dishwashing habits | The author argues against following the latest trends, so this is also incorrect. |
| (C) *Dishwashers Tonight*, a respected third-party consumer reporting podcast | Correct. This matches the prediction. It's a podcast rather than a magazine, but the key is that it is respected for its consumer reporting and is unaffiliated with a manufacturer. |
| (D) The expert, noncommissioned salespeople in a department store's home appliances section | This could be tempting, as salespeople who are not on commission might be less biased toward closing a sale, but that's not the same as "unbiased." The author never suggests the warning about salespeople is limited to those on commission, so this choice doesn't fit with what is known about the author's opinion. |

Now practice answering some questions on your own. After reading and mapping the passage and answering the questions, check your work against the explanations that follow.

**Questions 1–2 refer to the following stimulus.**

It is a common belief among writers that great art is born from experience. An overused example is the purported similarity of Ernest Hemingway with the protagonist of his celebrated novel *A Farewell to Arms*. Yet some of the greatest writers in literary history have had a very limited knowledge of the world.

Novelist Jane Austen, for example, did not venture far beyond her circle of family and friends. Yet, just by observing the people around her, she was able to write acclaimed comedies about love and marriage. And Robert Louis Stevenson, the author of classic adventures such as *Treasure Island* and *Kidnapped*, wrote many of his stories without having had similar experiences.

William Faulkner wrote, "A writer needs three things: experience, observation, and imagination, any two of which, at times any one of which, can supply the lack of the others." This is clearly true for great writers.

1.  How would the author of the passage above most likely feel about science fiction novels set on other planets?

    (A)  A writer with keen enough observation and imagination could write great stories in these settings.
    (B)  Childish adventure tales, like pirate tales set in space, would be the limit of what this genre could produce.
    (C)  Only a former astronaut could write such stories and achieve high literary quality.
    (D)  These stories mark the future of truly artful literature, as only the greatest writers go beyond their own experiences.

## Explanation

**Step 1:**

Topic: great writers
Scope: does life experience = great art?
Purpose: to argue life experience is not necessary to produce great art
¶ 1: Common belief: art from life
¶ 2: Austen and Stevenson: great writers with minimal experience
¶ 3: Author: for great writers, experience is not always necessary

**Step 2:** The question asks what the author's opinion would be of science fiction not set on Earth.

**Step 3:** The author seeks to persuade readers that not all great writers base their work on personal experience. The author uses the examples of Austen and Stevenson and quotes Faulkner in support of this conclusion.

**Step 4:** The author would feel that, though no one alive today has had experience living on other planets, science fiction in such a setting could achieve literary greatness.

**Step 5:** Answer choice **(A)** is a match for the prediction. Choice (B), with its negative tone indicated by words like "[c]hildish" and "limit," is not correct. Choice (C) contradicts the author's belief that experience is not always necessary. Choice (D) is too extreme. The author argues that writers without personal experience can still create great work, not that *only* writers without personal experience can create great work.

2.  What is the purpose of this passage?

    (A)  To provide information about several great classical authors
    (B)  To argue that Hemingway, though great, fell short of his more influential predecessors
    (C)  To argue that there is more than one approach to producing great literature
    (D)  To share several opinions about where great art comes from

## Explanation

**Step 2:** The question asks for the author's purpose in writing the passage.

**Step 3:** The passage is persuasive, and the author's opinion is that life experience is not always necessary for writers to produce great work.

**Step 4:** Predict that the author's purpose is to argue this point of view.

**Step 5:** The prediction matches answer choice **(C)**. The author believes that while some writers draw on personal experience to produce great literature, others do not. (A) is not correct; while the author does provide information about several authors, the author does so to make a point, not simply to inform the reader. (B) is also incorrect, as the author never compares the quality of Hemingway's work to that of other authors. The author dismisses the argument about Hemingway as "overused" but says nothing negative about Hemingway himself. (D) is incorrect; although the author does share some beliefs (a "common belief" in paragraph 1 and Faulkner's view in paragraph 3), the author's purpose is to argue for one over the other.

## KEY IDEAS

- An author's primary purpose can be to inform, to persuade, to tell a story, or to entertain.
- An author can reveal a point of view in both persuasive and informative texts through word choice, structure, and sources.
- To answer questions about what the author would think about something not mentioned in the stimulus, you need to understand the author's point of view.

# Understanding the Author's Purpose and Point of View Practice Questions

**Questions 1–4 refer to the following passage.**

Few immigrants just before the turn of the 20th century found life in America easy. Many of those who lacked professional skills and did not speak English found themselves living in slums in the busy cities of the Northeast, exploited by their employers and trapped in poverty. Around this time, a number of organizations tried to help these newly arrived immigrants adapt to American life. While many groups emerged as leaders in these efforts to aid immigrants, one organization put forward a much harsher recipe for adapting to America.

The Daughters of the American Revolution (DAR) approached immigrants with the expectation that newcomers should completely adopt American customs and culture. Consequently, this organization supported laws that required immigrants to take oaths of loyalty and to pass English language tests. Members of the DAR also tried to discourage the use of languages other than English in schools. While there were some scattered protests, most immigrants resigned themselves to being second-class citizens in areas where this brand of legislation held sway.

1. What purpose does this passage serve?

   (A) It describes the living conditions and political environment for immigrants to America around 1900.
   (B) It argues for more stringent immigration requirements for those wanting to come to the United States.
   (C) It argues for providing greater support and a warm welcome to new future Americans.
   (D) It provides an overview of the Daughters of the American Revolution, including its origins and accomplishments.

2. What term would the author most likely use to describe the Daughters of the American Revolution?

   (A) Heroic
   (B) Unsympathetic
   (C) Patriotic
   (D) Warm

3. Which of the following statements best aligns with the author's point of view?

   (A) Immigrants could have improved their situation, but they came from cultures that did not value personal ambition.
   (B) Though most immigrants struggled, they were fortunate to benefit from the generosity of American business owners.
   (C) As difficult as life as a new immigrant was, it was an improvement over the life most immigrants left behind in their home countries.
   (D) On the whole, new immigrants to the United States were not treated fairly compared to native-born citizens.

4. Which of the following is potentially a factual statement rather than an opinion?

   (A) The Daughters of the American Revolution was an anti-American organization.
   (B) Conservative groups unfairly persecuted new immigrants to the United States.
   (C) Most immigrants to the United States near the end of the 19th century were poor.
   (D) Most native-born Americans continue to look down upon new immigrants.

**Review your work using the explanations in Part Six of this book.**

# LESSON 2

# Using Text Structure and Features

## LEARNING OBJECTIVES

- Identify examples of the different modes of writing
- Recognize the different features that a text can contain and identify their purpose

There are many reasons why a writer might choose to write a passage. The passage might be intended to persuade the reader to follow a recommendation or adopt a position on some issue, it might seek to explain a situation or phenomenon, or its purpose may be entertain. No matter the **mode**, or passage type, all texts contain **key words** that signal the author's intent or other features—including headings and subheadings, footnotes, glossaries, illustrations, and italics—to help the reader understand the text.

## Modes of Writing

Some texts are written to persuade the reader. The mode of such passages is **persuasive** or argumentative. (Note that **argument** here does not necessarily mean a dispute but rather the writer's attempt to convince the reader that some assertion is true or false or that some action is advisable or inadvisable. See Chapter 3, Lesson 3: Evaluating an Argument for more information about arguments.) To achieve this goal, the writer provides different pieces of evidence to support the argument, including facts, examples, data, anecdotes, and details. The writer may also make use of rhetorical devices or word choices to help persuade the reader. There are many words or phrases that signal an author's opinion, so watch for them. Some examples include *clearly, without a doubt, undeniably, most importantly, I believe, I question*, and so on.

One common structure for a persuasive passage is problem/solution. As the name indicates, such a passage outlines a problem and argues for a possible solution or solutions. Besides *problem* and *solution*, other signal words include *because* and *the reason for* (which signal evidence) and *as a result* and *this will lead to* (which signal a conclusion).

Another mode of writing is **expository**. An expository text explains a process or phenomenon. It does not contain opinions but instead relies on facts and examples. Such writing sometimes resembles a persuasive text in that it presents evidence or analysis, but an expository passage is objective and does not promote the author's point of view. There are several structures for expository passages, including these:

- *Cause/effect:* In a causal relationship, one thing (the cause) is the reason why another (the effect) happens. Look for language like *due to, as a consequence, responsible for, as a result*, and *if . . . then*.
- *Compare/contrast:* Two (or more) things are compared to identify similarities or contrasted to highlight differences. Key words include *similarly, have in common*, and *in the same way* (for similarities) or *on the contrary, compared to*, and *in spite of* (for contrasts).

- *Steps in a process/procedure:* Look for words indicating some kind of sequence (*first, next, then, finally, in closing*). (See Chapter 1, Lesson 4: Understanding Sequences of Events for more information on this type of passage.)

Finally, some texts are **narrative** in mode. They can be structured like persuasive or expository texts and may use some of the same key words, but here the writer is trying to entertain or inform by telling a story. These passages might feature anecdotes (personal stories) and devices like foreshadowing.

Follow along as a TEAS expert analyzes a passage.

| Question | Analysis |
|---|---|
| The Czech composer Josef Suk (1874–1935) is arguably the leading figure in the Czech Modernist movement. Much influenced by his father-in-law, Antonin Dvorak, Suk wrote mostly instrumental music for orchestra, chamber ensembles, and piano. His output was admired by the Austrian composers Gustav Mahler and Alban Berg. Suk retired from composition in 1933, but he continued to be an inspirational figure to his fellow Czechs. | **Steps 1 and 3:** The passage provides information about a composer. The first sentence contains the word "arguably," which indicates that the statement about Suk's importance in Czech music is the author's opinion. What follows is a series of facts that support that opinion. Note that the positive words "admired" and "inspirational" relate to other people's reactions to Suk, which could be documented by referring to things these people wrote or said. Thus, they do not reflect the author's opinion. |
| Which sentence expresses an opinion? | **Step 2:** The question asks you to identify the statement that expresses an opinion. Be on the lookout for key words or phrases that signal opinion. |
| | **Step 4:** Predict that the first sentence expresses an opinion. |
| (A)  The first | **Step 5:** Correct. The first sentence states the opinion that Suk was the most important figure in the Czech Modernist movement. |
| (B)  The second | This is an objective statement, not an opinion, about Suk's music. |
| (C)  The third | This is an objective statement, not an opinion, about some of Suk's admirers. |
| (D)  The fourth | This is an objective statement, not an opinion, about Suk's reputation. |

Now try a question on your own.

The Battle of Vimy Ridge was a military engagement that took place between the Canadian Corps and the German Sixth Army, on April 9–12, 1917, during the First World War. The Canadian Corps wanted to take control of German-held high ground on a ridge at the northernmost end of the Arras offensive because the Canadian command was worried that advance troops would be exposed to German fire. The Canadian Corps captured most of the ridge during the first day of the attack, protecting the advance guard. The loss of Vimy Ridge forced the German command to reassess its defensive strategy, and the battle is considered a turning point in Canadian self-identity.

In this passage, what role does the statement "The Canadian Corps captured most of the ridge during the first day of the attack, protecting the advance guard" play?

    (A)    It identifies a problem that needs a solution.
    (B)    It identifies the solution to a problem.
    (C)    It is evidence in support of an argument.
    (D)    It is the author's conclusion.

## Explanation

**Step 1:** This is an expository passage, explaining a battle from World War I. As you read the passage, locate the statement quoted in the question statement. Pay attention to its context and look for any words that indicate its function in the passage. Don't worry about understanding details, such as "the Arras offensive," that aren't relevant to answering the question.

**Step 2:** The quoted statement is the third sentence in the passage. It says that after the ridge was captured, the advance troops could be protected. The previous sentence says that the Canadian command "was worried" that their advance troops would be exposed to German fire.

**Step 3:** Considering these two sentences together, it is clear that a problem and its solution are identified. Look for a choice that says the quoted statement is a solution to a problem.

**Step 4:** The passage states that the Canadian command was worried about protecting its troops from German fire. This was the problem, indicated by the word "worried," so (A) is not the correct choice. The solution was capturing most of the ridge and thus protecting the advance guard; therefore, **(B)** is the correct choice. The author makes no argument but is merely citing objective facts, so (C) is incorrect. The author's conclusion, (D), is the final sentence of the passage, which states the battle's ramifications for the future.

## Text Features

Text features are parts of the text that stand apart from regular text. They can highlight the location of certain content, provide information supplementary to the main body of the material, or accentuate the structure of the text. Their purpose is to guide the reader through the text.

Common text features include **titles, tables of contents, bold print, italics, quotations, sidebars, map legends, illustration captions, footnotes, headings,** an **index,** and so on. You are probably familiar with most of these from your experience with books and other printed materials. The TEAS may require that you identify these elements.

## KEY IDEAS

- Authors have different goals in writing, such as to persuade, to inform, or to entertain.
- No matter its mode, a passage will contain clues that help readers understand it.
- Features outside the main body of the text can help comprehension by highlighting important ideas or providing a guide to finding certain information.

# Using Text Structure and Features Practice Questions

**Questions 1–2 refer to the following passage.**

The Academy of Motion Picture Arts and Sciences (AMPAS) has had a separate category for Best Foreign Language Film at the Academy Awards since 1956 and has presented this award every year following. Every country is invited to submit a film to the AMPAS. After each country has submitted a film as its official entry, all submitted films, subtitled in English, are screened by the Foreign Language Film Award Committee. The committee decides by secret ballot the five official nominations. Final voting is conducted by those Academy members who have attended exhibition screenings of all Foreign Language Film entries. Questions and concerns had been occasionally raised about the fairness and representativeness of the process; subsequently, the process changed somewhat in 2006.

1. What kind of passage is this?

    (A) Problem/solution
    (B) Persuasive
    (C) Procedural
    (D) Narrative

2. The author of this passage is revising it. Which of the following words would best begin the second sentence?

    (A) First
    (B) Clearly
    (C) Generally
    (D) Finally

3. Which of the following would be most useful to help a reader understand a map?

    (A) Legend
    (B) Endnotes
    (C) Index
    (D) Sidebars

American novelist Anne Tyler has won numerous awards for her work, including the Pulitzer Prize. Born in Minneapolis, Minnesota, in 1941, to Quaker parents and raised in Raleigh, North Carolina, Tyler attended Duke University. She published her first novel, If Morning Ever Comes, when she was twenty-two.

4. Which of these terms should be italicized in the passage above?

    (A) Anne Tyler
    (B) Pulitzer Prize
    (C) Duke University
    (D) If Morning Ever Comes

5. Which of the following would be the most likely place to find supplementary or supporting information about a subject a writer is addressing?

    (A) Heading
    (B) Footnote
    (C) Subheading
    (D) Text in bold print

**Review your work using the explanations in Part Six of this book.**

# LESSON 3
# Determining Word Meaning

## LEARNING OBJECTIVES

- Derive the meanings of words from outside sources and from context
- Distinguish among denotative, connotative, and figurative meanings of words

Words can have different meanings depending on **context**. A word can be used with its **denotative**, or dictionary, meaning. A word can also be used **connotatively** or **figuratively**; these meanings are based on context and can be more complex to discern. Writers choose words carefully to make an impact on the reader or to signal tone, purpose, or point of view.

The TEAS will include questions that test your ability to comprehend the appropriate way to use a word and the meaning of words in context.

## Denotative Meaning

One way to determine what a word means is with a **dictionary**, whether in book form or online. A dictionary will give you the denotative meaning or meanings of a word. As well, a dictionary can tell you how to pronounce a word, and many dictionaries provide an etymology, or a description of a word's origin. This can be helpful, because if you know the meaning of the root or suffix or prefix of a word, the meaning of the entire words can frequently be approximated. For example, if you know *chronos* refers to time and *meter* to measurement, then you can surmise that a *chronometer* is something that measures time (it is a very precise clock or watch).

Another source for assisting in word usage is a **thesaurus**, which provides **synonyms**, or words with similar meanings. Be careful, though. Words grouped together in a thesaurus can have subtle differences in meaning or tone and can't always be perfectly substituted for one another. Consider that "incident," "event," and "situation" are synonyms but are not interchangeable.

You might not need a dictionary or other outside source to determine the meaning of an unfamiliar word. Frequently a word's meaning can be deduced by the way it is used in a sentence or passage.

Sometimes a word's definition will be clearly provided:

- The last known specimen of quagga, a kind of zebra once found in southern Africa, was exhibited at the London Zoo before the species went extinct.

Other times, a sentence will indicate if a word is an example, illustration, or type of something:

- Franz Schubert also wrote music for stringed instruments, some still in common use today, like the violin or cello, and others obsolete, like the arpeggione.

This sentence tells you that an arpeggione is an obsolete stringed instrument.

Key words can also distinguish meaning in context. Sometimes context clues will tell you whether the unknown word has a positive or negative charge.

- Despite his history of reckless behavior, Howard had the reputation of being a circumspect individual.

Here, the contrasting key word "despite" tells you that "circumspect" must have an opposing meaning to "reckless." In fact, it's a synonym for *prudent* or *cautious*.

Follow along as a TEAS expert tackles a question that tests word meaning.

| Question | Analysis |
| --- | --- |
| After all Sam's bragging about her cooking skills, I was expecting some delicious food, but the dinner she prepared was unpalatable. | **Step 1:** Look at the context in which "unpalatable" is used for clues to help you derive its meaning. |
| What does the word "unpalatable" mean in this sentence? | **Step 2:** Sam was "bragging" about her cooking, so the author must have been "expecting" good food. The contrast key word "but" signals that the dinner was *not good*. Even if you can't elicit any other meaning, knowing whether a word has a positive or negative charge can help you eliminate some wrong choices, improving your odds of getting the correct answer. |
| (A)  Delectable | **Step 3:** "Delectable" means "highly pleasing." If Sam had managed to deliver on her bragging and serve a delectable meal, the author would not have been disappointed. |
| (B)  Bad-tasting | Correct. This is the only choice with a negative charge. |
| (C)  Delicate | "Delicate," meaning "fine in texture, quality, etc.," does not convey a negative charge. |
| (D)  Attractive | This choice is also a positive word, not a negative one. |

## Figurative and Connotative Word Usage

A word's denotative or dictionary meaning is different from its figurative usage. Consider the expressions "a stormy day" and "a stormy personality." In the first example, the word "stormy" indicates the day had inclement weather, perhaps heavy rain and high winds. In the second example, the individual in question could be bad-tempered or easy to anger. The first is denotative use, while the second is figurative.

The TEAS will also test your understanding of writer's tone depending on word choice. A writer might select words that have a connotation associated with a particular image or feeling. Think of the different connotations of "sound," "noise," or "din."

Writers frequently use words in creative ways to make their meaning more vivid or evocative. Instead of writing, "The trapeze artist performed above our heads," a writer might choose to say, "The trapeze artist floated like a cloud above our the heads." Here, the trapeze artist's grace is signaled in an imaginative way. An understanding of how words can be used figuratively is vital for better reading comprehension.

When words deviate from their dictionary definitions, this usage is called *figurative language*. A **figure of speech** is figurative language in the form of a word or phrase. Some common figures of speech are these:

- Simile
- Metaphor
- Personification

Figurative language can be used to compare two different things. Sometimes the comparison is signaled by the words *like* or *as*, such as in the example of the trapeze artist above, in which case the figure of speech is a **simile**. The writer could have expressed the same image using a **metaphor**, which does not use *like* or *as* and implies that the two elements are equivalent: "The trapeze artist was a cloud floating above our heads." The result, though, is much the same.

Another common figure of speech is **personification**, in which human traits are ascribed to something nonhuman, like a *cowardly lion* or *friendly skies*.

Fiction writers and poets make much use of figurative language, but so do many other kind of writers: advertising copywriters, political speechwriters . . . anyone who wants to make her language more evocative, compelling, descriptive, or powerful.

## KEY IDEAS

- Word meaning can be determined by an external source, like a dictionary, or by context.
- Cues like key words can help you determine the meaning or tone of a word in context.
- Figurative language is commonly used in both literary and everyday writing.

# Determining Word Meaning Practice Questions

Walter de Coutances was a medieval bishop of Lincoln and an archbishop of Rouen. Although he held a number of political appointments and served as vice chancellor for Henry II, he also accumulated numerous ecclesiastical appointments, including canon of Rouen and archdeacon of Oxford. Coutances died in 1207 and was buried in his cathedral.

1. What is the meaning of "canon" as used in this passage?

   (A)  A kind of priest
   (B)  A diplomat
   (C)  A large gun
   (D)  A politician

The community center put on its summer carnival last weekend. There were sporting events and crafts available for sale. The children made costumes for their parade, and the police closed the street to traffic. Some people with culinary skills brought delicious treats for a bake sale. It was such a beehive of activity, I expected to find a jar of honey!

2. The author states that the community center was "was such a beehive of activity, I expected to find a jar of honey!" Which of the following is the most accurate interpretation of that sentence?

   (A)  The police closed the street to protect children from bee stings.
   (B)  There was so much activity at the center that people resembled bees working in a hive.
   (C)  The author was disappointed that none of the cooks brought homemade honey to the bake sale.
   (D)  An apiarist gave a demonstration to show people how bees make honey.

Keen to gain his manager's approval, Winston worked assiduously to complete all of his tasks.

3. Which of the following is a synonym for "assiduously" in the above sentence?

   (A)  Industriously
   (B)  Carelessly
   (C)  Needlessly
   (D)  Anonymously

4. Which of the following is a metaphor?

   (A)  The wind whistled.
   (B)  The lion roared.
   (C)  The icy road was like a sheet of glass.
   (D)  The politician thundered.

5. Which of the following would be least useful to have on hand if you were writing an essay and thinking about word choice?

   (A)  A dictionary
   (B)  A thesaurus
   (C)  A biography of a well-regarded writer
   (D)  A collection of famous poems

The governor talked about an important matter to the attentive audience.

6. Which of the following would be a more descriptive substitute for the word "talked" in the context of the above sentence?

   (A)  chatted
   (B)  gossiped
   (C)  orated
   (D)  mumbled

**Review your work using the explanations in Part Six of this book.**

# CHAPTER THREE

# INTEGRATING IDEAS TO DRAW CONCLUSIONS

## LEARNING OBJECTIVES

- Compare and contrast themes from multiple sources, identifying points of agreement and disagreement between the authors
- Make logical inferences and predictions based on information in a work of fiction
- Analyze an argument, including identification of the author's claim and supporting evidence and evaluation of the strength of the author's reasoning
- Synthesize data from textual and graphical sources to answer a question

Of the 47 scored *Reading* questions, 11 (23%) will be in the sub-content area of *Integration of knowledge and ideas*. With these questions, the TEAS tests your ability to compare different treatments of themes and ideas in various written works, including work in different formats such as text and graphics and work in nonfiction and fiction genres. You will also be asked to evaluate the strength of arguments.

This chapter addresses these skills in four lessons:

**Lesson 1:** Comparing and Contrasting Multiple Sources

**Lesson 2:** Making Inferences About Fiction

**Lesson 3:** Evaluating an Argument

**Lesson 4:** Integrating Data From Different Formats

**Reading Questions by Sub-content Area**

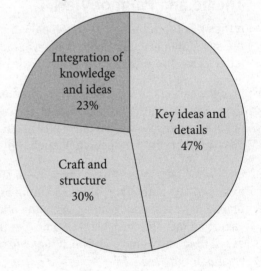

# LESSON 1

# Comparing and Contrasting Multiple Sources

## LEARNING OBJECTIVES

- Compare and contrast themes from multiple sources
- Identify points of agreement and disagreement between authors
- Distinguish between primary and secondary sources

As you already know from your own reading, multiple authors can write about the same themes from different points of view. One may write about the benefits of exercise, while another may focus on the dangers of excessive exercise. Both, however, are writing about exercise. Similarly, one author may write a poem on wildflowers while another writes a treatise on the conservation of natural flora. Again, both are writing on the same theme: native plants. On the TEAS, you may be given two stimuli, such as two passages or a passage and a graphic, and asked to compare and contrast their themes and their authors' points of view.

## Theme and Point of View

A **theme** is the subject or central idea of a piece of work. A visual representation and a text may concern the same theme. For example, Mathew Brady's graphic Civil War photos could be paired with a soldier's letter home about casualties at the Battle of Antietam.

In some cases, the shared theme is obvious, as it would be with the photos and letter above. Other times the shared theme is more subtle. A newspaper account of the maiden voyage of a new supertanker might be paired with a fictional story about fishing in a local pond. Despite their disparate settings, both passages concern how people interact with water.

Even when two sources have the same or similar themes, the authors may disagree with each other. For example, one author may write about the benefits of video games for hand-eye coordination, reaction time, and stress management, while the other draws a cartoon about how video games waste a student's valuable time. The theme is the same, but the conclusions are quite different. On the TEAS, you may be asked to identify points on which the two authors both agree and disagree, so note which author has what **point of view**.

## Primary and Secondary Sources

A **primary source** is written by a person who actually witnessed the event. Examples include a journalist writing about a battle for a newspaper or a soldier describing that battle in a letter home, a film critic reviewing a movie, or a scientist documenting an experiment. Primary sources can be written in the first person (using the pronoun *I*) or in the more neutral third person.

A **secondary source** is at least one step removed from a primary source. Often it is an interpretation of the primary source, a commentary on it, or a quote from it. Examples of secondary sources are a history textbook, a paper for school that analyzes President Franklin Roosevelt's speeches, or a government publication that analyzes data on housing starts and home ownership patterns.

Follow along as a TEAS expert answers two questions about a pair of passages.

**Passage 1:** The new high school exit exam is unfair. It assumes a higher level of science knowledge than is taught in our local public high schools. In order for high school students to pass the exit exam, high schools must upgrade their science education.

**Passage 2:** In this technological world, it is imperative that high school students receive a thorough education in science. This will not only allow them to enter a science career but also enable this country to compete with other countries that excel in the sciences and technology.

| Question | Analysis |
|---|---|
| | **Step 1:** The first passage starts with a problem, then offers the solution of better science education. The second passage is also about science education, focusing on its importance for careers and international competition. Note the author's topic, scope, and purpose for each passage. |
| Which of the following best captures the two paragraphs' shared theme? | **Step 2:** This question asks you to identify a theme shared by both passages. |
| | **Step 3:** If you had read the passages without taking notes, different details might stand out in your memory, making it difficult to identify the main topic they have in common. Because you jotted down a passage map, however, you can easily identify the authors' shared interest. |
| | **Step 4:** Predict that the answer will concern the value of a good high school science education. |
| (A)   The new high school exit exam is unfair. | **Step 5:** This answer refers to passage 1 only. |
| (B)   Science education is important in today's world. | Correct. This is a stated theme in both passages, so it matches the prediction. |
| (C)   Public school science teachers are not well trained. | Neither passage refers to teacher training. |
| (D)   Private schools provide excellent science education. | Private schools are not mentioned in either passage. |

| Question | Analysis |
|---|---|
| Identify the primary difference between the content in passage 1 and that in passage 2. | **Step 2:** This question asks how the passages differ. |
| | **Step 3:** Again, check your passage map to confirm your understanding of the difference in the passages' scope. Both passages deal with the importance of science education. However, the author of passage 1 is concerned with helping students pass the high school exit exam, while the author of passage 2 cares about individuals' future career opportunities and the nation's competitiveness. |
| | **Step 4:** Predict that the major difference is the reasons the authors give for providing strong science education. |
| (A) The passages express different opinions about how important science is today. | **Step 5:** This answer is the opposite of the prediction. Both authors agree on the importance of a good science education. |
| (B) The first passage is concerned with a biased test, while the second assumes that the test is fair. | The test—the high school exit exam—is only mentioned in the first passage. There is no way to know the second author's opinion of the exam. |
| (C) The second passage refutes the claim that science education is more important than technology education. | Neither passage claims that technology education is more important than science education. |
| (D) The passages differ in the support they provide for the importance of science education. | Correct. As predicted, the authors support their claims with different reasons. |

Now practice answering two questions on your own. After reading and mapping the passage and answering the questions, check your work against the explanations that follow.

**Passage 1:** When we were kids, Teresa was the bane of my life. She tormented me in school with nasty comments about my clothes, hair, attitude, and, most especially, the fact that I was smart. Today I make an excellent living as an architect, and my buildings are landmarks all over the world. Teresa, on the other hand, lives in obscurity in the same little town in which we grew up. Is it any wonder that it gave me great pleasure to greet her at our 20th high school reunion?

**Proverb:** Revenge is a dish best served cold.

The author of the passage and someone who quoted the proverb would agree that

(A) bullying should be prohibited in schools.
(B) delayed retaliation is the most satisfying.
(C) cold foods are tastier than hot foods.
(D) bullies always get their punishment sooner or later.

## Explanation

**Step 1:**

Topic: revenge
Scope: pleasure gained after a long time
Purpose: to support delayed revenge
Passage 1: description of bullying and the victim's revenge 20 years later
Proverb: highlights the satisfaction from delayed vengeance

**Step 2:** This question asks you to select the statement supported by both parts of the stimulus.

**Step 3:** Research your passage map, looking for a common theme.

**Step 4:** Both the passage and the proverb speak of the pleasure derived from delayed vengeance.

**Step 5:** The only answer that reflects the shared theme is choice **(B)**. Though it uses the word "retaliation" instead of "revenge," the meaning is the same. "Bullying" in choice (A) is discussed in the first passage only, and it does not say that bullying should be prohibited. Choice (C) incorrectly focuses on food rather than on revenge; passage 1 does not mention food, and the proverb uses food as a metaphor. Choice (D) is extreme ("always"), and "punishment" is not discussed by either stimulus.

> Which of the two sources is/are a primary source?
> - (A) The first
> - (B) The second
> - (C) Both
> - (D) Neither

## Explanation

**Step 2:** This question asks which of the two statements, or conceivably both, is a primary source, meaning it was written by a person who experienced the event described.

**Step 3:** Note who authored passage 1 and the proverb and their relationship to any event discussed.

**Step 4:** Only the passage is a primary source. It is a first-person account written by the individual who was bullied and went on to become a successful architect. A proverb has no known author and is simply a widely quoted piece of wisdom. The correct answer will include only the passage.

**Step 5:** Only the first statement, choice **(A)**, is a primary source.

### KEY IDEAS

- When presented with multiple stimuli, be prepared to identify any overlap between their themes as well as points of contrast.
- Two authors cannot be assumed to agree or disagree about something unless both mention it.
- Primary sources are written by a person who experienced the event described; secondary sources are at least one step removed from primary sources.

# Comparing and Contrasting Multiple Sources Practice Questions

**Questions 1–2 refer to the following poem and letter.**

## In Flanders Fields

In Flanders fields the poppies blow
Between the crosses, row on row,
That mark our place; and in the sky
The larks, still bravely singing, fly
Scarce heard amid the guns below.

We are the Dead. Short days ago
We lived, felt dawn, saw sunset glow,
Loved and were loved, and now we lie
In Flanders fields.

Take up our quarrel with the foe:
To you from failing hands we throw
The torch; be yours to hold it high.
If ye break faith with us who die
We shall not sleep, though poppies grow
In Flanders fields.

*by John McCrae, a Canadian physician who served in World War I, May 1915*

## Eve of the Battle of the Somme

We go up to the attack tomorrow. This will probably be the biggest thing yet. We are to have the honor of marching in the first wave. I will write you soon if I get through all right. If not, my only earthly care is for my poems. I am glad to be going in first wave. If you are in this thing at all it is best to be in to the limit. And this is the supreme experience.

*Excerpt from a letter by American poet Alan Seeger, writing about his participation in the WWI Battle of the Somme, June 28, 1916*

1. Both the letter and the poem share the themes of

   (A) disgust at the human cost of war.
   (B) bravery in battle.
   (C) a glorious death on the battlefield.
   (D) the contrast between the beauty of flowers and the horror of battle.

2. A partial quote from Marcus Luttrell, a US Navy Seal who was the inspiration for the film *Lone Survivor*, states, "There's nothing glorious about war. There's nothing glorious about holding your friends in your arms and watching them die" (January 15, 2014). How might Seeger and McCrae respond to this statement?

   (A) With disgust at an expression of cowardice
   (B) By questioning the writer's firsthand experience with war
   (C) By disagreeing that death is painful to watch
   (D) By arguing that fighting for a cause can be worthwhile

**Testimonial:** I am very pleased with my new Sportmax SUV. In particular, I feel it is designed for safety, and I know that today most car companies are very focused on manufacturing reliable vehicles and spend a considerable portion of manufacturing costs on quality control. This gives me assurance that my family and I will not suffer an accident in this vehicle.

**Newspaper article:** The manufacturer of the Sportmax SUV today issued a recall based on evidence that the gears may shift into reverse without warning. Several accidents have been reported by people whose Sportmax SUVs suddenly reversed, causing collisions and, in one case, the death of a child standing behind the car. The auto manufacturer's CEO has admitted that quality control measures may not have kept pace with the company's growth.

3. Based on the two statements, with which statement would the authors likely disagree?

   (A) Quality control for the Sportmax SUV is inadequate.
   (B) Other SUVs have the same problem as the Sportmax SUV, so its defect is an unfortunate result of the styling of the vehicle.
   (C) Most SUVs are safer than sedans.
   (D) Automobile manufacturers strive to make their products safe.

**Review your work using the explanations in Part Six of this book.**

# LESSON 2

# Making Inferences About Fiction

## LEARNING OBJECTIVES

- Make logical inferences based on information in a story or poem and personal knowledge and experience
- Make predictions based on information in a story or poem and personal knowledge and experience

## Inferences

An **inference** is an implied conclusion. As you learned in Chapter 1, Lesson 3: Making Inferences, inferences are not stated directly in the passage but must be supported by evidence in the passage, flowing logically from the information provided. To draw an inference, think not only about what the author has actually written but also about what else must be true. Consider, too, what you know from your own experience.

>    *Example:* "Alejandro was upset after taking the final exam."

You can infer that Alejandro thought he did not do well on the test. This conclusion is not stated in the sentence, but it is fully supported based on what the author writes and your own experience when you or a friend didn't do well at something.

Inference questions about fiction may ask you to draw conclusions about actions, characters' motives and feelings, the passage's theme, and the author's point of view. When answering inference questions about fiction, think about the implied meaning of the characters' words, actions, and feelings as well as the author's choice of words and details.

## Predictions

Both in life and in reading, **predictions** are assumptions about something that has happened or will happen. A story may start in the middle of something—a conversation, memory, action, or the like. A question may ask you to infer what happened beforehand, what will probably happen afterward, or what the author is likely to write about next. Based on clues in the passage and your personal experience, you can make a good prediction.

## Scope

When making inferences and predictions, it's important to remember to stay within the context of the passage. Don't go out of **scope**, thinking beyond what the author has written. For example, if a story is about a narrator's experience with a difficult family member, infer what is indicated about that relationship but don't assume without warrant that the narrator has trouble with other members of her family or that other people have similar problems with their relatives. Both ideas would be out of scope.

Follow along as a TEAS expert answers first an inference question and then a prediction question.

| Question | Analysis |
|---|---|
| Luisa and her twin sister had always been mirror images of each other. They chose the same clothes, got the same grades in school, had the same likes and dislikes (they both hated mashed potatoes), and even, when they were 16, fell in love with the same boy. That's when the mirror was smashed. | **Step 1:** The passage is about twin sisters and how similar they were ("mirror images"). The metaphor of a "smashed" mirror implies that the last event, falling in love with the same boy, disrupted their relationship. |
| What can be inferred from the sentence "That's when the mirror was smashed"? | **Step 2:** This is an inference question, asking for a conclusion that is unstated but must be true based on the given information. |
| | **Step 3:** Research your passage map and reread the sentence in context. |
| | **Step 4:** Predict that the twins no longer felt close. |
| (A)  The twins began to have violent disagreements. | **Step 5:** Though it can be inferred that the twins were no longer close, concluding that they fought violently goes too far. |
| (B)  Luisa and her sister no longer had the same likes and dislikes. | This answer is not supported by the passage. Luisa and her sister may still have had the same likes and dislikes—they probably still hated mashed potatoes— and they certainly had the same preferences in boys. |
| (C)  The closeness the twins had experienced was disrupted. | Correct. This is a good match for the prediction. |
| (D)  Luisa and her sister experienced difficult teenage years. | As with choice (B), this is not supported by the passage. You know there was a particular conflict, but you can't infer that all their teenage years were difficult. |

| Question | Analysis |
|---|---|
| Which of the following is the author likely to include in the next paragraph? | **Step 2:** This is a prediction question. |
| | **Step 3:** Consider what the author has already written and how he ends the paragraph. He establishes a pattern of a close relationship, then dramatically announces it ended. Logically, the next paragraph will give more details about this situation. |
| | **Step 4:** Predict an explanation of how falling in love with the same boy changed the twins' relationship. |
| (A)  What the sisters were doing before they met the boy | **Step 5:** The question asks you to predict what comes next, not what came before. |
| (B)  The folly of falling in love | This would be out of scope. The author is not critiquing falling in love in general but narrating a specific love triangle. |

K

| Question | Analysis |
|---|---|
| (C) Whether the sisters eventually reconciled as adults | The resolution of the sisters' relationship will likely come at the end of the passage, not in the second paragraph. Be aware of how an author logically organizes his narrative. |
| (D) A description of the boy and how he met the sisters | Correct. It would make sense for this information to follow as part of the opening of a complicated love story. |

Now practice answering an inference question and a prediction question on your own. After reading and mapping the passage and answering the questions, check your work against the explanations that follow.

In the lazy, sweet-smelling summer of my childhood, the sloping expanse of green behind our vacation bungalow was a vast playground for my older brother Peter and me. Our father had hung a simple swing on the low-hanging branch of a tree, and my brother and I would argue over who would get to swing first, and who would do the pushing. My mother sat nearby in her beloved, faded Adirondack chair, a book open on her lap. But she wasn't reading; she had closed her eyes and tilted her face up to the sun. Even so, she always seemed to have a sense of what her two rambunctious boys were up to.

When my turn came to swing, I urged my brother to push harder, higher, faster. I was almost up into the leaves of the tree when my mother softly said, "Peter, don't push your brother so high. He'll fly off into the sky!" Peter slowed down with a vengeance, pushing me so gently that I moved only a few inches with each push. I could never understand why my mother wouldn't let me go as high as I could; flying off into the sky sounded wonderful—exactly what I'd always dreamed I could do.

From the passage it can be inferred that

(A) the brothers argued frequently.
(B) the younger brother was disobedient.
(C) Peter's brother was an adventurous dreamer.
(D) swinging was the brothers' favorite activity.

## Explanation

### Step 1:

Topic: narrative about two brothers playing
Scope: swinging in the backyard
Purpose: to relate an incident in the narrator's life
P1: describes narrator and brother swinging in the backyard
P2: younger brother wants to fly high, but mom won't let him

**Step 2:** The word "infer" makes this an inference question.

**Step 3:** The question is open-ended, so you cannot research a specific part of the story. Make a mental inventory of what you know about this family, especially the narrator, who is the younger brother of Peter. Then check each answer choice against your understanding of the passage.

**Step 4:** You cannot make an exact prediction. However, the correct answer will reflect evidence provided in the passage. Here is what you know: this seems to be a close family, in which dad builds a swing for his sons, mom watches over them carefully, and the two brothers play together. The only point of conflict is in the younger brother's (the narrator's) desire to swing high and his mother's protectiveness. The correct answer will reflect these facts.

**Step 5:** The only answer choice supported by the passage is **(C)**, which refers to the narrator's desire to swing as high as possible, even off into the sky ("flying off into the sky sounded wonderful—exactly what I'd always dreamed I could do"). Choice (A) is unsupported; just because the narrator was frustrated when Peter only pushed him a little doesn't mean the brothers argued frequently. (B) is unsupported; wanting to do something mom forbids is not the same as actually being disobedient. (D) is unsupported; the brothers liked to swing, but there is no information about whether this was the boys' favorite activity.

> As the story continues, the reader can reasonably expect that the boys' mother will
>
> (A) lose interest in her sons' activities as they grow up.
> (B) quietly exert authority over her children.
> (C) pursue her passion for reading books.
> (D) live in constant fear that her son will be hurt.

## Explanation

**Step 2:** The words "reasonably expect" indicate that you need to make a prediction based on the information present in the passage.

**Step 3:** Research your passage map for notes you've made about the narrator's mother and research the passage for what is stated about her. The narrator describes the mother as sunning herself in her favorite chair, but alert enough to realize that Peter is swinging his brother too high. Her response is to gently admonish him, speaking "softly."

**Step 4:** The correct answer will reflect one or all of the mother's relaxed demeanor, concern for her children, and soft-spoken approach to discipline.

**Step 5:** Choice **(B)** is a match. The last sentence of paragraph 1 states: "Even so, she always seemed to have a sense of what her two rambunctious boys were up to." You can expect that her soft-spoken concern for their safety will be a constant feature of her character. Choice (A) is the opposite of her attitude now, and there is no reason to think her feelings will change in the future. Choice (C) is also counter to the information provided; the author writes that mother wasn't reading. Choice (D) is extreme, since while she was concerned enough to urge Peter to slow down, her gentle tone and whimsical words do not indicate fear, nor is there any reason to believe she fears for his safety during any other activities.

## KEY IDEAS

- In fiction as in nonfiction, inferences and predictions are unstated conclusions that must be true based on evidence in the passage and personal knowledge.
- Paying attention to characters' words, actions, and feelings as well as the author's choice of words and details will help you make supported inferences.
- An understanding of how stories typically proceed from beginning to development to conclusion will help you make predictions.

# Making Inferences About Fiction Practice Questions

**Questions 1–3 refer to the following passage.**

Johnny was already late—his fault entirely. He'd been so tired last night that he'd set the alarm for half an hour later than he meant to. He now regretted cramming until 1:00 AM, but the day had slipped away from him without his notice, just as it always did. Suddenly there were only a few hours left to prepare for what might be the most important meeting of his career. He'd prepared a detailed, persuasive presentation of course—he always did—but too little sleep and too much stress didn't bode well for the rest of the day.

Johnny poured a take-away cup of coffee, finally found his car keys (he was always misplacing them), and quickly backed the car out of the car port, hoping for a quick drive to work. Just as he hit yet another red light, his cell phone began to ring. Reaching for his phone, he knocked over his drink, spilling piping hot coffee all over his lap. He screamed loudly and frantically tried to mop up his soaking trousers. "Perfect," thought Johnny. "Why do these things always happen to me?"

1. Based on the author's description of Johnny, it can be inferred that Johnny is

   (A) lazy and apathetic.
   (B) a young man on the rise in his career.
   (C) a victim of bad luck.
   (D) a disorganized procrastinator.

2. It is likely that in the next few paragraphs, the author will

   (A) provide more examples of Johnny's clumsiness.
   (B) describe Johnny's arrival at the office and the upcoming meeting.
   (C) relate Johnny's reaction to what was said in the meeting.
   (D) detail how Johnny relaxes after a stressful day.

3. Which of the following is probably true of the protagonist?

   (A) He is unprepared for his meeting.
   (B) He blames others for his misfortunes.
   (C) He is not fully aware of his actions and their consequences.
   (D) He is usually too tired to do his job well.

**Review your work using the explanations in Part Six of this book.**

# LESSON 3

# Evaluating an Argument

---

## LEARNING OBJECTIVES

- Identify the author's claim in an argument
- Identify the evidence used to support a claim
- Evaluate how well the evidence supports a claim
- Evaluate what evidence would strengthen or weaken the claim

---

As you learned in Chapter 2, Lessons 1 and 2, on the TEAS, an **argument** is not a heated debate but a logical statement of an author's claim and the evidence he or she uses to support it. Several questions on the TEAS will ask you to determine how an author has constructed an argument and how valid that argument is. To answer these questions, It is helpful to mentally reword the argument as "the author claims X (conclusion) because of Y (evidence)." This will help you identify the author's claim and the stated evidence for it, then think about the unstated assumptions the author has made to connect the evidence and conclusion. You can then determine how valid the argument is. When you make your passage map, jot down brief summaries of the author's claim (conclusion), evidence, and unstated assumptions.

## Claims and Support

An author's claim is her argument's **conclusion**—the opinion with which she wants the reader to agree. Occasionally, an author will make this very clear with words such as "I believe" or "in my opinion," but generally a claim will be more subtle, signaled by phrases such as "without a doubt" or "it is clear that." Sometimes authors make claims by using contrast key words to refute someone else's claim. Such terms include "however," "but," and "on the other hand." Claims can also be made simply as if they were factual statements, with no reference to the author's feelings or opinions.

All well-constructed arguments require support. Support is **evidence**, which can take several forms. Evidence can be examples that support the claim or counterexamples that undermine someone else's claim with which the author disagrees. Evidence can also be analogies, comparing the author's conclusion to something else using the words "like" or "as." Appeals to authority make use of quotes or references to experts, personal attacks focus on the person making the claim rather than the claim itself, and eliminating possibilities provides evidence that there is only one possible reason for a claim. Support can also take the form of appeals to emotions, such as fear, or references to the argument's popularity (e.g., "Everybody believes this is so").

## Assumptions

While support in the form of evidence is explicit in the text, the author will also make **assumptions**, which are implicit evidence. For example, if the author says, "The girl is holding an empty dog leash and crying. Therefore, she must have lost her dog," the author is assuming that the evidence (the leash and the tears) can mean only one conclusion (the dog is lost). The author doesn't say, "And an empty leash and tears can only mean a lost dog," but this must be true for the author's conclusion to follow from the evidence. This is a reasonable assumption, but because it is not necessarily true, it is still an *assumption*. It could also be that the girl thought her family would be adopting a dog today, but then the dog was adopted by someone else first. Now the author's conclusion is in error. Thus, an author's assumptions are closely related to potential flaws in the argument.

There are two categories of assumptions: mismatched concepts and overlooked possibilities. Consider this argument:

> This year our company introduced a new line of shoes. Sales of our company's shoes have increased this year as compared to last year. Thus, customers must like our new shoes better than our old shoes.

The argument makes two assumptions. First, the author assumes that increased *sales* indicate *customer preference*, but these are not necessarily the same thing. After all, you have probably bought one thing when you would have preferred another, perhaps because you needed to buy the more affordable item. This is a mismatched concept. Second, the author assumes there is only one reason sales increased (customers like our shoes better). The author overlooks other possible reasons for the increased sales; perhaps the economy improved, allowing more shoe purchases, or a major competitor went out of business.

## Question Types

- **Conclusion questions:** These questions ask you to identify the author's claim, which he explicitly states in the argument. Incorrect answers may be evidence used in support of the claim.
- **Evidence questions:** Like conclusion questions, these ask you about an explicit part of the argument, but they require you to identify something the author has said in support of her claim. Incorrect answers may be the author's conclusion instead of evidence, irrelevant evidence, or evidence that other people use to support alternate claims.
- **Assumption questions:** These ask you to think about what unstated evidence must be true in order for the author's conclusion to logically follow.
- **Strengthen/Weaken questions:** You may be asked what evidence would strengthen or weaken the author's claim, in which case each answer choice will present a new piece of evidence. To strengthen a claim, look for evidence that helps to bridge the gap between the evidence already provided and the author's conclusion. To weaken it, choose evidence that undermines the claim; often this is information that shows the author made a faulty assumption. Note that an incorrect answer to a strengthen question may weaken the argument or may just be irrelevant to the argument, neither strengthening nor weakening it. Incorrect answers to weaken questions may strengthen the argument or, again, simply be irrelevant.

Follow along as a TEAS expert maps a passage and answers a question about an argument.

| Question | Analysis |
|---|---|
| Four years ago, the governor came into office seeking to change the way politics were run in this state. Now, it appears he has been the victim of his own ambitious political philosophy. Trying to do too much has given him a reputation of being pushy, and the backlash both from other legislators and voters has let him accomplish little. As a result, he will probably not be reelected. | **Step 1:** Conclusion: The governor may lose the election. Evidence: The way he has done his job and the voters' and legislators' reaction to it. Assumption: Voters and legislators will respond a certain way, probably negatively, to the governor's reputation and ineffectiveness. |
| What does the author assume about the governor's reelection? | **Step 2:** This question asks for the author's assumption. Be careful not to predict that it will be difficult for the governor to be elected: this is the author's stated conclusion. The assumption is some fact or idea the author does *not* state that must be true for the conclusion to be true. |
|  | **Step 3:** Predict that the author's assumption is that the governor's attitude and accomplishments are something voters consider in their decision. |
| (A) Voters based their decisions on their perceptions of an officeholder's personality and effectiveness. | **Step 4:** Correct. Choice **(A)** is a perfect match for your prediction. |
| (B) Politicians always promise more than they can deliver. | What politicians always do is outside the scope of the argument. The author bases her conclusion on evidence about this particular politician, and the assumption must connect that evidence to the conclusion. |
| (C) The governor's opponent in the next election would be a better state leader. | How good a leader the governor's opponent would be, if elected, is outside the scope of the argument, which is entirely about how voters will respond to the governor's record. |
| (D) Voters prefer a candidate who seeks compromise over pushing an agenda and therefore will not reelect the governor. | The author does assume that voters will react negatively to the governor's reputation as "pushy." However, the author's conclusion does not depend on whom voters would prefer instead. Indeed, the argument only discusses voters' opinion of the governor, so any other candidate is outside the scope. |

Now practice answering question about an argument yourself. After reading and mapping the passage and answering the question, check your work against the explanation that follows.

Contrary to popular belief, time spent playing video games is not wasted time. Studies show that playing video games can help increase reaction time, hand-eye coordination, and good decision making. Of course, parents should monitor the amount of time children spend on games, as well as the types of games children play, but adults should also recognize that there are benefits to what may seem at first glance like pure, and even unproductive, play.

What evidence is provided in support of playing video games?

(A)    They offer opportunities for shared play.
(B)    They increase the ability to choose proper words and grammar.
(C)    They increase hand-eye coordination.
(D)    They allow children to relax.

## Explanation

### Step 1:

Conclusion: video games are beneficial
Evidence: three specific benefits
Assumption: drawbacks do not outweigh the benefits

**Step 2:** This question asks you to identify evidence for the author's claim.

**Step 3:** Predict that the evidence is at least one or more of the benefits the author lists.

**Step 4:** The only answer that reflects a stated benefit is choice **(C)**. Although some of the other choices would be benefits, none of them is stated in the passage.

Which of the following, if true, would most strongly support the author's argument about video games?

(A)    Studies show that airplane pilots who have consistently played video games react faster and more appropriately to unexpected events because of their gaming experience.
(B)    Video game developers are more concerned with the plot and characters of the games than they are with the benefits of playing the games.
(C)    Engineers who worked on complicated designs complete their work more slowly if they are addicted to video games.
(D)    Teachers discourage parents from letting their children play video games because this activity interferes with students getting homework done on time.

## Explanation

**Step 2:** This question asks for additional information that would support the author's argument.

**Step 3:** Predict that the answer will confirm some of the proffered evidence in the argument is actually true.

**Step 4:** If playing video games increases a pilot's speed and effectiveness of reaction to unexpected events, this qualifies as a benefit of playing the games, a match for choice **(A)**. Choice (B) is out of scope; the interests of game developers are irrelevant to the argument. Choices (C) and (D) would weaken the argument.

## KEY IDEAS

- In an argument, the author states a conclusion and supports it with evidence.
- Most arguments include one or more assumptions, which are unstated facts or ideas that are necessary for the conclusion to follow from the evidence.
- Claims can be strengthened or weakened by new evidence.

# Evaluating an Argument Practice Questions

**Questions 1–4 refer to the following passage.**

It is without question a travesty that our children are no longer given healthy, nutritious food options for lunch in our public schools. Hamburgers, pizza, and chocolate are giving our kids bigger waistlines. For example, one piece of milk chocolate contains 107 calories, 9 grams of fat, and no calcium (an essential mineral for strong bones), while one apple contains 53 calories, 2 grams of fat, and 6.1 mg of calcium. Junk foods are most assuredly helping teach our children poor eating habits. It is imperative that we change the mindset that any food is good food. Otherwise, a new generation of obese Americans is a given.

1. Which of the following statements would support the author's conclusion that "a new generation of obese Americans is a given"?

   (A) Exercise can counteract obesity.
   (B) Students prefer nutritious meals over junk food.
   (C) Home meals consist of similarly unhealthy choices.
   (D) The price of school meals is the major determinant of what is served.

2. The author constructs the argument by use of

   (A) example.
   (B) appeal to authority.
   (C) opposition to another argument.
   (D) analogy.

3. Which of the following is an accurate restatement of the author's argument?

   (A) There are no healthy foods in school lunches.
   (B) Hamburgers, pizza, and chocolate are fattening.
   (C) It is important for children to eat a variety of foods.
   (D) School lunches are unhealthy and result in overweight children.

4. The author's argument would be weakened if it were true that

   (A) the hamburgers are made with extra-lean meat.
   (B) most children bring healthy lunches from home.
   (C) school lunch chefs are aware of what makes a healthy meal.
   (D) school lunches are more nutritious than the snacks available in campus vending machines.

**Review your work using the explanations in Part Six of this book.**

# LESSON 4

# Integrating Data From Different Formats

## LEARNING OBJECTIVES

- Organize and synthesize data from textual and graphical sources
- Select relevant data from various sources in order to answer a question

It will sometimes be necessary to consider not only textual information within a stimulus but also information presented in a graphical format, most commonly a type of chart, such as a **table** or **graph**, but also potentially in a map, **flowchart**, or other visual representation. This information will be related to what's discussed in the text. For example, a passage about divorce rates in the United States might include a table showing percentages of adults who were divorced each decade from 1950 to 2010, or it might include a pie chart showing what proportion of the population is currently divorced and single, divorced and remarried, never married, married and never divorced, and so on.

When a stimulus includes graphical information, you can expect to answer the same kinds of questions already discussed in previous *Reading* lessons: detail, global, inference, evaluation of arguments, and so forth. The difference is that you will be expected to research both text and graphics to find the answer, sometimes combining information from both. When you map a stimulus with graphical elements, summarize the information in the text as well as in the graphic, including any relationships or trends.

Follow along as a TEAS expert maps a passage and answers two questions using data from multiple formats.

Don't be misled by recently published data on patients at our hospital, specifically the chart of raw patient release numbers. It's important to note that the hospital has not been releasing patients at a higher rate or keeping them for a shorter period of time. Through January, which typically starts out slower in terms of total patients, the average hospitalization time for patients remained between four and five days, with about 70% of total patients being released the same week they were admitted, the same as in the previous three months. This is not a hospital that rushes its patients out the door, nor will it ever be.

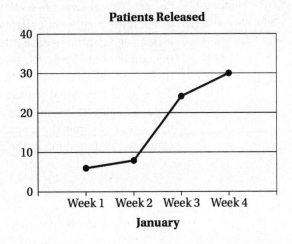

| Question | Analysis |
|---|---|
| | **Step 1:** The passage consists of a graph and a paragraph discussing patient release data from a hospital. According to the author, the average time each patient stays in the hospital has not changed recently, and neither has the rate at which patients have been released. The graphic, however, shows the actual number of patients being released has been increasing each week of January. |
| Which of the following can be concluded from the passage? | **Step 2:** This is an inference question. The answer will be something that follows logically from the data but hasn't already been stated in the stimulus. |
| | **Step 3:** The implied conclusion will follow from either the information in the paragraph, the graph, or both. Research your passage map, which should capture the key ideas of both: (a) patients are not being released at a higher rate (as a percentage), and (b) more patients are being released as time goes on (in raw numbers). |
| | **Step 4:** Predict that the correct answer will follow logically from the information in the stimulus. Given the apparent contradiction between the chart and paragraph text, odds are also good that the inference will resolve the discrepancy. |
| (A) February will have lower raw patient release numbers. | **Step 5:** This is incorrect. The trend shown in the graph is an increase, not a decrease. If the trend continues, February will have even higher numbers. |
| (B) The patient release percentage rate will increase. | The percentage rate is given in the paragraph, where it is described as holding steady at 70%. There is no indication that it will increase, despite the uptick in raw numbers shown in the graph. |
| (C) The lower average hospitalization time is the result of an influx of patients with minor medical concerns. | This statement contradicts information given in the paragraph: the average hospitalization time has remained steady. |
| (D) The total number of patients admitted to the hospital has been steadily increasing throughout the month. | Correct. This answer fits with the information already given. If the number of patients in the hospital has been increasing, and the release rate has been constant, then the number of patients released must also increase. Higher patient intake numbers explain the apparent disparity of a constant release rate but higher raw release numbers. It's also possible to select this answer by process of elimination, since every other choice contradicts information in the passage. |

| Question | Analysis |
|---|---|
| During which week in January did the hospital have its biggest increase in patient releases? | **Step 2:** This is a detail question. The answer will be stated in the stimulus. |
| | **Step 3:** The chart provides information about patient releases for each week of January. The text discusses only rates and average hospitalization time in the month as a whole rather than week by week. |
| | **Step 4:** The chart shows that total patient releases jumped from about 8 in week 2 to about 25 in week 3. This was the biggest increase. |
| (A)  Week 1 | **Step 5:** The graph doesn't show what the numbers were before week 1, but even if there were 0 releases, week 1 would have an increase of fewer than 10 patients. |
| (B)  Week 2 | Week 2 saw an increase of less than 2. |
| (C)  Week 3 | Correct. The number of releases in week 3 is over 15, the largest increase in January. |
| (D)  Week 4 | This week saw an increase of fewer than 10. |

Now practice answering two questions on your own. After reading and mapping the stimulus and answering the questions, check your work against the explanations that follow.

> While the United States never formally adopted the metric system, leaving the average American citizen rather befuddled when traveling to Canada or most Latin American and European countries, American scientists and engineers are quite comfortable with it. It's not simply a question of having an international standard to foster easier collaboration between scientists of different countries. No, the system first championed in Revolutionary France is simply very convenient when making calculations involving weights and measures.
>
> Even nontechnically minded citizens are now becoming more comfortable with the system of metric prefixes, however, because of the technologies that affect their daily lives. In hospitals and pharmacies, tiny doses are measured precisely in milligrams, deciliters, and the like. At big-box stores, consumers compare laptops and PCs by their RAM and hard drive space, which were once measured in mere kilobytes, then in megabytes and later gigabytes, and today are measured in terabytes. And who signs onto a smartphone plan without first considering their monthly data usage, measured the same way?

| Prefix | Symbol | Value relative to base unit |
|---|---|---|
| mega | M | $10^6$ or 1,000,000 |
| kilo | k | $10^3$ or 1,000 |
| hecto | h | $10^2$ or 100 |
| deka | da | $10^1$ or 10 |
| base (no prefix) | — | 1 |
| deci | d | $10^{-1}$ or $\frac{1}{10}$ or 0.1 |
| centi | c | $10^{-2}$ or $\frac{1}{100}$ or 0.01 |
| milli | m | $10^{-3}$ or $\frac{1}{1,000}$ or 0.001 |
| micro | μ (the Greek letter mu, to avoid confusion with "mega") | $10^{-6}$ or $\frac{1}{1,000,000}$ or 0.000001 |

Which of the following, if true, would call into question the passage author's conclusion that US citizens have increased familiarity with the metric system?

(A)   A higher proportion of the US population works in the information technology industry.
(B)   A recent survey shows that most Americans think *megabyte* and *gigabyte* are interchangeable terms.
(C)   Smartphone use has exploded in African countries already using the metric system, like Zimbabwe.
(D)   Most state educational standards include some coverage of the metric system in science curricula.

## Explanation

### Step 1:

Topic: the metric system
Scope: its use and popularity in the United States
Purpose: to inform about the history of metric system in the US; to show public knowledge is changing
¶ 1: metric is efficient; US scientists use it, but public does not
¶ 2: technology is leading US citizens to become more familiar with metric
Table: common metric prefixes

**Step 2:** This question asks you to evaluate what new information would weaken the argument. The argument seems accurate and reasonable. Nevertheless, new information could put the conclusion into question.

**Step 3:** The conclusion (that citizens are more familiar with the metric system) can be weakened either by presenting counterexamples that show US consumers actually have less exposure to metric measurements or by attacking the structure of the argument itself, questioning whether the conclusion about familiarity follows from the evidence of increased use.

K

**Step 4:** Predict the correct answer will introduce evidence that shows Americans have decreased exposure to the metric system or that their increased exposure to it is not leading to greater understanding of it.

**Step 5:** Match your prediction with correct answer choice **(B)**. While the author suggests greater familiarity with terms like *megabyte* or *gigabyte* is leading to better public understanding of the metric system, if the average American does not understand what these terms mean, the conclusion that "citizens are now becoming more comfortable with the system of metric prefixes" is questionable. The statement in answer choice (A) would, if anything, increase the likelihood that more Americans understand the metric system, since it's been established that science and technology use that system. Choice (C) is out of scope, since the argument does not concern countries other than the United States; this also confuses cause and effect, indicating that use of the metric system might result in greater smartphone use rather than the other way around. The statement in (D) would, if anything, support the conclusion that understanding is likely increasing.

> Based on the above information, a gigabyte is
>
> (A)   computer slang for what should have been designated a millibyte.
> (B)   between 1000 and 1,000,000 bytes.
> (C)   1,000,000 bytes.
> (D)   more than 1,000,000 bytes.

## Explanation

**Step 2:** This is an inference question, because *gigabyte* is not explicitly defined in the passage or table.

**Step 3:** The second paragraph discusses kilobytes, megabytes, gigabytes, and terabytes. The table includes the prefixes *kilo-* and *mega-*.

**Step 4:** The context of the description of the units of computer power in the second paragraph implies that that *kilo-*, *mega-*, *giga-*, and *tera-* are listed in order of increasing size, since these measurements were used in this order over time beginning with "mere kilobytes." According to the table, *mega-* represents 1,000,000. You can safely predict that a gigabyte is more than a megabyte, or more than 1,000,000 bytes.

**Step 5:** Choice **(D)** is the correct answer. Answer choices (B) and (C) are inconsistent with the minimum value implied by the passage. There is no support for (A) being true.

## KEY IDEAS

- Include both text paragraphs and graphics in your passage map and include both when researching an answer.
- Combine data from paragraphs and graphics to draw conclusions not explicitly stated in the stimulus.
- Note any obvious trends or patterns in the data.

# Integrating Data From Different Formats Practice Questions

Scientific tools and medical instruments display important information. Being able to interpret this information is vital. The kinds of instruments and tools that you will find in medical professions vary. This chart lists some common instruments and what they are used for in a medical setting.

| Instrument | Purpose |
|---|---|
| Scales | • To measure weight<br>• To measure medication |
| Blood pressure monitor | • To measure diastolic and systolic blood pressure<br>• To measure pulse rate |
| Thermometers | • To measure body temperature<br>• To measure air temperature |

1. Which of the following is an example of a medical instrument that is used only with healthcare clients?

   (A) Blood pressure monitor
   (B) Scale
   (C) Barometer
   (D) Thermometer

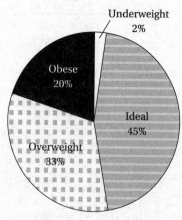

**Body Mass Index**

While the pie chart displays the proportion of citizens in different weight categories in our state today, a similar chart from the 1930s would tell a different story. During the Dust Bowl era, more than 50% of the population was underweight, and indeed, American citizens really did starve to death, and not infrequently. Public health concerns have certainly undergone a dramatic shift, with the obese and overweight categories essentially switching places with the underweight category.

2. Given the information above, approximately what percentage of Americans were overweight or obese during the Dust Bowl era?

   (A) 2%
   (B) 20%
   (C) 33%
   (D) 53%

It doesn't show up on most maps, but the tiny town of Star Point, with its somewhat spread-out cluster of 15 houses, predates Oak Ridge by over 50 years. When the local section of Route 29 was expanded into a four-lane highway, Star Point's government-run grocery and post office were demolished to make room. Today, Starries (as the town's 40-odd members call themselves) drive 18 miles east to the outskirts of Oak Ridge for their basic needs.

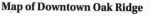

**Map of Downtown Oak Ridge**

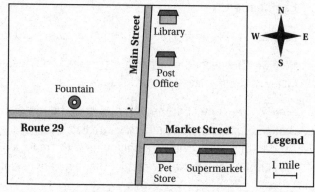

3. When a Starry drives to Oak Ridge to send a letter, which way does she turn once she reaches the town?

   (A) She doesn't turn.
   (B) She turns right onto Market Street, then right onto Main Street.
   (C) She turns right onto Main Street, then left on Market Street.
   (D) She turns left onto Main Street.

**Review your work using the explanations in Part Six of this book.**

# Review and Reflect

Think about the questions you answered in these lessons.

- Were you able to approach each question systematically, using the Kaplan Method for Reading?
- Were you able to read the passage strategically, using key words to find important facts and ideas? Did you take brief notes as needed to map the passage?
- Did you feel confident that you understood what the question was asking you to do?
- How well were you able to predict an answer before looking at the answer choices?
- Could you match your prediction to the correct answer?
- If you missed any questions, do you understand why the answer you chose is incorrect and why the right answer is correct? Could you do the question again now and get it right?

Use your thoughts about these questions to guide how you continue to prepare for the TEAS. If you feel you need more review and practice with reading for main ideas and details and making inferences, you should study this chapter some more before taking the online Practice Test that comes with this book. Also, consider using **Kaplan's ATI TEAS® Qbank**, which contains over 500 practice questions, to increase your mastery of the *Reading* content area.

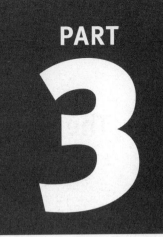

# Mathematics

As a nursing or health science program student, and later in your career as a healthcare professional, you will need to interpret data, perform calculations, and translate real-world situations into math to respond appropriately. You might be reading test results presented as numbers or a graph, calculating medication dosages, interpreting research study results, or planning client care. The TEAS *Mathematics* content area tests your ability to perform arithmetic and algebra. You will apply these skills to solving word problems; interpreting charts and graphs; using descriptive statistics to characterize data sets; understanding relationships between numbers; calculating geometric values; and using measurements appropriately, including by converting from one unit of measure to another.

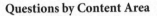

**Questions by Content Area**

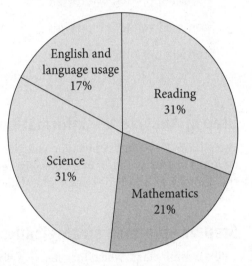

## The TEAS Mathematics Content Area

Of the 170 items on the TEAS, 36 will be in the *Mathematics* content area, and you will have 54 minutes to answer them. Thus, you will have 54 minutes ÷ 36 questions = 1.5 minutes per question.

Of the 36 *Mathematics* questions, 32 will be scored and 4 will be unscored. You won't know which questions are unscored, so do your best on every question.

The 32 scored *Mathematics* questions come from two sub-content areas:

| Sub-content Areas | # of Questions |
|---|---|
| Number and algebra | 23 |
| Measurement and data | 9 |

To help you prepare for these questions, this part of your book is divided into two chapters:

- Chapter 1: Arithmetic and Algebra
- Chapter 2: Statistics, Geometry, and Measurements

# The Kaplan Method for Mathematics

Approaching every *Mathematics* question on the TEAS in a systematic way will help you solve efficiently.

## KAPLAN METHOD FOR MATHEMATICS

**Step 1:** Analyze the information provided.

**Step 2:** Approach strategically.

**Step 3:** Evaluate the answer choices.

**Step 4:** Confirm your answer.

## Step 1: Analyze the information provided.

Every TEAS *Mathematics* question will give you the information you need to solve it. This information may be in the question and/or in a table, figure, or other information supplied above the question. The answer choices may also provide useful information, so analyze those as well.

## Step 2: Approach strategically.

Unlike a math class, which focuses on a single subject such as algebra, the TEAS tests many types of math. When you look at a new question, pause briefly—give yourself the time it takes to take a deep breath—and think about what type of math you will use to solve. Is the question testing arithmetic? Algebra? Geometry? Call to mind the math rules you use to solve this type of question.

In addition, make sure that you have clearly stated in your mind what you are solving for. It's a shame to do all the math right only to choose the wrong answer because you solved for $x$ when the question was asking for $x - 2$, or because you solved for a possible solution when the question asked for a value that *cannot* be a solution. Make sure you are solving for the right thing.

Finally, use the answer choices to your advantage. For example, if there are two negative numbers and two positive numbers in the answers, then if you can quickly determine that the answer must be negative (or must be positive), you can immediately rule out two choices. If the values in the answers are far apart, then estimating an approximate value may be an efficient approach. If you can tell that the answer must be a little less than 1, and only one answer choice fits that description, then you can choose that answer without doing any calculations.

## Step 3: Evaluate the answer choices.

Choose the correct answer from the answer choices. If no choice matches the value you arrived at, then revisit Steps 1 and 2 to see if you overlooked any information or made an error in solving.

## Step 4: Confirm your answer.

You're not done yet! Double-check that you've answered the right question. For example, you don't want to choose the time it takes to load one truck if the question asks for the time to load two trucks. Also, make sure your answer makes sense. For example, if a coat cost $100 and it's now on sale, the sale price should be less, not more, than $100.

# CHAPTER ONE

# ARITHMETIC AND ALGEBRA

## LEARNING OBJECTIVES

- Perform operations with rational numbers, including fractions, decimals, and percentages
- Isolate and calculate the value of a variable
- Translate word problems into math and solve for an unknown value
- Determine a value using a proportion and calculate percent change and rate of change
- Convert measurements between different metric units
- Use rounding and estimating to solve problems efficiently

Of the 32 scored *Mathematics* questions, 23 (72%) will be in the sub-content area of *Number and algebra*. With these questions, the TEAS tests your ability to use arithmetic and algebra to solve questions presented with numbers, variables, and words. Some questions will concern percentages, proportions, and rates. In addition, you'll solve some questions more easily by using estimation and rounding than by calculating an exact value.

This chapter addresses these skills in five lessons:

**Lesson 1:** Arithmetic

**Lesson 2:** Algebra

**Lesson 3:** Solving Word Problems

**Lesson 4:** Ratios, Percentages, and Proportions

**Lesson 5:** Estimating and Rounding

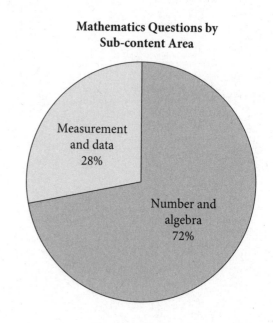

**Mathematics Questions by Sub-content Area**

Measurement and data 28%

Number and algebra 72%

# LESSON 1

# Arithmetic

---

## LEARNING OBJECTIVES

- Compare and order rational numbers
- Convert among non-negative fractions, decimals, and percentages
- Perform arithmetic operations with rational numbers

---

## Place Value and the Number Line

The value of a digit (the digits are the integers 0−9) depends on its place or position in the number. This is the **place value**. In this place value chart, which shows the number 679.32815, the digit on the left (6) has the greatest value.

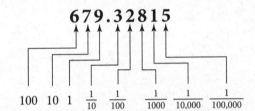

To order numbers, align the place values of the numbers being compared. Start at the left and compare the value of the first digit of each number. Here is how an expert would answer a question about place value.

| Question | Analysis |
|---|---|
| Place the numbers 253, 87, and 216 in order from least to greatest. | **Step 1:** You are given three numbers and asked to put them in order from least to greatest. |
| (A) 87, 253, 216<br>(B) 253, 216, 87<br>(C) 216, 253, 87<br>(D) 87, 216, 253 | **Step 2:** Compare using a place values chart.<br><br>Hundreds   Tens   Ones<br>   2        5      3<br>   0        8      7<br>   2        1      6<br><br>The least (smallest) number is the one whose leftmost digit has the smallest place value. This is 87. Now compare the first digit of the remaining numbers. Both numbers have the same digit in the hundreds place, so compare the digits in the tens place. Because 1 is less than 5, 216 is less than 253. |

| Question | Analysis |
|---|---|
| | **Step 3:** The correct answer is **(D)**. |
| | **Step 4:** Double-check that you made valid, accurate comparisons and you ordered the numbers as asked. Choice (B) is a trap; the numbers are ordered greatest to least. |

You can also use a **number line** to compare numbers. Beginning with zero, numbers increase in value to the right (0, 1, 2, 3, . . .) and decrease in value to the left (–3, –2, –1, 0, . . .). The order in which numbers are placed on the number line will determine which are greater and which are less than other numbers.

A **signed number** tells you two things: the sign tells you the direction from zero, and the number tells you the distance from zero. For example, −3 is three spaces to the left of zero, and +5 is five spaces to the right of zero.

Try this question.

What is the correct order of the numbers 2, −10, and −4, from least to greatest?

- (A)  2, −4, −10
- (B)  −4, −10, 2
- (C)  −10, −4, 2
- (D)  2, −10 −4

## Explanation

**Step 1:**  You are given three numbers and asked to put them in correct order, from least to greatest.

**Step 2:**  Compare the numbers: −10 lies ten spaces to the left of zero, −4 lies four spaces to the left of zero, and 2 lies two spaces to the right of zero.

**Step 3:**  The correct answer choice is **(C)**.

**Step 4:**  Double-check that you made accurate comparisons and ordered the numbers as asked. Choice (A) is a trap; the digits 2, 4, and 10 are in order from least to greatest, but when the signs are taken into account, the numbers are in order from greatest to least.

# Operations With Positive and Negative Numbers

Use a number line to help add signed numbers. For example:

$2 + (−5) = −3$    Begin at +2; move 5 steps in the negative direction (left); end at −3.

$−3 + (−4) = −7$    Begin at −3; move 4 steps in the negative direction (left); end at −7.

K

To add without a number line, follow these steps:

- If numbers have like signs, add the numbers and keep the same sign.
- If the numbers have different signs, find the difference between the two numbers and write the difference (the answer) with the sign of the larger number.

For example, add $2 + (-5)$. Because the numbers have different signs, subtract: $5 - 2 = 3$. Then use the sign from the larger number—here that's the negative sign with the 5—to get $-3$.

You can rewrite a subtraction problem as an addition problem. Change the operation symbol to addition and change the sign on the number you are subtracting. Then apply the rules for adding signed numbers.

Here is how the TEAS would ask about operations with positive and negative numbers. See if you can answer this one.

$$-22 + (-13) - (-11) + 27 = ?$$

- (A) $-19$
- (B) 3
- (C) 7
- (D) 73

## Explanation

**Step 1:** You are given an expression that involves the addition and subtraction of numbers with unlike signs and asked to find its value.

**Step 2:** Rewrite the subtraction as addition and change the sign of the following number:
$-22 + (-13) + 11 + 27$.
Add the positive terms: $11 + 27 = 38$.
Add the negative terms: $22 + 13 = -35$.
Combine the result: $38 + (-35) = 3$.

**Step 3:** The correct answer is **(B)**.

**Step 4:** Double-check your arithmetic, making sure you handled each sign correctly, including when adding numbers with mixed signs in the final step.

Multiplying and dividing signed numbers is no different from other multiplication and division, except that you need to determine whether the solution will be positive or negative. Count the number of negative numbers. If the number of negatives is odd, the answer will be negative. If you have an even number of negative numbers, the answer will be positive.

So for example, to multiply $6(-3)(2)$, first multiply the numbers only: $6 \times 3 \times 2 = 36$. Then, because there is one negative term, the answer is negative: $6(-3)(2) = -36$.

Now you try this example:

$$-(5)(5)(-1)(-3)(2) =$$

- (A) $-150$
- (B) $-2$
- (C) 16
- (D) 150

## Explanation

**Step 1:** You are given an expression that involves multiplying numbers with unlike signs and asked to find its value.

**Step 2:** Multiply the numbers only: $5 \times 5 \times 1 \times 3 \times 2 = 150$. Now, because there are three negative terms and 3 is an odd number, the product is negative: $-150$.

**Step 3:** The correct answer is **(A)**.

**Step 4:** Double-check that your multiplication is correct and that you counted the number of negative signs accurately. Choice (D) has the correct number but the wrong sign.

# Fractions, Decimals, and Percents

## Fractions

A **fraction** is part of a whole. The top number, the **numerator,** is the number of parts you are working with. The bottom number, the **denominator,** is the number of equal parts in the whole.

There are eight equal parts in this rectangle. Because three are shaded, $\frac{3}{8}$ of the rectangle is shaded.

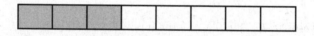

In a **proper fraction**, the numerator is less than the denominator (i.e., $\frac{2}{3}$). A proper fraction represents a quantity less than 1. An **improper fraction** has a numerator with a greater magnitude than that of denominator (i.e., $\frac{9}{8}$). The value is greater than 1. A **mixed number** consists of a whole number and a proper fraction. Its value is greater than 1 (or less than −1 if the improper fraction is negative). Thus, the shaded portion of the following figure represents $\frac{11}{8}$ (written as an improper fraction) or $1\frac{3}{8}$ (written as a mixed number).

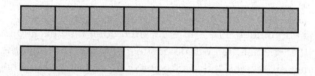

When two fractions have the same denominator, the fraction with the smaller numerator is smaller.

$$\frac{5}{8} < \frac{7}{8}$$

When two fractions have the same numerator, the fraction with the smaller denominator is larger.

$$\frac{5}{6} > \frac{5}{10}$$

When fractions have different numerators and different denominators, a comparison can be difficult. The X method can be used to compare fractions. To compare two positive fractions:

- Draw lines as shown to form an X.
- Multiply denominator × numerator for each line and record the result above each fraction.

$$3 \times 4 = 12 \quad 5 \times 2 = 10$$
$$\frac{4}{5} \diagtimes \frac{2}{3}$$

The fraction beneath the greater product is the greater fraction. For instance, because 12 > 10 in the example above, $\frac{4}{5} > \frac{2}{3}$.

## Decimals

**Decimals** are numbers that use place value to show amounts. The number 2.375 is a number between 2 and 3. Read "and" in place of the decimal point. After reading the decimal part, say the place value of the last decimal digit. This number would be read "two and three hundred seventy-five thousandths."

## Percentages

**Percent** means "per hundred" or "out of one hundred." Because percent is a way of showing part of a whole, it has much in common with fractions and decimals. For example, 75% is 0.75 in decimal form. More, 75% can be written as $\frac{75}{100}$, which is $\frac{3}{4}$ when reduced to its simplest form (by dividing the top and bottom of the fraction by 25).

## Conversion of Numbers to Different Forms

Percents, fractions, and decimals are all ways to show part of a whole.

Change fractions to decimals by dividing. For example, to express $\frac{3}{8}$ as a decimal, divide 3 by 8: $\frac{3}{8} = 0.375$.

You can change a decimal to a fraction by using place value. For example, to express 0.25 as a fraction, consider that the last digit, 5, is in the hundredths column. So, write 25 over 100 $\left(\frac{25}{100}\right)$. Then reduce by dividing the top and bottom of the fraction by 25: $\frac{25}{100} = \frac{1}{4}$.

Now use your understanding of percents, fractions, and decimals to try two questions on your own.

Express 65% as a fraction in its simplest form.

(A) $\frac{13}{200}$

(B) $\frac{13}{20}$

(C) $\frac{6}{5}$

(D) $6\frac{1}{2}$

## Explanation

**Step 1:** You are given a percent and asked to convert it to a fraction. The answer choices range from tiny, $\frac{13}{200}$, to quite a bit larger, $6\frac{1}{2}$.

**Step 2:** One way to approach this question is with estimation. If you know that 50% is $\frac{1}{2}$, and you know that 100% is 1, then you know that 65% must be greater than $\frac{1}{2}$ but less than 1. Only one answer choice fits this description.

Another way to solve is through calculating the conversion. Write the percent over 100 and reduce to its simplest form: $65\% = \frac{65}{100} = \frac{13}{20}$.

**Step 3:** The correct answer is **(B)**.

**Step 4:** Double-check that you performed the operations accurately and that your answer makes sense. To confirm, you can divide 13 by 20: $\frac{13}{20} = 0.65 = 65\%$. Choice (A) is a trap for those who divided 65 by 1000.

# Arithmetic Operations

## Operations With Whole Numbers

Addition, subtraction, multiplication, and division are **operations**. If there are more than two operations in a single expression, they *must* be performed in a specific manner called the **order of operations**. Use the made-up word PEMDAS to remember the order in which to perform the operations in an expression. PEMDAS stands for:

- **P**arentheses
- **E**xponents
- **M**ultiplication and **D**ivision (from left to right)
- **A**ddition and **S**ubtraction (from left to right)

Write out your calculations step-by-step. Perform each operation one at a time and then simplify before you move on. Here is how you would use PEMDAS to answer a question on the TEAS.

| Question | Analysis |
|---|---|
| What is the value of $(3+4)\times2+6$? | **Step 1:** You are given an expression involving addition and multiplication and asked to find its value. |
| (A) 15<br>(B) 17<br>(C) 20<br>(D) 56 | **Step 2:** Use PEMDAS. $(3+4)\times2+6$. Start with parentheses: $7\times2+6$. Next, multiply: $14+6$. Now, add: 20. |

| Question | Analysis |
|---|---|
| | **Step 3**: The correct answer is **(C)**. |
| | **Step 4**: Double-check that you performed the operations in the right order and that your calculations are correct. Choice (B) results from disregarding the parentheses and multiplying $4 \times 2$ first. |

Practice working on PEMDAS with this example.

What is the value of $4 + 6 \times (7 - 2)$?

(A) 34
(B) 44
(C) 50
(D) 68

## Explanation

**Step 1:** You are given an expression with different operations and asked to find its value.

**Step 2:** Solve, keeping in mind the order of operations (PEMDAS).

$4 + 6 \times (7 - 2)$

Start with parentheses: $4 + 6 \times 5$

Next, multiply: $4 + 30$

Now, add: 34

**Step 3:** The correct answer is **(A)**.

**Step 4:** Did you perform the operations in the correct order and do the arithmetic correctly?

## Operations With Fractions

To add or subtract fractions that have the same denominator, just add or subtract the numerators and use the common denominator for the result.

$$\frac{3}{7} + \frac{2}{7} = \frac{3+2}{7} = \frac{5}{7}$$

If the denominators are not the same, then you must find a **common denominator**.

For example, to add $\frac{1}{2}$ and $\frac{1}{3}$, you need equivalent fractions with a common denominator, which is really just the **least common multiple** (LCM) of the given denominators.

- The multiples of 2 are 2, 4, 6.
- The multiples of 3 are 3, 6.
- The LCM is 6, and the common denominator of $\frac{1}{2}$ and $\frac{1}{3}$ is 6.

For each fraction, multiply the denominator by the other denominator to get the new common denominator. Then, multiply the numerator by the same number (whatever you do to the bottom of a fraction, you must do to the top, and vice versa).

$$\text{Change } \frac{1}{2}: \quad \frac{1}{2} \times \frac{3}{3} = \frac{3}{6}$$

$$\text{Change } \frac{1}{3}: \quad \frac{1}{3} \times \frac{2}{2} = \frac{2}{6}$$

Once you have a common denominator, you can continue with the addition.

$$\frac{1}{2} + \frac{1}{3} = \frac{3}{6} + \frac{2}{6} = \frac{5}{6}$$

| Question | Analysis |
|---|---|
| What is the value of $\frac{1}{3} - \frac{1}{4}$ ? | **Step 1:** You are given an equation with fractions with different denominators and asked to subtract. |
| (A) $\frac{7}{12}$ <br> (B) $\frac{1}{7}$ <br> (C) $\frac{1}{12}$ <br> (D) $-\frac{1}{1}$ | **Step 2:** The common denominator of $\frac{1}{3}$ and $\frac{1}{4}$ is 12 (the LCM of 3 and 4). <br><br> $$\frac{1}{3} \times \frac{4}{4} = \frac{4}{12} \qquad \frac{1}{4} \times \frac{3}{3} = \frac{3}{12}$$ <br> Now you can subtract: <br><br> $$\frac{4}{12} - \frac{3}{12} = \frac{1}{12}$$ |
| | **Step 3:** The correct answer is **(C)**. |
| | **Step 4:** Double-check that you correctly multiplied the top and bottom of each fraction and then subtracted the numerators. |

To multiply fractions, multiply the numerators straight across and the denominators straight across.

$$\frac{2}{5} \times \frac{2}{3} = \frac{2 \times 2}{5 \times 3} = \frac{4}{15}$$

To divide fractions, multiply the first fraction by the **reciprocal** (the numerator and denominator change places) of the second fraction.

$$\frac{1}{8} \div \frac{3}{4} = \frac{1}{8} \times \frac{4}{3} = \frac{4}{24}$$

You can first convert mixed numbers to improper fractions by multiplying the denominator by the whole number, adding the numerator to that product, and placing the sum over the denominator.

To convert $2\frac{1}{4}$ to an improper fraction:

- Multiply the whole number part by the denominator of the fraction part: $2 \times 4$.
- Add this product to the numerator: $(2 \times 4) + 1$.
- Record this result as the numerator: $(2 \times 4) + 1$.
- Keep the denominator the same as in the fraction part: $\frac{(2 \times 4) + 1}{4}$.
- Simplify: $2\frac{1}{4} = \frac{(2 \times 4) + 1}{4} = \frac{8 + 1}{4} = \frac{9}{4}$.

Practice using mixed numbers with this problem.

What is the value of $2\frac{1}{4} \times 3\frac{2}{3}$, converted to a mixed number?

(A)   1

(B)   $\frac{15}{12}$

(C)   $6\frac{1}{6}$

(D)   $8\frac{1}{4}$

## Explanation

**Step 1:** You are given an expression with mixed numbers and asked for its value as a mixed number.

**Step 2:** Convert the mixed numbers to improper fractions before multiplying the values. The final step is to simplify the equation.

$$2\frac{1}{4} \times 3\frac{2}{3} = \frac{(4 \times 2) + 1}{4} \times \frac{(3 \times 3) + 2}{3} = \frac{9}{4} \times \frac{11}{3} = \frac{99}{12} = 8\frac{3}{12} = 8\frac{1}{4}$$

**Step 3:** The correct answer is **(D)**.

**Step 4:** Double-check that your arithmetic is correct and your answer makes sense. Because $2 \times 3 = 6$ and $3 \times 4 = 12$, it makes sense that $2\frac{1}{4} \times 3\frac{2}{3}$ is about halfway between 6 and 12.

## KEY IDEAS

- A number line is a tool that helps you compare and order rational numbers.
- Be alert for the effect of negative numbers in multiplication and division.
- Any number can be represented as a fraction, decimal, or percent.
- The key to evaluating an expression is the order of operations (PEMDAS).

# Arithmetic Practice Questions

1. Convert 0.32 to a fraction and percent.

   (A)  $\dfrac{4}{25}$, 0.32%

   (B)  $\dfrac{8}{25}$, 3.2%

   (C)  $\dfrac{8}{25}$, 32%

   (D)  $\dfrac{4}{25}$, 32%

2. What is the least common multiple of 4, 8, and 10?

   (A)  10
   (B)  20
   (C)  40
   (D)  80

3. Order the following fractions from least to greatest:
   $\dfrac{3}{8}, \dfrac{2}{5}, \dfrac{1}{4}$.

   (A)  $\dfrac{1}{4}, \dfrac{2}{5}, \dfrac{3}{8}$

   (B)  $\dfrac{1}{4}, \dfrac{3}{8}, \dfrac{2}{5}$

   (C)  $\dfrac{3}{8}, \dfrac{1}{4}, \dfrac{2}{5}$

   (D)  $\dfrac{2}{5}, \dfrac{3}{8}, \dfrac{1}{4}$

4. What is the sum of $1\dfrac{5}{8}$ and $\dfrac{7}{12}$?

   (A)  $2\dfrac{1}{24}$

   (B)  $2\dfrac{5}{24}$

   (C)  $2\dfrac{7}{24}$

   (D)  $2\dfrac{11}{24}$

5. What is the value of $81 + 324 \div 27 - 18 + 17(12)$.

   (A)  143
   (B)  195
   (C)  201
   (D)  279

6. What is the value of $8 + (2 + 5) \times 6$?

   (A)  21
   (B)  40
   (C)  50
   (D)  90

**Review your work using the explanations in Part Six of this book.**

**K**

# LESSON 2

# Algebra

> ## LEARNING OBJECTIVES
>
> - Recognize a variable in an algebraic expression
> - Use the correct arithmetic operations to isolate a variable
> - Efficiently calculate the value of a variable

A **variable** is a letter used to represent a numerical value that is unknown. The value of a specific variable (such as $x$) will be the same throughout a given problem, but it can differ from one problem to another.

A **constant** is a value that doesn't change, typically a number. For example, in the expression $x + 6$, $x$ is the variable and 6 is the constant.

A **term** is a variable, constant, or the product of a constant and a variable. A term containing only a number is called a **constant term** because it contains no variables. The following are all terms: $y$, 42, and $7a$.

**Like terms** are terms that can be combined. Simplify algebraic expressions by combining like terms.

## Isolating a Variable

The key to solving an equation is to do the same thing to both sides of the equation until you have the variable by itself on one side of the equation and all of the numbers on the other side.

Use **inverse operations** to move terms from the side of the equation containing the variable to the other side. Inverse operations are arithmetic operations that are used to cancel or "undo" each other:

- Addition and subtraction cancel each other.
- Multiplication and division cancel each other.

Here's an example of how an expert combines like terms to simplify an expression.

| Question | Analysis |
|---|---|
| $y + 7 + 3y + 10$<br><br>Which of the following is equivalent to the above expression? | **Step 1:** The question gives you an expression containing like terms, constant terms, and terms with the variable $y$. It asks you to find the equivalent value among the answer choices, which also contain constant terms and terms with $y$. |
| (A) $4y + 3$<br>(B) $2y + 7$<br>(C) $3y + 70$<br>(D) $4y + 17$ | **Step 2:** Simplify by combining like terms.<br><br>First, combine $y$ and $3y$: $y + 3y = 4y$.<br><br>Next, combine 7 and 10: $7 + 10 = 17$.<br><br>Then, add the unlike terms: $4y + 17$. |
| | **Step 3:** The correct answer is choice **(D)**. |
| | **Step 4:** Check that you've performed the arithmetic correctly. |

Now study how a test expert uses inverse operations to isolate a variable.

| Question | Analysis |
|---|---|
| $x + 6 = 9$<br><br>In the above equation, what is the value of $x$? | **Step 1:** The question presents an equation and asks you to solve for the value of $x$. In this equation, $x$ is added to 6. |
| (A) 0<br>(B) 3<br>(C) 6<br>(D) 15 | **Step 2:** To get the variable $x$ alone on one side, you must undo the addition with the inverse operation. The inverse of adding 6 is subtracting 6. Therefore, subtracting 6 from the left side of the equation will cancel out the $+6$.<br><br>Make sure that whatever you do to one side of the equation, you also do to the other, so subtract 6 from both sides: $x + 6 - 6 = 9 - 6$.<br><br>Next, simplify both sides: $x = 3$. |
| | **Step 3:** The correct answer is **(B)**. |
| | **Step 4:** Check your answer by plugging it in for $x$ in the original equation: $3 + 6 = 9$. |

Now you try a question. This one involves multiplication and division.

$$5a = 20$$

In the above equation, what is the value of $a$?

    (A)   4
    (B)   5
    (C)   15
    (D)   25

## Explanation

**Step 1:** The question asks for the value of $a$. In this equation, $a$ is multiplied by 5.

**Step 2:** To get the variable $a$ alone on one side, you must undo the multiplication with the inverse operation. The inverse of multiplying by 5 is dividing by 5, so dividing the left side of the equation by 5 will cancel out the multiplier 5. Whatever you do to one side of the equation, you must also do to the other, so divide by 5 on both sides, then simplify.

$$\frac{5a}{5} = \frac{20}{5}$$
$$a = 4$$

**Step 3:** The correct answer is **(A)**.

**Step 4:** Check your answer by plugging it in for $a$ in the original equation: $5 \times 4 = 20$.

Note that a variable sometimes appears on both sides of an equation; however, you'll still use inverse operations to isolate the variable. Try this one.

$$7y + 4 = 3y + 12$$

In the above equation, what is the value of $y$?

    (A)   1.6
    (B)   2
    (C)   4
    (D)   8

### Explanation

**Step 1:** The question asks for the value of $y$. The variable $y$ appears on both sides of the equation. There is both addition and multiplication on each side.

**Step 2:** To get the variable $y$ alone on one side, you must undo both the addition and the multiplication with the appropriate inverse operations. Start by subtracting 4 from both sides: $7y + 4 - 4 = 3y + 12 - 4$. And simplify: $7y = 3y + 8$.

Subtract $3y$ from both sides: $7y - 3y = 3y + 8 - 3y$. And simplify: $4y = 8$.

Divide both sides by 4: $y = 2$.

**Step 3:** The correct answer is **(B)**.

**Step 4:** Check your answer by plugging it in for $y$ in the original equation.

$$(7 \times 2) + 4 = (3 \times 2) + 12$$
$$14 + 4 = 6 + 12$$
$$18 = 18$$

---

## KEY IDEAS

- Simplify algebraic expressions by combining like terms.
- Use inverse operations to isolate the variable on one side of an equation, with all the numbers on the other side.
- Always do the same thing to both sides of an equation.

# Algebra Practice Questions

1. $2x + 16 = 30$

   Solve for $x$ in the equation above. Which of the following is correct?
   (A) 7
   (B) 14
   (C) 23
   (D) 46

2. $5y - 11 + 9y + 81$

   Simplify the expression above. Which of the following is correct?
   (A) $4y - 92$
   (B) $4y + 70$
   (C) $14y + 70$
   (D) $14y + 92$

3. $10b - 21 = 9$

   Solve for $b$ in the equation above. Which of the following is correct?
   (A) $-11$
   (B) $-10$
   (C) 3
   (D) 30

4. Find the sum of the expressions $44x - 1$ and $12x + 5$.

   Which of the following is correct?
   (A) $32x + 4$
   (B) $32x - 6$
   (C) $56x - 6$
   (D) $56x + 4$

5. $\dfrac{5a}{2} = 2a + 5$

   Solve for $a$ in the equation above. Which of the following is correct?
   (A) $\dfrac{5}{3}$
   (B) $\dfrac{10}{3}$
   (C) 5
   (D) 10

**Review your work using the explanations in Part Six of this book.**

# LESSON 3

# Solving Word Problems

## LEARNING OBJECTIVES

- Translate problems described in words into math expressions, equations, and inequalities
- Solve word problems that describe real-world scenarios

Word problems, by definition, require you to translate English into math. Therefore, a key to solving word problems is knowing how to translate various words and phrases into their mathematical equivalents.

The following table lists words and phrases that commonly appear in word problems, along with their mathematical translations.

| When you see: | Think: |
|---|---|
| sum, plus, more than, added to, combined, total | $+$ |
| minus, less than, difference between, decreased by | $-$ |
| is, was, equals, is equivalent to, is the same as, adds up to | $=$ |
| times, product, multiplied by, of, twice, double, triple | $\times$ |
| divided by, quotient, over, per, out of, into | $\div$ |
| what, how many, how much, a number | $x$, $a$, etc. |

Try translating the following English phrases into the equivalent math.

**English**                                                    **Math**

1. $b$ is 7 more than $a$.                                    _____

2. $y$ is half of $x$.                                        _____

3. $m$ decreased by 3 is twice $n$.                           _____

4. Malia earns 20 percent more than Lola.                     _____

5. The product of $a$ and $b$ is twice their sum.             _____

6. There are at least three times as many carrots as tomatoes. _____

Now check how you did:

1. $b = a + 7$
2. $y = \dfrac{x}{2}$
3. $m - 3 = 2n$
4. $M = 1.2L$
5. $ab = 2(a + b)$
6. $c \geq 3t$ or $t \leq \dfrac{1}{3}c$

Word problems on the TEAS sometimes include information that is unnecessary to solve the problem. Be sure to distinguish between important and irrelevant information.

See how a test expert uses the relevant information in a word problem to answer this question.

| Question | Analysis |
|---|---|
| Kendra has just purchased an exercise tracker. She also has an app to analyze the data and calculate how many calories she burns. Kendra's step length is 2 feet 3 inches. Which of the following is the distance she will travel if she walks 3500 steps? | **Step 1:** The question provides Kendra's step length and the number of steps she walks, and it asks for the distance she travels. The first two sentences about Kendra's exercise tracker and her app are irrelevant to answering the question. |
| (A) 3500 feet <br> (B) 7350 feet <br> (C) 7875 feet <br> (D) 8050 feet | **Step 2:** Because the answer choices are given in feet, convert the step length of 2 feet 3 inches into decimal form. Three inches is one-fourth of a foot, or 0.25 feet. Thus, 2 feet 3 inches = 2.25 feet. <br><br> Next, multiply the length of each step by the number of steps: 2.25 feet × 3500 steps = 7875 feet. |
| | **Step 3:** The correct answer is **(C)**. |
| | **Step 4:** Check your answer by dividing it by the number of steps: 7875 ÷ 3500 = 2.25. This is the length of each step. |

Try this one yourself. Identify the relevant information and translate from English into math.

A medical seminar is being held as part of a yearly science and technology conference. The seminar is attended by a total of 210 doctors, nurses, and scientists. One-fifth of the attendees are nurses, and one-third of the attendees are doctors. How many attendees are neither doctors nor nurses?

(A) 42
(B) 70
(C) 98
(D) 112

## Explanation

**Step 1:** The relevant information is the total number of seminar attendees, the three different types of attendees, and the fraction of the total who are nurses and the fraction of the total who are doctors. You need to find the number of attendees who are not doctors or nurses.

**Step 2:** First, translate "one-fifth of the attendees are nurses" as $210 \times \frac{1}{5} = 42$. There are 42 nurses.

Translate "one-third of the attendees are doctors": $210 \times \frac{1}{3} = 70$. There are 70 doctors. Therefore, the

total number of doctors and nurses is $42 + 70 = 112$. Subtract this from the total attendees to find the number who are neither doctors nor nurses: $210 - 112 = 98$.

**Step 3:** The correct answer is **(C)**.

**Step 4:** Check that you applied the correct fractions to the correct groups and that you performed your calculations correctly.

Sometimes, a word problem on the TEAS won't require you to solve for a value. Instead, it will ask you to identify the expression among the answer choices that correctly matches the language in the question stem. Try the following question.

A dog groomer charges $x$ dollars for each small dog and $y$ dollars for each large dog. Which of the following expressions correctly represents the amount of money the groomer will charge in dollars for three small dogs and two large dogs?

(A)  $3x + 2y$
(B)  $5(x + y)$
(C)  $5xy$
(D)  $6(x + y)$

## Explanation

**Step 1:** The question provides the prices the groomer charges for small and large dogs and a variable to represent each, as well as the number of dogs of each size. You're asked to find the expression that represents how much the groomer will charge in the scenario described.

**Step 2:**  Because each small dog is represented by $x$, and there are three small dogs, multiply $x$ by 3 to yield $3x$. The large dogs are represented by $y$, and there are two of them, so multiply $y$ by 2 to yield $2y$. Now add the two parts to determine the total: $3x + 2y$.

**Step 3:** The correct answer is **(A)**. Choice (B) incorrectly combines both prices charged and multiplies by the total number of dogs. Choice (C) incorrectly multiplies the prices and multiplies that product by the total number of dogs. Choice (D) incorrectly combines the two prices and multiplies this sum by the product of the dogs of both sizes.

**Step 4:** Check your answer by plugging in real dollar values for *x* and *y* (for example, *x* = 5 and *y* = 10) and then calculating the total amount the groomer will charge as described in the question stem: (3 × $5) + (2 × $10) = $35. Now plug $5 for *x* and $10 for *y* into the answer choices to see which equals $35.

---

## KEY IDEAS

- Be sure to distinguish between important and unimportant information within word problems.
- Don't be intimidated by lengthy word problems; translate the English into mathematical expressions step-by-step.
- Determine whether you actually need to solve the problem or only identify which mathematical expression it represents.

# Solving Word Problems Practice Questions

1. Karina buys lunch at the cafeteria for herself and her son. They both get a soda for $1.50. Karina gets an $8.00 sandwich for herself, and her son has the mac 'n' cheese for $4.75. How much does Karina spend altogether on lunch?

   (A) $12.75
   (B) $14.25
   (C) $15.75
   (D) $28.50

2. Jamal just received a promotion at work, and now he wants to begin saving money. His new salary is $2,875 a month, and his bills come to $2,360 a month. He also wants to have some fun, so he plans to save half of what's left over after paying his bills. How much will he save each month?

   (A) $207.50
   (B) $257.50
   (C) $515.00
   (D) $1030.00

3. A teacher is handing out crayons to students that they will use in an art project, drawing either a landscape scene or a portrait of a family member. Of the students, 9 have chosen to draw a landscape, and 3 have chosen to draw a portrait. The teacher has 60 crayons and wants to distribute them equally. How many crayons should she give each student?

   (A) 5
   (B) 6
   (C) 10
   (D) 20

4. Tyler makes $80 of profit on every six pallets of strawberries he sells at his roadside stand. It takes two bales of straw to grow each pallet of strawberries. How many bales of straw will Tyler need to earn a $400 profit?

   (A) 15
   (B) 30
   (C) 50
   (D) 60

5. Kaitlyn lives 10 miles from her work. Each day, she travels at an average speed of 40 miles per hour to get to work in the morning. In the afternoon, due to heavier traffic, she averages only 30 miles per hour on the trip home. How much time does Kaitlyn spend traveling to and from work each day?

   (A) 30 minutes
   (B) 35 minutes
   (C) 40 minutes
   (D) 1 hour 10 minutes

6. A therapist is considering jobs at two different clinics. Clinic A pays therapists $25 per client treated plus a flat weekly salary of $200, and each therapist is assigned 30 clients a week. Clinic B pays therapists $40 per client treated, with no additional salary. What is the minimum number of clients per week the therapist would need to treat at Clinic B to exceed the income he'd make at Clinic A?

   (A) 23
   (B) 24
   (C) 30
   (D) 31

7. A highway on-ramp contains a traffic light to regulate the flow of traffic onto the highway. The light allows one car to pass every 10 seconds, one car to pass every 15 seconds, or one car to pass every 20 seconds, depending on the flow of traffic on the highway. Which of the following expressions represents the number of cars, $n$, that can pass through this light in 15 minutes, assuming a continuous flow of cars?

   (A) $10 \geq n \geq 20$
   (B) $10 \leq n \leq 20$
   (C) $45 \leq n \geq 90$
   (D) $45 \leq n \leq 90$

8. Each day, 36 gallons of water are applied to a garden. One-fourth of this amount is used to grow vegetables. The water applied to the vegetables must first pass through a filter. The filter can process 360 gallons of water before being replaced, and it is only used to filter the water applied to the vegetables. After how many days will the filter need to be replaced?

   (A) 4
   (B) 10
   (C) 18
   (D) 40

**Review your work using the explanations in Part Six of this book.**

# LESSON 4

# Ratios, Percentages, and Proportions

## LEARNING OBJECTIVES

- Relate the value of different quantities as a ratio or percentage
- Calculate percentage changes
- Determine the value of an unknown quantity using proportions
- Solve problems using rates

## Ratios

**Ratios** are representations of the relationship of one quantity to another. They can be expressed verbally (for example, "The ratio of cats to dogs is 3 to 4") or by separating the two quantities with a colon (as in 3:4). Ratios can also be written as fractions (e.g., $\frac{3}{4}$). In order to perform calculations using ratios, you will use this format. Because it is common practice to reduce ratios to their lowest terms, ratios do not necessarily specify the actual quantities. For instance, if there are 9 cats and 12 dogs in a pet store, the ratio $\frac{9}{12}$ can be simplified to $\frac{3}{4}$ by dividing both the numerator and denominator by 3.

Ratios can be either "part to part" or "part to whole." The example above is a **part-to-part ratio** because it compares cats to dogs. This situation could also be expressed in terms of a **part-to-whole ratio** of cats to total animals. The numerator would still express the number of cats, but the denominator would come from the sum of cats and dogs: $\frac{9}{9+12} = \frac{9}{21}$, which simplifies to $\frac{3}{7}$.

Study how an expert would approach a ratio question.

| Question | Analysis |
|---|---|
| There are 35 staff members at a meeting. Fifteen of the staff members are nurses, and the rest are doctors. What is the ratio of doctors to nurses? | **Step 1:** The question gives the number of staff members and how many of them are nurses, and asks for the ratio of doctors to nurses. |
| (A) $\frac{3}{7}$ <br><br> (B) $\frac{3}{4}$ <br><br> (C) $\frac{4}{3}$ <br><br> (D) $\frac{7}{3}$ | **Step 2:** This question is asking about a part-to-part ratio, doctors:nurses. Determine the number for each of the parts and express the ratio as a fraction. Since there are 35 total staff and 15 are nurses, there are $35 - 15 = 20$ doctors. The ratio of doctors to nurses is thus $\frac{20}{15}$. |

| Question | Analysis |
|---|---|
| | **Step 3:** Although none of the answer choices is $\frac{20}{15}$, choice **(C)** is $\frac{20}{15}$ reduced to its simplest terms. |
| | **Step 4:** Be certain you calculated the ratio that was asked for and check your calculations. Choice (B) is the ratio of nurses to doctors. |

## Percentages

**Percentages** are the ratio of a quantity to 100. If 4% of the parts made by a factory are defective, then 4 out of every 100 or $\frac{4}{100}$ are defective. It is possible to have values greater than 100%. For instance, this year's sales for a store could be 120% of last year's. As you learned in Lesson 1: Arithmetic, converting between percentages and decimal values is merely a matter of moving the decimal two places to the left when converting from percent to decimal or to the right when converting from decimal to percent. For instance, 27% = 0.27 and 1.13 = 113%.

Test questions and real-world situations may require calculating percentage increase or decrease using the formula $\frac{\text{new amount} - \text{old amount}}{\text{old amount}} \times 100\%$. If the change is a decrease, the result will be negative. Study this example.

| Question | Analysis |
|---|---|
| Jack's doctor increased the dosage of his medication from 80 milligrams to 100 milligrams. What was the percentage increase of the dosage? | **Step 1:** The problem describes an increase from 80 to 100 and asks for the percentage increase. |
| (A) 20%<br>(B) 25%<br>(C) 80%<br>(D) 125% | **Step 2:** Using the applicable formula, the percent increase is $\frac{100 - 80}{80} \times 100\%$. This simplifies to $\frac{20}{80} \times 100\%$, which is 25%. |
| | **Step 3:** Choice **(B)** is correct. |
| | **Step 4:** Check to be certain you answered the correct question and that your calculations are correct. Choice (A) is a typical trap answer since it is 20 ÷ 100 rather than 20 ÷ 80. Choice (D) might be tempting because the new dosage is 125% of the original dosage, but the *increase* is only 25%. |

Pay close attention to the exact wording of percentage change questions. Had the question above asked "The new dosage is what percentage of the previous dosage?" the correct answer would have been 125% rather than 25%.

# Rates

**Rates** are ratios with units in the numerator and denominator, such as the price of corn in dollars/bushel or speed measured in kilometers/hour. Ratios can have units as well, but the units in rates have a fixed relationship. The number of cats in the pet store in the ratio example above could be increased without affecting the number of dogs. However, if the number of bushels of corn is increased, then the dollar cost will increase proportionately.

Another way to describe rates is to use the **constant of proportionality**, often represented by the letter $k$. For instance, if corn costs \$4/bushel, then $k = 4$ and the total price of any amount of corn is $k(b)$, where $b$ is the number of bushels.

If it takes 30 minutes for 150 cc of a solution to drip from an IV bag, then the *rate* of infusion is $\dfrac{150 \text{ cc}}{30 \text{ minutes}}$. **Unit rates** are rates that are restated so that the value of the denominator is 1. In this example, that would be $5\dfrac{\text{cc}}{\text{min}}$. Unit rates can be very useful because they show the rate of change of the quantity in the numerator per single unit change in the quantity of the denominator. Try applying this principle in the question below.

A certain IV solution drips at the rate of $5\dfrac{\text{cc}}{\text{min}}$. If there are 300 cc of solution remaining in the IV bag, how much longer will the bag last, assuming the rate remains constant?

   (A)   30 minutes
   (B)   60 minutes
   (C)   300 minutes
   (D)   1500 minutes

## Explanation

**Step 1:** The question provides a drip rate and a quantity and asks how long that quantity would last at the given rate.

**Step 2:** The bag empties at the rate of $5\dfrac{\text{cc}}{\text{min}}$ and contains 300 cc, so it would take $\dfrac{300}{5} = 60$ minutes to deplete the contents of the bag.

**Step 3:** Choice **(B)** is correct. Choice (D) is a trap answer obtained by multiplying the rate times the amount of fluid. If the rate were $5\dfrac{\text{cc}}{\text{min}}$ and the solution were dripping for 300 minutes, then a total of 1500 cc would be administered.

**Step 4:** Check your math and your units. Here, you want to end up with minutes (the unit in the answer choices), and you get that by dividing the cc by cc so those units cancel out, leaving just the minutes: $\text{cc} \div \dfrac{\text{cc}}{\text{min}} = \text{cc} \times \dfrac{\text{min}}{\text{cc}} = \text{min}$.

In complex ratio and rate problems, paying close attention to the units (as was done in Step 4 above) can be the key to determining whether to divide or multiply.

Some rate questions may involve algebra and graphical information displayed on a **coordinate grid**. As shown on the graph with the question below, the coordinate grid is composed of a horizontal $x$-axis and a vertical $y$-axis. The place where they meet is called the origin.

The points on a coordinate grid represent horizontal and vertical distances from the origin. The values increase from left to right on the $x$-axis and from bottom to top on the $y$-axis. Negative values of $x$ are to the left of the origin; negative values of $y$ are below the origin. Any point can be located on the coordinate grid by its $x$ and $y$ values, conventionally written as $(x, y)$. The line that passes through any two points on a coordinate grid can be defined by the equation $y = m(x) + b$, where $m$ represents the **slope** of the line and $b$ is the value of $y$ where the line crosses the $y$-axis. The slope represents the change in the $y$ value per unit change in the $x$ value. Thus, $m$ represents the value of a ratio; if the units of the $y$- and $x$-axes are proportionately related, then $m$ is also a rate.

Study how this information applies to a question.

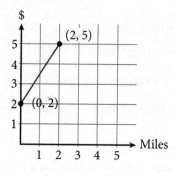

| Question | Analysis |
|---|---|
| If the graph shows the taxi fare in dollars on the $y$-axis and the miles traveled on the $x$-axis, and the cost per mile does not vary, what would be the fare for a 10-mile trip? | **Step 1:** The question refers to a line on a coordinate grid showing miles and taxi fares and asks what the fare would be for 10 miles. |
| (A) $10 <br> (B) $12 <br> (C) $15 <br> (D) $17 | **Step 2:** Because the rate will help to answer the question, determine the slope of the line. Compare the two points on the line, (0, 2) and (2, 5). The fare increased by $3 (5 − 2), and the mileage increased by 2 miles (2 − 0). Therefore, the slope is $\frac{3}{2} = 1.50$, and the units are $\frac{\$}{\text{mi}}$. The $y$-intercept on the graph is $2, which is the charge just to get into the taxi. The additional charge to travel 10 miles is $1.50 \times 10 = \$15$ for a total fare of $17. |
| | **Step 3:** Choice **(D)** is correct. |
| | **Step 4:** Check that you have answered the question that was asked and confirm your calculations. |

# Proportions

A **proportion** is an equation that sets two ratios equal to each other, for instance, $\frac{1}{3} = \frac{4}{12}$. Proportions can be used to solve for an unknown quantity when three of the values of a proportion are known, such as when $\frac{1}{3} = \frac{4}{x}$. The most efficient way to solve proportions is to **cross multiply** the numerator of each ratio by the denominator of the other ratio and set the products equal to each other. For this example, that would be $1 \times x = 3 \times 4$, which simplifies to $x = 12$. Study this example to see how cross multiplying is used in a word question:

| Question | Analysis |
|---|---|
| James has a storage tank to collect rainwater for household use. Unfortunately, there was a severe dry spell where he lives, and the tank ran dry. James added 12 gallons of water to the empty tank, and the gauge on the tank read 5% full. What is the capacity of the tank? | **Step 1:** The problem states that 12 gallons is 5% of the capacity of a tank and asks for the full capacity. |
| (A) 60 gallons<br>(B) 100 gallons<br>(C) 120 gallons<br>(D) 240 gallons | **Step 2:** Set up a proportion to solve this, remembering that a percent is a ratio with 100 in the denominator: $\frac{5}{100} = \frac{12}{C}$, where $C$ is the capacity of the tank. Each ratio in the proportion represents how "full" the tank is. Cross multiply to obtain $5C = 1200$. Divide both sides by 5, so $C = 240$ gallons. |
| | **Step 3:** Choice **(D)** is correct. |
| | **Step 4:** Verify that you set up the proportion correctly and check your calculations. |

Some questions may ask you to calculate an unknown percentage or to derive a number that is a certain percentage of another number. Proportions are an ideal tool to use to solve such problems. Try this one on your own.

What percent of 5 is 4?

(A) 4%
(B) 45%
(C) 80%
(D) 125%

**Explanation**

**Step 1:** The question asks you to determine what percentage 4 is of 5.

**Step 2:** Because percent is the ratio of a quantity to 100, you can set up a proportion: $\dfrac{4}{5} = \dfrac{x}{100}$. Cross multiply to get $400 = 5x$. Divide both sides by 5 to find that $x = 80$.

**Step 3:** Choice **(C)** is correct. Notice that you could have answered this question without doing any math. Logic dictates that $\dfrac{4}{5}$ is greater than $\dfrac{1}{2}$ but less than 1, so the answer must be between 50% and 100% and **(C)** is the only choice that falls within this range.

**Step 4:** Double-check that you set up the correct proportion and that your math is correct.

## KEY IDEAS

- Ratios show the relationship between two quantities; the values in the ratio may or may not be the actual amounts of the quantities.
- Percentages are ratios that express the number or rate of something per 100 of that thing.
- Percentage change is always calculated relative to the original amount.
- A proportion, which is an equation setting two ratios equal to each other, is a good tool to use with percentage questions.

# Ratios, Percentages, and Proportions Practice Questions

1. Juanita made an investment in the stock market. The value of her investment declined by 20%, but then it increased by 50% from that reduced value. What was the overall percent change in the value of her investment?

   (A)  30% decrease
   (B)  No change
   (C)  20% increase
   (D)  30% increase

2. Sixty is 15% of what number?

   (A)  180
   (B)  400
   (C)  600
   (D)  900

3. Mary is restocking the inventory of first-aid supplies. The ratio of ointment to bandages to swabs should be maintained at 2:5:8. The current inventory is 6 tubes of ointment, 10 bandages, and 20 swabs. How many of which two types of supplies does she have to add to bring the ratio to its specified value?

   (A)  5 bandages and 4 swabs
   (B)  2 tubes of ointment and 6 swabs
   (C)  4 bandages and 5 swabs
   (D)  10 bandages and 8 swabs

4. A hospital maintenance department is installing new sanitary molding at the junction of the floor and the wall along both sides of a hallway. The plan drawing for the hallway has a scale of $\frac{1}{4}$ inch :1 foot. The hallway measures $7\frac{3}{4}$ inches long on the plan.

   How many pieces of 8-foot-long molding should the maintenance department order?

   (A)  4
   (B)  6
   (C)  7
   (D)  8

5. A medication is being administered to a client intravenously via a solution that has a 5% concentration of medication by volume of solution. At 8:00 AM, Alicia checked the remaining contents of the client's IV drip bag and noted that there were 780 cc of solution remaining. When she returned at 10:00 AM, there were 300 cc of the solution left in the IV bag. Which of the following correctly expresses the unit rate at which the medication is being dispensed?

   (A)  $\dfrac{240 \text{ cc}}{\text{hour}}$

   (B)  $\dfrac{24 \text{ cc}}{2 \text{ hours}}$

   (C)  $\dfrac{2 \text{ cc}}{\text{minute}}$

   (D)  $\dfrac{0.2 \text{ cc}}{\text{minute}}$

**Review your work using the explanations in Part Six of this book.**

# LESSON 5

# Estimating and Rounding

## LEARNING OBJECTIVES

- Convert measurements between various metric units
- Round given quantities to a specified degree of precision
- Determine when estimating is an appropriate problem-solving strategy
- Use estimating to efficiently solve problems

## Metric Units

The metric system of measurements has been widely adopted in medicine. The base units of measurement in the metric system are **meter** for length and **gram** for weight. A meter is about 10 percent longer than a yard, and a paper clip weighs about 1 gram. To have units that are appropriate to what is being measured, prefixes are used that correspond to the base unit times various powers of 10, as shown in this table.

| Prefix | Power of 10 | Unit Value |
|---|---|---|
| mega | $10^6$ | 1,000,000 |
| kilo | $10^3$ | 1000 |
| hecto | $10^2$ | 100 |
| deca | $10^1$ | 10 |
| deci | $10^{-1}$ | 0.1 or $\frac{1}{10}$ |
| centi | $10^{-2}$ | 0.01 or $\frac{1}{100}$ |
| milli | $10^{-3}$ | 0.001 or $\frac{1}{1000}$ |
| micro | $10^{-6}$ | 0.000001 or $\frac{1}{1,000,000}$ |

By using a prefix, you can specify the exact unit of measurement. Because the different metric units are related by multiples of 10, converting from one unit to another is merely a matter of moving the decimal point and, if necessary, adding zeroes. For instance, to convert 1.75 kilograms to grams, multiply by 1000, which is $10 \times 10 \times 10$.

1.75 kilograms $\times$ 10 = 17.5 hectograms

17.5 hectograms $\times$ 10 = 175 decagrams

175 decagrams $\times$ 10 = 1750 grams

Similarly, to convert 23 millimeters to meters, multiply by $10^{-3}$, an operation that is the same as dividing by 10 three times.

23 millimeters $\div$ 10 = 2.3 centimeters

2.3 centimeters $\div$ 10 = 0.23 decimeters

0.23 decimeters $\div$ 10 = 0.023 meters

Remember, when converting from larger units to smaller, there will be more of the smaller units, so you multiply; when converting from smaller units to larger ones, divide.

Metric area and volume measurements use the same units as length. Becuase area is, in its simplest terms, length times width, areas are expressed in units such as square meters ($m^2$). Similarly, volume is described in cubic units. A common such unit is cubic centimeters (abbreviated as $cm^3$ or cc). One measure of volume that is frequently used is the **liter**, which is 1000 cubic centimeters.

## Rounding

Some questions on the TEAS will specifically direct you to round a given quantity or the results of calculations to a certain degree of accuracy. The rule for **rounding** is straightforward: if the digit following the one being rounded is 5 or greater, change it to 0 and add 1 to the previous digit. If the digit is less than 5, merely round down to 0. For example, to round 75 to the nearest multiple of 10 (the tens place; see Lesson 1: Arithmetic for a review), change the 5 to 0 and add 1 to the previous digit, 7, to obtain 80. To round 166.3 to the nearest whole number, just roll the 3 down to 0 to get 166.0, which is 166 to the nearest whole number.

When rounding by more than one digit, consider the whole amount that is being rounded. If you are rounding 847 to the nearest hundred, do not round the 7 up to get 850 and then round that up to 900. The digit actually being rounded is 4, so round down to 800.

Occasionally, rounding can involve quantities that are not decimal based. Pay close attention to the units involved. A common example is time. To round 3 hours 41 minutes to the nearest hour, don't just round down to 3 hours because 41 is less than 50. Instead, recall that an hour is 60 minutes so the quantity you are rounding is actually $3\frac{41}{60}$; because 41 is more than half of 60, round up to 4 hours.

This is the same technique that is used for rounding fractions. If the numerator is less than half the denominator, round down. If the numerator is greater than or equal to half the denominator, round up. For example, rounded to the nearest whole number, $3\frac{19}{32} \approx 4$ because 19 is greater than half of 32, but $3\frac{19}{46} \approx 3$ because 19 is less than half of 46.

## Estimating

**Estimating** is a way to obtain approximate values for expressions by using rounding or other techniques to simplify the calculations. It is not guessing! The judicious use of estimating can save time and reduce errors. Rounding is a technique frequently used in estimating. If, for instance, a question required you to calculate the value of $37 \times 53$, you could estimate by rounding 37 to 40 and 53 to 50. Multiplying 40 times 50 gets 2000, very close to the actual value of 1961.

There are a few clues that you can use to decide whether estimating is an appropriate strategy. If you encounter a question with rather complex calculations that might be a candidate for estimating, take a glance at the answer choices to see if they are spaced far apart. For instance, if the choices for the above multiplication were 1224, 1611, 1961, and 2335, you could readily determine that 1961 was correct based on the estimated result of 2000. If, however, the choices were 1855, 1922, 1961, and 2013, merely estimating would not result in a correct answer. The question itself may also suggest when estimating is a good strategy. Wording such as "approximately," "closest to," or "about" might be a clue that you can arrive at the correct answer using estimating.

Study how an expert would apply these concepts to a test question.

| Question | Analysis |
|---|---|
| Crystal has several pieces of pipe. She has 3 pieces that are 2.1 meters long, 5 that are 2.9 meters long, and 6 that are 4.1 meters long. How long would these pieces be if laid end to end? | **Step 1:** The question lists the lengths of several pieces of pipe and asks for their total length. A glance at the answer choices shows that they are spaced far enough apart that you can estimate the answer. |
| (A)  41.2 meters<br>(B)  45.3 meters<br>(C)  48.2 meters<br>(D)  50.3 meters | **Step 2:** Round the lengths of the pipes. The total length will be about $(3 \times 2) + (5 \times 3) + (6 \times 4) = 6 + 15 + 24 = 45$ meters |
| | **Step 3:** The estimate of 45 meters is very close to the correct answer choice **(B)**, 45.3 meters. |
| | **Step 4:** Check your rounding and calculations and that you properly used the data in the question. |

Be careful when using several rounded numbers to estimate, particularly in multiplication calculations. If a set of calculations required you to calculate $17 \times 8 \times 16$ and you estimated by rounding up all three numbers to 20, 10, and 20, your estimate would be 4000. However, the actual value is 2176. This big difference is due to the cumulative effect of multiplying three numbers that are all rounded up. However, if you used rounding to estimate $27 \times 23$ as $30 \times 20 = 600$, this would be a good approximation of the actual value, 621, because one number was rounded up and the other was rounded down.

Estimating can use techniques other than rounding. One such technique is to choose "compatible" numbers, that is, numbers that are easier to work with when calculating. For instance, to estimate $365 \div 73$, rather than just rounding to 370 and 70, use nearby compatible numbers of $350 \div 70$ to obtain an estimated value of 5.

Another technique that can be used either in combination with estimating or alone is rearranging. Look for opportunities to group sums into pairs that are easy to combine mentally. The most helpful rearrangements give you zeroes (through addition or subtraction) or multiples of 10.

Here's how an experienced test taker would use rearranging to simplify answering a question.

| Question | Analysis |
|---|---|
| What is the value of $67 + 79 + 33$?<br><br>(A) 169<br>(B) 170<br>(C) 178<br>(D) 179 | **Step 1:** The question adds three 2-digit numbers. |
| | **Step 2:** You are asked to find the sum of those numbers. Before you begin adding, see whether any pairs of numbers might be added to get a nice round number; 67 and 33 end with digits that add up to 10. Indeed, 67 and 33 sum to 100. Now you can add the remaining number more easily: $100 + 79 = 179$. |
| | **Step 3:** Choice **(D)** matches. |
| | **Step 4:** Double-check the $67 + 33$ calculation to be certain that your tens digit is correct. |

Rearranging requires a bit of extra thought up front, but you will increase your speed overall and reduce the chance of making a mistake. Avoid rearranging numbers in expressions that involve a combination of different operations and always follow PEMDAS.

Now you try an estimating question:

Paula's car is low on gasoline, so she stops at a convenience store on her way home to buy gas and a few other items. She purchases a bottle of water for $1.69, 3 candy bars at 60¢ each, a sandwich for $2.29, and tissue for $2.69. Gasoline costs $2.49 per gallon. Paula only has $20 to spend. This particular store dispenses gasoline only by the gallon. How much gas can she add to her tank?

(A) 3 gallons
(B) 4 gallons
(C) 5 gallons
(D) 6 gallons

## Explanation

**Step 1:** The question provides the prices of a few items and how much money is available to spend and asks how much will be left over to purchase gasoline. The answer will be stated to the nearest gallon, and the price per gallon is given.

**Step 2:** Due to the number of calculations required and the fact that the answer will be "to the nearest gallon," estimating is a good strategy. Rounding the prices, Paula will spend $1.70 + (3 \times 0.60) + 2.30 + 2.70$. Use PEMDAS and rearrange to get $1.70 + 2.30 + 1.80 + 2.70 = 4 + 4.50 = \$8.50$. Therefore, Paula will have about $11.50 left over to buy gasoline at about $2.50 per gallon. Try 5 gallons as a possible answer: $5 \times (2 + 0.50) = 10 + 2.50 = \$12.50$. Now try 4 gallons: $4 \times (2 + 0.50) = 8 + 2 = \$10.00$.

**Step 3:** Even though the $11.50 that Paula has available to buy gas is closer to the price of 5 gallons than to the amount needed to buy 4 gallons, the pump only dispenses by the gallon, so the most Paula could buy is **(B)**, 4 gallons. Choice (C) is a trap answer that ignores this detail.

**Step 4:** Double-check your logic, rounding, and calculations.

## KEY IDEAS

- The metric system is decimal based, thus facilitating easy conversion between units.
- Rounding follows straightforward rules and can simplify calculations.
- Techniques that help solve problems include estimating, using compatible numbers, and rearranging.

# Estimating and Rounding Practice Questions

1. What is the volume of 2753 cubic centimeters to the nearest liter?

   (A)  2
   (B)  3
   (C)  27
   (D)  28

2. What is the value of $(61 - 40) \times (36 - 18)$?

   (A)  189
   (B)  378
   (C)  641
   (D)  738

3. A leaky faucet drips water at a rate of 22 mL/hr. How much water drips from this faucet in 2 days?

   (A)  528 mL
   (B)  792 mL
   (C)  1056 mL
   (D)  1326 mL

4. There are 30 chocolate chip cookies in each package. A case consists of 24 packages. If the average breakage rate for these cookies is 1.72%, what would be the expected number of broken cookies per case, expressed as the nearest whole number?

   (A)  6
   (B)  10
   (C)  12
   (D)  15

5. What is the value of $27 \times 43$?

   (A)  1161
   (B)  1172
   (C)  1183
   (D)  1194

**Review your work using the explanations in Part Six of this book.**

# CHAPTER TWO

# STATISTICS, GEOMETRY, AND MEASUREMENTS

## LEARNING OBJECTIVES

- Identify values and draw conclusions about relationships between variables based on line graphs, bar graphs, circle graphs, and scatterplots
- Describe data sets using the shapes of graphs, trendlines, and measures of central tendency and spread
- Distinguish between independent and dependent variables and identify positive and negative covariance
- Calculate perimeter and area of triangles, rectangles, circles, and irregular shapes
- Convert measurements within and between the standard and metric system

Of the 32 scored *Mathematics* questions, 9 (28%) will be in the sub-content area of *Measurement and data*. Your ability to use graphs and tables to identify relevant data will be tested, as will your ability to describe data statistically. In addition, the TEAS tests plane geometry, the concepts of correlation and causality, and your ability to use measurement systems appropriately.

This chapter addresses these skills in five lessons:

**Lesson 1:** Graphs and Tables

**Lesson 2:** Statistics

**Lesson 3:** Covariance and Causality

**Lesson 4:** Geometry

**Lesson 5:** Converting Measurements

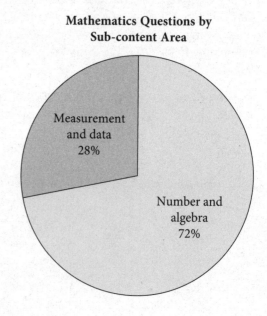

**Mathematics Questions by Sub-content Area**

Measurement and data 28%

Number and algebra 72%

# LESSON 1

# Graphs and Tables

## LEARNING OBJECTIVES

- Extract values from a graph that uses Cartesian coordinates
- Draw conclusions about relationships among variables using line and bar graphs
- Convert between percentages and quantities using data from circle graphs

Numerical information is sometimes depicted in a graph or table. Presenting data in this manner makes it easier to see patterns in the data and to interpret relationships within the data.

A **table** organizes and displays values in columns and rows. A **graph** is a diagram that represents interrelations among two or more things (two is most common). Tables and graphs are both considered types of **charts**.

## Cartesian Coordinates

Named after the 17th-century French mathematician Rene Descartes, **Cartesian coordinate** graphs display values in two dimensions. The **x-axis** is horizontal, and values increase from left to right; the **y-axis** is vertical, and values increase from bottom to top. Thus, any point on such a graph is **bivariate**, consisting of an $x$ value and a $y$ value. Any bivariate point can be expressed as an **ordered pair** in parentheses with the $x$ value followed by the $y$ value. The ordered pair (3, 5) defines a point with an $x$ value of 3 and a $y$ value of 5.

Ordered pairs, like many forms of data, can be displayed in a table. This table shows the data points $A = (4, 4)$, $B = (-2, 3)$, $C = (0, 0)$, $D = (1, -3)$, and $E = (-2, -1)$.

| Point | x value | y value |
|-------|---------|---------|
| A | 4 | 4 |
| B | -2 | 3 |
| C | 0 | 0 |
| D | 1 | -3 |
| E | -2 | -1 |

The same data could be displayed on a Cartesian coordinate graph.

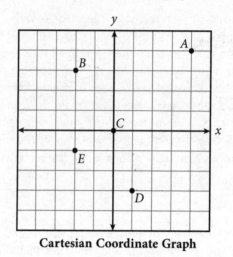

**Cartesian Coordinate Graph**

Notice that point $C$ at (0, 0) is where the two axes intersect. This point is called the **origin**.

Some graphs and other pictorial representations, such as blueprints and models, may use a **scale** that depicts the ratio of values on the graphic to actual quantities. For instance, if the scale of the graph above were that the length of 1 increment ("box") represented 1 meter, then point $A$ would be 4 meters to the right and 4 meters above the origin.

## Scatterplots

**Scatterplots** are collections of individual data points plotted by their values so that any pattern can be observed. A simple scatterplot is shown here as an example. The use of scatterplots in data analysis will be discussed in Lesson 2: Statistics.

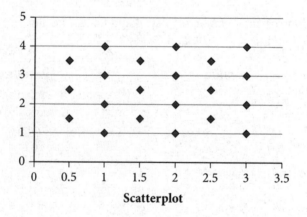

**Scatterplot**

# Line Graphs

The graph in the "Cartesian Coordinates" section showed five points with *x*- and *y*-values that had no particular relationship to each other. Graphs can be used to show situations in which the two variables are related to each other. One such type of graph is the **line graph**, which simply connects the known points with a line. The values of any point on the line can be determined by going across horizontally to the *y*-axis and up or down vertically to the *x*-axis. If two quantities have a cause-and-effect relationship, the variable that is the "cause" is called the **independent variable** and is usually depicted on the *x*-axis. The variable whose value depends upon the value of the independent variable is called the **dependent variable** and is usually shown on the *y*-axis. One common use of line graphs is to show how some dependent variable, shown on the *y*-axis, changes over time, as shown on the *x*-axis.

Inferences about the relationship between the variables can often be made by observing the shape and placement of the line in a line graph. Study this question about a line graph, which shows temperature and daily water usage in a certain municipality, to see how conclusions can be drawn.

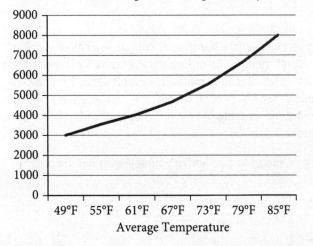

| Question | Analysis |
|---|---|
| Based on the information in the graph, which of the following describes the relationship between temperature and water usage? | **Step 1:** The question refers to a line graph showing water usage on the *y*-axis and average temperature on the *x*-axis and asks which of the answer choices describes the relationship between temperature and water usage. |
| (A) There is no relationship between temperature and water usage.<br><br>(B) Water usage decreases as temperatures rise.<br><br>(C) Water usage increases as temperatures rise but at a slower rate when temperatures are warmer.<br><br>(D) Water usage increases as temperatures rise and at a faster rate when temperatures are warmer. | **Step 2:** The data imply that, quite logically, consumption depends at least partly upon temperature. As temperature increases, so does usage. |

| Question | Analysis |
|---|---|
| | **Step 3:** The initial analysis showed that water usage increased as temperatures rose. Eliminate choices (A) and (B). Selecting between (C) and (D) will require a closer look at the graph. Notice that, as temperatures rise, the slope of the line becomes steeper. In other words, for each 6° increase in temperature, the water usage increased by a greater amount than for the previous 6° increase. Therefore, choice **(D)** is correct. |
| | **Step 4:** Check that your logic in interpreting the line graph is correct. |

## Bar Graphs

Another commonly used type of chart is a **bar graph**, sometimes called a *column graph* because values are displayed as columns rather than points or lines. Bar graphs can be particularly useful when the data consist of more than two variables. Because multiple variables may be depicted, sometimes a **legend** or key is included with these graphs to show how different variables are represented on the graph. A **histogram** is a bar graph with one variable in which the bars of different heights display the frequency of each value or range of values.

Try answering the following question to familiarize yourself with bar graphs.

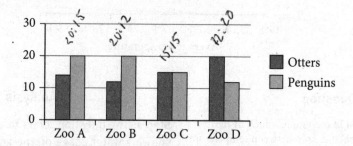

Which of the four zoos in the bar graph above has the highest ratio of penguins to otters?

(A)   Zoo A
(B)   Zoo B
(C)   Zoo C
(D)   Zoo D

## Explanation

**Step 1:** The question refers to a bar graph showing the numbers of otters and penguins at four zoos and asks which zoo has the highest penguin:otter ratio.

**Step 2:** Check the legend to see which bar shading represents which animal. The bars on the left represent the number of otters and the ones to their right show the numbers of penguins. Since the question asks for the highest ratio of penguins to otters, look for the zoo that has a penguin bar that is much taller than its otter bar. Choice (C)'s bars are equal; choice (D) has more otters than penguins. Eliminate these choices. The numbers for Zoo A and Zoo B look fairly similar, but a close examination reveals that both have the same number of penguins but Zoo A has more otters. Therefore the penguin:otter ratio is the greatest at Zoo B.

**Step 3:** Choice **(B)** is correct. Choice (D) is a trap answer because that zoo has the highest ratio of otters to penguins.

**Step 4:** Check that you correctly interpreted the legend and that you answered the question that was asked.

# Circle Graphs

**Circle graphs,** sometimes called *pie charts*, are used to display parts of a whole. The individual quantities can be shown either as numbers or percentages. The size of each sector of the circle shows that item's proportion of the whole. Study the following question to see how circle graph concepts can be tested.

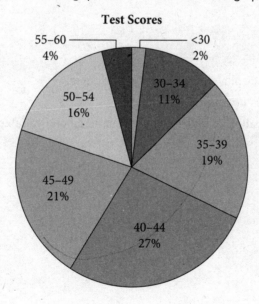

**Test Scores**

55–60
4%

<30
2%

50–54
16%

30–34
11%

45–49
21%

35–39
19%

40–44
27%

| Question | Analysis |
|---|---|
| A skills test was administered to a nursing school class. The percentage distribution of student scores is shown on the circle graph above. If 30 students scored 50 or above, how many students took the test? | **Step 1:** A circle graph shows the percentage distribution of scores on a test. The question states that 30 students scored 50 or above on the test and asks how many students took the test. |
| (A) 100<br>(B) 120<br>(C) 150<br>(D) 180 | **Step 2:** The total percentage of students scoring 50 or above is contained in the two sectors "50–54" and "55–60," which represent 16% and 4% of the test takers respectively. Adding these together, 20% scored 50 or above. If 20% of the total is 30 students, set up the proportion $\dfrac{20}{100} = \dfrac{30}{T}$, where $T$ is the total number of test takers. Cross multiply to get $20T = 3000$ and divide by 20 to obtain $T = 150$. |
| | **Step 3:** Answer choice **(C)** is correct. |
| | **Step 4:** Check that you extracted the correct values from the circle graph and that your calculations are correct. |

## KEY IDEAS

- Tables organize and display data in rows and columns.
- Graphs display values in a pictorial manner.
- Graphs help you visualize relationships between or among variables.

# Graphs and Tables Practice Questions

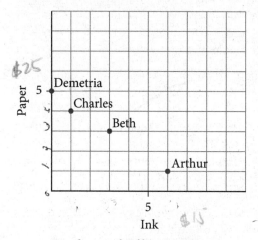

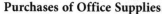

**Purchases of Office Supplies**

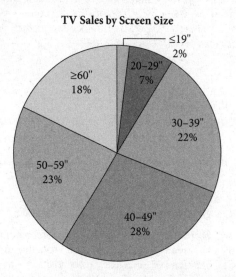

1. The graph above shows the numbers of ink cartridges and cases of paper purchased by four different people. If ink cartridges cost $15 each and paper is priced at $25 per case, which person spent the most money?

   (A) Arthur
   (B) Beth
   (C) Charles
   (D) Demetria

2. The circle graph above shows the sales of television sets at a store, categorized by screen size. Which of the following statements could be true?

   (A) More TVs were sold with screens 39" or smaller than those with screens 50" or larger.
   (B) There were as many sets smaller than 47" sold as there were sets larger than 47".
   (C) The smallest screen size sold was 21".
   (D) Less than half the TVs sold had screen sizes between 40" and 59" inclusive.

**City Hospital Emergency Room Cases**

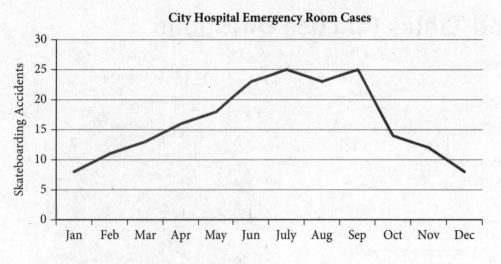

3. What conclusion can you infer from the graph?

(A) There is a seasonal pattern for skateboarding.
(B) The trend of emergency room visits due to skateboard injuries is increasing.
(C) The trend of emergency room visits due to skateboard injuries is decreasing.
(D) People should wear a helmet when skateboarding.

**Drug Sales Comparison**

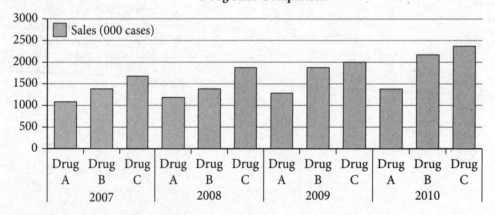

4. Use the graph above to correctly complete this statement: When the year-to-year sales changes of all three drugs are compared, drug _____ had the greatest increase in cases sold between _____ and _____.

(A) A, 2007, 2008
(B) B, 2008, 2009
(C) B, 2009, 2010
(D) C, 2009, 2010

**Review your work using the explanations in Part Six of this book.**

# LESSON 2

# Statistics

## LEARNING OBJECTIVES

- Identify data characteristics by examining the shapes of graphs
- Quantify the relationship between variables using trendlines
- Calculate measures of central tendency and measures of spread

To determine effective treatment, healthcare professionals must be able to answer questions such as "Is the client's blood sugar within a healthy range?" "Is the client's respiratory rate trending up or down?" or "Does the client's pain follow a pattern?" Consequently, it is important to understand some concepts of data interpretation.

## Shape

In the previous lesson, five types of graphs were discussed: Cartesian coordinates, line graphs, bar graphs, circle graphs, and scatterplots. These are all related to each other. Raw data are often collected in the form of a scatterplot (in Cartesian coordinates), which can be used to characterize any pattern in the data. If multiple observations of a single variable are made and identical values are "stacked" on top of each other in a scatterplot, the results would look like the example, which also shows the same data in bar graph and line graph formats.

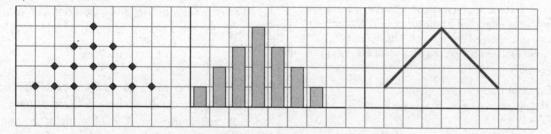

By observing the **shape** of the distribution of data values in any of these formats, you can identify certain characteristics. (For simplicity's sake, many of the illustrations that follow will be line graphs, but the same principles apply to all the formats.) One such characteristic is **symmetry**. The data in the graphs above are symmetrical; that is, the left side of the distribution looks the same as the right side.

Another parameter that can be easily observed from a graph is the number of peaks in the data. The first graphs have one clear peak in the data, so they are classified as **unimodal**. The next graph has two peaks, so it is **bimodal**. Notice that although the height of the two peaks is slightly different, there are still two clearly evident peaks; bimodal does *not* imply that the peaks are equal.

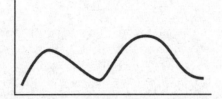

Another observable characteristic of graphs is **skewness**. Some distributions that are not symmetrical clearly have more data points on one side or the other of the graph. These illustrations show that skewness is directional.

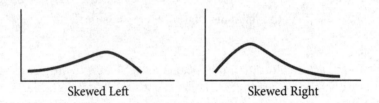

Skewed Left                    Skewed Right

Data distributions can also be uniform, as shown in this illustration.

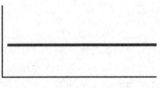

| Question | Analysis |
|---|---|
| A certain road is used primarily by commuters in the morning and the afternoon and is more lightly traveled the rest of the day. If the number of vehicles for both directions combined during each half-hour period of the day were plotted on a graph, what would be the shape of that graph? | **Step 1:** The question states that a certain road is used mostly for morning and afternoon commuting and asks for the shape of a graph of total traffic counts. |
| (A)  Uniform<br>(B)  Spiral<br>(C)  Bimodal<br>(D)  Bilateral | **Step 2:** Since the traffic count is for both directions combined, there would be a peak level in the morning and another peak level in the afternoon. Thus, a graph of these values would have two peaks. This is a bimodal distribution. |
|  | **Step 3:** Answer choice **(C)** matches the prediction and is correct. Since there are peaks, choice (A), uniform, is incorrect. Choice (B), spiral, makes no sense in terms of this data. Choice (C), bilateral, is not a term used to describe data distribution. |
|  | **Step 4:** Check that you answered the question that was asked and that your logic is sound. |

# Trends

In broad terms, the **trend** of data is the general relationship between the variables, addressing questions such as "Do they both rise or fall together, or do they move in opposite directions?" and "Does the rate of increase or decrease get larger or smaller?" A **trendline** shows this relationship more precisely; with an independent variable on the *x*-axis and the related dependent variable on the *y*-axis, the slope of the trendline is determined by the relationship between the two variables. When data are plotted in this manner, either as a scatterplot or a line graph, they show the trend.

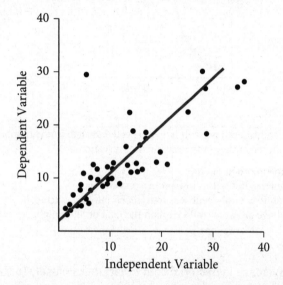

The trendline shown can be calculated, but to do so would require using a complex formula. Instead, trendlines can be approximated by sketching them in on a graph. The slope of the trendline shows the relationship between the two variables. A line drawn straight up from the point on the *x*-axis where the independent variable is 10 would intersect the trendline at a point where the dependent variable, on the *y*-axis, is about 11. At a value of 20 on the *x*-axis, the trendline value of the dependent variable is about 19. Thus, for every 10 increase in the *x*-axis value, the *y*-axis value increases by about 8.

Notice the value at the top left; it is far from the trendline and the other data points. Based on the grouping of the data points, the **expected value** of the dependent variable when the independent variable is 6 or 7 would be within a range (*y* value) of approximately 4 to 12. However, that point at the top left of the graph is about 28; hence, it is referred to as an **outlier**. Outliers can be due to extreme random variation, errors in making or recording measurements, or some underlying change in conditions. In real-life situations, it can be important to identify the cause of the outlier data point.

Trends do not have to be a straight line. Try applying logic and what you have learned about trends to answer this question.

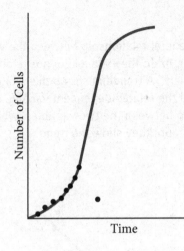

The S-shaped trendline shown on the graph is the expected growth in the number of bacteria in a petri dish. What would explain the outlier in the recorded observations?

(A)    The data were recorded in error.
(B)    The lab technician did not follow proper procedures.
(C)    A powerful antibacterial agent was introduced into the petri dish.
(D)    Any of the above answers could explain the data on the graph.

## Explanation

**Step 1:** The graph shows an increase in bacterial count that tracks closely to the expected growth curve until partway up the curve, where one data point is well below the curve. The question asks which of the answer choices could explain the outlier.

**Step 2:** Outlier data points can be the result of errors in measurement or in the recording of data, unexplained extreme randomness, or a change in the underlying conditions. Look for these possibilities in the answer choices.

**Step 3:** Choice (A) is one of the predicted reasons for the outlier. If the technician did not follow proper procedures, as in choice (B), that too could distort the data. Certainly the introduction of an antibacterial substance per choice (C) could slow or even reverse the growth of bacteria. Since (A), (B), and (C) are all reasonable explanations, choice **(D)** is correct.

**Step 4:** Check that you answered the question that was asked and that your logic is correct.

The growth curve in the previous question has a common trendline shape. It applies to other phenomena in real life such as sales of a new product, growth of chickens, or acquisition of new knowledge, just to cite a few examples.

## Measures of Central Tendency and Spread

One characteristic of data sets that statistics describe is the "middle" or "typical" value. There are several **measures of central tendency.**

- The **mean,** also called the **arithmetic average,** is the sum of all the individual values in the group divided by the number of values. For instance, the mean of {8, 0, −3, 9, 2}, is $\dfrac{8 + 0 - 3 + 9 + 2}{8} = \dfrac{16}{8} = 2$.

- The **median** is simply the middle number. In the example above, first rearrange the numbers in order from least to greatest: {−3, 0, 2, 8, 9}. The middle number is 2, so that is the median. If the group of numbers has an even number of values, such as {−3, 0, 2, 4, 8, 9}, the median is the average of the two numbers in the middle. Here, 2 and 4 are the numbers in the middle; their average is 3, so that is the median.

- The **mode** of a set of numbers is the number that appears most frequently. The mode of {−20, 2, 3, 10, 10} is 10. Although mode is classified as a measure of central tendency, this example shows that such classification could be misleading. Here, the mode is much greater than either the mean of 1 or the median of 3.

Another characteristic of data sets is how "spread out" the values are. There are two commonly used measures of **spread.**

- **Range** is the absolute difference between the highest and lowest values. For the set of numbers {−3, 0, 2, 8, 9}, the range is $9 - (-3) = 9 + 3 = 12$.

- A more complex measure of the distribution of numbers is **standard deviation**. Standard deviation is a measurement that is often associated with a "bell curve," also called a "normal" distribution. As shown on this graph, the bell curve is symmetrical with its mean at the highest point and most values falling close to the mean.

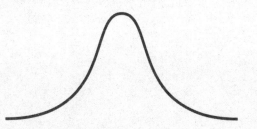

Apply these statistics concepts to this question.

Given the set of data {1, 0, 8, 0, −2, 4, 3}, if $R$ is the range and $A$ is the mean, what is the value of $R - A$?

(A)  4
(B)  6
(C)  8
(D)  10

## Explanation

**Step 1:** The question provides a set of numbers and asks for the difference between the range and the mean (arithmetic average) of those numbers.

**Step 2:** The range is the largest number in the group minus the smallest number. Rearrange the numbers in order, $\{-2, 0, 0, 1, 3, 4, 8\}$ to identify the extremes. The range ($R$) is $8 - (-2) = 10$. The mean ($A$) is $\dfrac{-2 + 0 + 0 + 1 + 3 + 4 + 8}{7} = \dfrac{14}{7} = 2$. So $R - A = 10 - 2 = 8$.

**Step 3:** Answer choice **(C)** is correct. Had you miscalculated the range as $8 - 2 = 6$, you would have selected choice (A). Choice (D) is the range rather than the difference between the range and the mean.

**Step 4:** Check that your calculations are correct and that you answered the question that was asked.

## KEY IDEAS

- The same data can be displayed in different types of graphs.
- Key characteristics of data can be identified by the visual interpretation of graphs.
- Trendlines depict the relationship between the variables plotted.
- Measures of central tendency and spread can be used to describe a set of data.

# Statistics Practice Questions

-6, -1, 1, 3, 4 5

1. What is the median of 3, −6, 5, 1, −1, and 4?

   (A)  0
   (B)  1
   (C)  2
   (D)  3

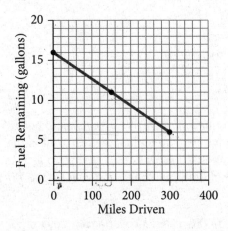

| Time Period | Airport Arrivals |
| --- | --- |
| 00:01 AM–1:00 AM | 6 |
| 1:01 AM–2:00 AM | 4 |
| 2:01 AM–3:00 AM | 3 |
| 3:01 AM–4:00 AM | 3 |
| 4:01 AM–5:00 AM | 5 |
| 5:01 AM–6:00 AM | 9 |
| 6:01 AM–7:00 AM | 18 |
| 7:01 AM–8:00 AM | 35 |
| 8:01 AM–9:00 AM | 60 |
| 9:01 AM–10:00 AM | 63 |
| 10:01 AM–11:00 AM | 58 |
| 11:01 AM–12:00 PM | 44 |
| 12:01 PM–1:00 PM | 37 |
| 1:01 PM–2:00 PM | 33 |
| 2:01 PM–3:00 PM | 32 |
| 3:01 PM–4:00 PM | 44 |
| 4:01 PM–5:00 PM | 52 |
| 5:01 PM–6:00 PM | 61 |
| 6:01 PM–7:00 PM | 64 |
| 7:01 PM–8:00 PM | 55 |
| 8:01 PM–9:00 PM | 40 |
| 9:01 PM–10:00 PM | 27 |
| 10:01 PM–11:00 PM | 14 |
| 11:01 PM–12:00 AM | 10 |

2. Ruby tracks the gallons of gasoline remaining in her car's tank and the miles that she drives. If she wants to refill her tank when there are two gallons remaining, how many total miles can she travel before she stops to refuel, assuming that the trend shown on the graph above continues?

   (A)  120 miles
   (B)  420 miles
   (C)  450 miles
   (D)  480 miles

3. The chart shows the number of arrivals at a major airport in each of 24 one-hour intervals. If these values were graphed, what would be the shape of the graph?

   (A)  Bimodal
   (B)  Bell curve
   (C)  Growth curve
   (D)  Uniform distribution

**Review your work using the explanations in Part Six of this book.**

# LESSON 3

# Covariance and Causality

## LEARNING OBJECTIVES

- Describe how changes in one quantity affect changes in another
- Define and identify positive and negative covariance
- Identify the relationship between independent and dependent variables
- Distinguish between covariance and causality

Understanding the connection between related values (often termed *variables*) is a key skill in health careers and for the TEAS. How does the quantity of food a person eats affect his weight? What is the relationship between someone's medication dosage and her condition? How does a change in a certain procedure relate to overall health outcomes? Does the amount of time you spend studying for the TEAS affect your score on the test?

One of the most important concepts to understand is **covariation** (also called **covariance**). Covariation is the change in the values of two related variables. For example, a study may find that there is a relationship between the amount of sugar people eat each day and their weight; the study finds that people who eat more sugar per day weigh more on average than people who eat less sugar. This is an example of **positive covariation** (or **positive covariance**); as one variable rises (the amount of sugar eaten), so does the other (weight). It is also possible for one value to rise as another falls. This is called **negative covariation** (or **negative covariance**). For example, as an animal shelter places more pets for adoption, the amount of money the shelter spends on pet food diminishes.

Another important concept is the difference between covariation and **causality**. An observable relationship between two variables does not necessarily mean changes in one are *caused by* changes in the other. Think about the example above regarding sugar consumption and weight. It may be that greater sugar consumption actually does cause greater weight. However, it's also possible that people who eat more sugar do so mainly by eating high-fat desserts. It could be that the difference in the amount of fat eaten or the difference in total calories consumed, rather than the amount of sugar eaten, is the cause of the difference in weight.

The scientific standard for proof of causality is quite high and depends on numerous separate studies establishing the same or similar results between variables. While a full discussion of this standard is beyond the scope of this lesson, it's important to understand that the results of a single study are never sufficient to establish proof of causality.

Earlier in this chapter, in Lesson 1: Graphs and Tables, you learned the terms **independent variable** and **dependent variable**. Recall that an independent variable is the value that is manipulated in an experiment and the dependent variable is the value that is observed in connection with the independent variable. Put another way, the independent variable is the factor that is hypothesized to affect the dependent variable. For example, say there is a hypothesis that higher altitude results in lower blood oxygen levels. A study is performed to measure the blood oxygen levels of people at different altitudes. Researchers measure the blood oxygen level of a group of people at sea level, at 500 meters above sea level, and at 1,000 meters above sea level. In this scenario, the independent variable is altitude and the dependent variable is blood oxygen level.

Study this question to see how a test expert solves a covariance question.

| Question | Analysis |
|---|---|
| A study of several hundred 50-year-old men finds that the more years of school the men attended, the lower their incidence of shoulder injuries in later life. Based on this information, which of the following is true? | **Step 1:** The question provides a scenario describing an apparent relationship between two values. The answer choices include words such as "causes" and "covariance." |
| (A) Attending school causes reduced shoulder injuries in men.<br>(B) This is an example of negative covariance.<br>(C) This is an example of positive covariance.<br>(D) A relationship between years of school attended and shoulder injuries in men cannot be determined. | **Step 2:** Use your knowledge of covariance and causality to correctly characterize the study. One variable decreases (the incidence of shoulder injuries) as the other variable increases (the number of years of school attended). This is an example of negative covariance. |
| | **Step 3:** The correct answer is choice **(B)**. (A) indicates causality, which has not been established by this study. (C) describes the opposite relationship. (D) is too extreme, since the information in the question indicates that a relationship has been observed. |
| | **Step 4:** Check that your answer correctly characterizes the scenario. |

Try the following question and then review the explanation.

Which of the following describes positive covariation?

(A) Rainfall amounts in New York City vary throughout the year.
(B) A decrease in oxygen in a pond is associated with a greater growth of algae.
(C) An increase in consumption of dark green vegetables by women has been associated with higher amounts of lean muscle mass.
(D) Human heart rates fall within a predictable range.

## Explanation

**Step 1:** The question asks you to identify the answer that is an example of positive covariation.

**Step 2:** Positive covariation occurs when two variables rise together or fall together. Find the answer choice that describes such a situation.

**Step 3:** The correct choice is **(C)**. Choices (A) and (D) do not show a rise or fall of two values in relation to each other. Choice (B) describes negative covariation.

**Step 4:** Be sure that the answer you've chosen matches the described relationship.

## KEY IDEAS

- Positive covariance describes a situation in which two values increase or decrease in the same direction in relation to each other.
- Negative covariance describes a situation in which two values move in opposite directions in relation to each other.
- Covariance, either positive or negative, does not necessarily indicate causality.

# Covariance and Causality Practice Questions

1. Researchers in Yellowstone National Park noticed that as wolf populations increased, stream water quality also increased. In areas with fewer wolves, water quality was consistently lower. Which of the following best describes the relationship between wolf populations and water quality?

   (A) There is a positive covariation between wolf populations and stream water quality.
   (B) Larger wolf populations result in higher stream water quality.
   (C) There is an inverse relationship between wolf populations and stream water quality.
   (D) There is a no relationship between wolf populations and stream water quality.

2. A study was performed to determine the relationship between the amount of pollen in the air and the frequency of asthma attacks. Researchers hypothesized that higher levels of pollen lead to an increase in asthma attacks. For three months, they measured pollen levels and the frequency of asthma attacks among 80 asthma sufferers. It was determined that on days when the pollen count was higher, there were more asthma attacks, and on days when the pollen count was lower, there were fewer asthma attacks. Which of the following describes this scenario?

   (A) Positive covariation; number of asthma attacks is the independent variable; pollen count is the dependent variable.
   (B) Negative covariation; number of asthma attacks is the dependent variable; pollen count is the independent variable.
   (C) Positive covariation; number of asthma attacks is the dependent variable; pollen count is the independent variable.
   (D) Causality has been established; number of asthma attacks is the dependent variable; pollen count is the independent variable.

3. Which of the following is NOT an example of negative covariance?

   (A) As altitude increases, temperature decreases.
   (B) The more a person works, the more fatigued he or she becomes.
   (C) As a dog's age increases, its muscle strength decreases.
   (D) The more kilometers an airplane travels, the less fuel it has in its tanks.

**Review your work using the explanations in Part Six of this book.**

# LESSON 4
# Geometry

## LEARNING OBJECTIVES

- Recognize commonly tested shapes
- Define geometric measures, including length, perimeter, and area
- Calculate the perimeter of triangles, rectangles, circles, and irregular shapes
- Calculate the area of triangles, rectangles, circles, and irregular shapes

The TEAS tests several fundamental concepts in geometry. You'll need to be familiar with certain principles and formulas to answer geometry questions effectively.

## Lines and Angles

To answer questions about lines and angles, you will need to know the following definitions:

- A **right angle** is an angle equal to 90 degrees.
- An **acute angle** is an angle less than 90 degrees.
- An **obtuse angle** is an angle greater than 90 degrees.

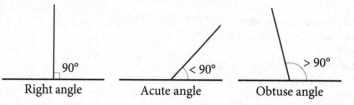

- **Parallel lines** never touch or intersect. When graphed on the coordinate plane, parallel lines have the same slope.
- **Perpendicular lines** intersect to form a 90-degree angle (a right angle).
- **Vertical angles** are directly across from each other when two or more lines intersect. Vertical angles are always equal to each other.
- A **transversal** is a line that crosses two other distinct lines in a plane. When a transversal crosses two or more parallel lines, all acute angles created are equal to each other, and all obtuse angles created are equal to each other.

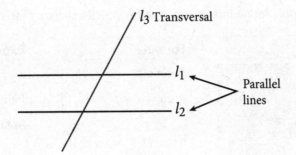

## Basic Shapes

There are a few basic shapes that are commonly tested on the TEAS.

- A **rectangle** is a four-sided shape that is made up of two pairs of parallel lines and has four right angles.
- A **square** is a type of rectangle with four sides of equal length.
- A **circle** is a curved, closed shape with all points equally distant from the center.
- A **triangle** is a three-sided shape that is made up of three straight lines.

These are not the only shapes that the TEAS may test; see the table in this lesson for others.

## Perimeter

**Perimeter** is the distance around the outside of a two-dimensional shape. Perimeter is calculated in units of length such as centimeters (cm), inches (in.), feet (ft), meters (m), and miles (mi). For example, the perimeter of a square is the length of all four sides added together. The perimeter of a circle is the distance once around the circle and is called the **circumference**.

## Area

**Area** is a measure of the surface space taken up by a two-dimensional shape such as a rectangle, triangle, or circle. Area is calculated in **square units** such as square inches ($in.^2$), square feet ($ft^2$), or square centimeters ($cm^2$).

The table contains the formulas for perimeter and area for various shapes that are tested on the TEAS.

| Shape | | Formula | Example |
|---|---|---|---|
| Square | | Perimeter = $4 \times s$<br><br>Area = $s \times s = s^2$ | $s = 5$ cm<br><br>Perimeter = $4 \times 5$ cm = 20 cm<br><br>Area = 5 cm $\times$ 5 cm = 25 cm² |
| Rectangle | | Perimeter = $(2 \times \text{Width}) + (2 \times \text{Length})$<br>Area = Length $\times$ Width | $W = 4$ ft<br>$L = 8$ ft<br><br>Perimeter = $(2 \times 4$ ft$) + (2 \times 8$ ft$) = 24$ ft<br><br>Area = 8 ft $\times$ 4 ft = 32 ft² |
| Triangle | | Perimeter = $a + b + c$<br>Area = $\frac{1}{2}(b \times h)$ | $a = 5$ in.<br>$b = 6$ in.<br>$c = 5$ in.<br>$h = 4$ in.<br><br>Perimeter = 5 in + 6 in + 5 in = 16 in<br><br>Area = $\frac{1}{2}(6$ in. $\times 4$ in.$) = 24$ in.² |
| Parallelogram | | Perimeter = $2a + 2b$<br>Area = $b \times h$ | $a = 5$ in.<br>$b = 8$ in.<br>$h = 4$ in.<br><br>Perimeter = $(2 \times 5$ in$) + (2 \times 8$ in$) = 26$ in<br><br>Area = 8 in $\times$ 4 in = 32 in² |
| Trapezoid | | Perimeter = $a + b_1 + b_2 + c$<br><br>Area = $\frac{1}{2}(b_1 + b_2) \times h$ | $a = 13$ m<br>$b_1 = 10$ m<br>$b_2 = 24$ m<br>$c = 15$ m<br>$h = 12$ m<br><br>Perimeter = 13 m + 10 m + 24 m + 15 m = 62 m<br><br>Area = $\frac{1}{2}(10$ m + 24 m$) \times 12$ m<br><br>$= 204$ m² |

| Shape | | Formula | Example |
|---|---|---|---|
| Rhombus | 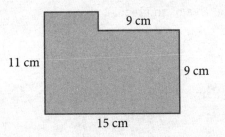 | Perimeter = $4 \times s$ <br> Length of diagonals = $d_1, d_2$ <br> Area $= \dfrac{1}{2}(d_1 \times d_2)$ | $d_1 = 20$ cm <br> $d_2 = 48$ cm <br> $s = 26$ cm <br><br> Perimeter $= 4 \times 26$ cm $=$ 104 cm <br><br> Area $= \dfrac{1}{2} \times 20$ cm $\times 48$ cm <br> $= 480$ cm$^2$ |
| Circle | | Radius $= r =$ distance from center to outer edge <br> Diameter $= d =$ distance across circle through the center <br><br> Circumference $= 2\pi r = \pi d$ <br><br> Area $= \pi r^2$ <br><br> $\pi =$ pi = approximately 3.14 | $r = 3$ <br><br> Circumference $= 2 \times 3 \times \pi = 6\pi$ <br><br> Area $= \pi \times 3^2 = 9\pi$ |

Take a look at how a test expert handles this question involving a perimeter.

9 cm

11 cm

9 cm

15 cm

| Question | Analysis |
|---|---|
| Which of the following is the perimeter of the figure above? (All angles in the figure are right angles.) | **Step 1:** The question provides a figure with four lengths specified and two lengths unspecified, and it asks for the perimeter of the figure. |
| (A) 44 cm <br> (B) 46 cm <br> (C) 50 cm <br> (D) 52 cm | **Step 2:** Use the known dimensions to calculate the unknown dimensions. To calculate the missing top dimension, subtract the known top dimension of 9 cm from the bottom dimension of 15 cm to yield 6 cm. To calculate the missing right dimension, subtract the known right dimension of 9 cm from the left dimension of 11 cm to yield 2 cm. Next, add all lengths to find the perimeter: 11 cm + 15 cm + 6 cm + 2 cm + 9 cm + 9 cm = 52 cm. |

| Question | Analysis |
|---|---|
| | **Step 3**: The correct answer is **(D)**. |
| | **Step 4**: Check that you've correctly calculated the unknown dimensions and that you added all six sides to get the perimeter. |

## Right Triangles

A triangle that contains a right angle (90 degrees) is a **right triangle.** You can calculate the perimeter and area of right triangles just as you do with other triangles. The longest side of a right triangle (which is opposite the 90-degree angle) is the **hypotenuse**. If any two of the side lengths of a right triangle are known, the unknown length of the third side can be calculated using the Pythagorean theorem. The Pythagorean theorem states that $a^2 + b^2 = c^2$, where $a$ and $b$ are the lengths of the sides and $c$ is the length of the hypotenuse, as in the figure shown.

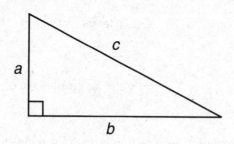

Now try this question involving the area of an irregular shape.

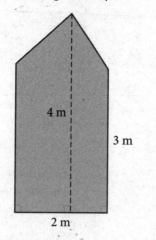

What is the area of the figure above?

- (A)  4 m²
- (B)  6 m²
- (C)  7 m²
- (D)  8 m²

## Explanation

**Step 1:** The question provides a figure with some dimensions specified and asks you to calculate the area of the figure.

**Step 2:** Break the figure into familiar shapes and calculate the area of each shape; then combine them. There is a triangular portion joined to a rectangular portion. The width of the rectangle is 2 m, and the length of the rectangle is 3 m, so the area of the rectangular portion is 6 m². To determine the height of the triangular portion, subtract the height of the rectangle from the total height: $h = 4\,\text{m} - 3\,\text{m} = 1\,\text{m}$. The base of the triangle is the same as the width of the rectangle, 2 m. Thus, the area of the triangle is $\frac{1}{2} \times 2\,\text{m} \times 1\,\text{m} = 1\,\text{m}^2$. Finally, combine the areas of the two portions: $6\,\text{m}^2 + 1\,\text{m}^2 = 7\,\text{m}^2$.

**Step 3:** The correct answer is **(C)**.

**Step 4:** Check that you've used the correct formula to calculate each area and combined them correctly.

## Circle Proportions

The length of an arc (a portion of a circle's circumference) can be calculated by multiplying the circumference by the fraction $\dfrac{\text{central angle measure}}{360}$. For example, the arc length of the figure shown is the circumference $\times \dfrac{70}{360}$.

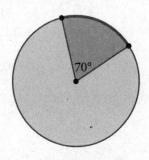

Try this one.

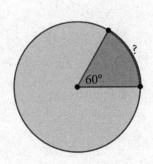

The circle above has a radius of 3 inches. What is the length, in inches, of the arc that has a central angle of 60 degrees?

    (A)   $\pi$
    (B)   $2\pi$
    (C)   $3\pi$
    (D)   $6\pi$

**Explanation**

**Step 1:** The question presents a circle with a radius of 3 and a sector with a central angle of 60 degrees. Your task is to find the sector's arc length.

**Step 2:** The arc length is part of the circumference, so begin by calculating circumference. Circumference $= 2\pi r = 2 \times \pi \times 3 = 6\pi$. To find the arc length, use the formula $\dfrac{\text{central angle measure}}{360} \times \text{circumference} = \dfrac{60}{360} \times 6\pi = \dfrac{1}{6} \times 6\pi = \pi$.

**Step 3:** The correct answer is **(A)**.

**Step 4:** Check each calculation to be sure you've applied the formulas correctly.

## KEY IDEAS

- Perimeter is calculated by determining the entire length around the outside of a shape.
- Area is calculated by determining the entire space taken up by a shape, expressed in square units.
- Irregular shapes can be broken into familiar shapes to calculate perimeter and/or area.

# Geometry Practice Questions

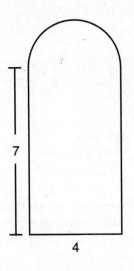

1. What is the perimeter of the figure above?

   (A)  $11 + 2\pi$
   (B)  22
   (C)  $18 + 2\pi$
   (D)  $18 + 4\pi$

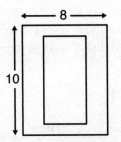

2. What is the area of the frame in the above diagram if the picture inside has a length of 8 and a width of 4?

   (A)  24
   (B)  32
   (C)  48
   (D)  56

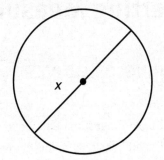

3. The diameter of the circle above has a length of $x$ inches. The area of the circle is $16\pi$ square inches. What is the value of $x$?

   (A)  2 inches
   (B)  $2\pi$ inches
   (C)  4 inches
   (D)  8 inches

**Review your work using the explanations in Part Six of this book.**

# LESSON 5

# Converting Measurements

## LEARNING OBJECTIVES

- Convert measurements within standard and metric systems
- Convert measurements between standard and metric systems
- Use dimensional analysis to efficiently solve math problems

Quantities or measurements (like length, weight, volume, time, and temperature) are expressed as a numerical quantity and often as a unit of dimension. For example, a person's weight is expressed as 165 pounds (lb) or 75 kilograms (kg). Just as important as the numerical value is the unit of measure attached to that number. Without units, the number is meaningless.

The exam may ask that you convert between units of measure (e.g., mL and L, fl oz and mL, lb and kg, mcg and mg, mg and g, tsp and L, oz and g, cm and m, Fahrenheit and Celsius).

## Conversion Rates in the Standard Measurement System

The **standard (customary) system** of measurement is the system of everyday measurements in the United States. Examples of standard units are inches, miles, cups, gallons, pounds, and tons. The wording of the question will give the conversion ratio between customary units, so you do not have to memorize them, but you should familiarize yourself with the ratios before test day.

Here is a list of common conversion ratios of the standard measurement system.

| Length | Volume | Weight | Time |
|---|---|---|---|
| 1 ft = 12 in. | 1 c = 8 fl oz | 1 lb = 16 oz | 1 min = 60 sec |
| 1 yd = 3 ft | 1 pt = 2 c | 1 ton = 2000 lb (US) | 1 hr = 60 min |
| 1 mi = 5280 ft | 1 qt = 2 pt | | 1 day = 24 hr |
| | 1 gal = 4 qt | | 1 week = 7 days |
| | | | 1 yr = 12 mo |

## Conversions Between Units

To convert between units, use the unit conversion method (i.e., multiply the given measurement by the appropriate **conversion ratio**). The results will be an equivalent measurement with a different unit. Use the four steps of **dimensional analysis** to make a conversion. This is similar to the work done in Math Chapter 1, Lesson 5: Estimation and Rounding.

1. Use the *units* given in the problem to identify the appropriate conversion ratio.
2. *Multiply* the original measurement by the conversion ratio, written as a fraction.
3. *Cancel* common units.
4. Record the result with the unit that did not cancel and *simplify* the numerical expression to find the answer.

Pay close attention to the units. Be sure that you write the conversion ratio the right way, so you can cancel like units when you finish. For example, say you are asked to convert 2 hours to minutes. The conversion ratio 1 hour = 60 minutes can be written $\dfrac{1 \text{ hr}}{60 \text{ min}}$ or $\dfrac{60 \text{ min}}{1 \text{ hr}}$. Writing the conversion ratio upside down produces this: $2 \text{ hr} \times \dfrac{1 \text{ hr}}{60 \text{ min}} = \dfrac{2 \text{ hr} \times 1 \text{ hr}}{60 \text{ min}}$, which does not allow for canceling. Done correctly: $2 \text{ hr} \times \dfrac{60 \text{ min}}{1 \text{ hr}} = \dfrac{2 \text{ hr} \times 60 \text{ min}}{1 \text{ hr}}$, and the hour units cancel.

Here is how an expert uses this approach to answer a test question.

| Question | Analysis |
| --- | --- |
| Which of the following is 3 feet in terms of inches? | **Step 1:** The question asks you to convert from feet to inches. |
| (A) 0.25 in.<br>(B) 0.36 in.<br>(C) 25 in.<br>(D) 36 in. | **Step 2:**<br><br>1. The conversion ratio: $\dfrac{12 \text{ in.}}{1 \text{ ft}}$<br><br>2. Multiply by conversion ratio: $3 \text{ ft} \times \dfrac{12 \text{ in.}}{1 \text{ ft}}$<br><br>3. Cancel the common units: $3 \times \dfrac{12 \text{ in.}}{1}$<br><br>4. Simplify: 36 in. |
|  | **Step 3:** The correct answer is **(D)**. |
|  | **Step 4:** Be sure that you set up the conversion ratio correctly. The denominator of the appropriate ratio must have the same unit as the measurement you are converting from. The common units will cancel, leaving you with the unit you set out to convert to. Choice (A) is the result if the wrong conversion ratio is used. |

Now you try one.

Joaquin is operating a lemonade stand. He has 3 pints of lemonade in one pitcher and 8 ounces of lemonade in another pitcher. How many cups of lemonade can he sell?

(A) $2\dfrac{1}{2}$

(B) 7

(C) $9\dfrac{1}{2}$

(D) 14

## Explanation

**Step 1:** The question provides a volume of liquid measured in pints and ounces and asks for the equivalent volume measured in cups.

**Step 2:** Convert the pints to cups and the ounces to cups separately. Then add the two amounts in cups together. The conversion ratio for pints to cups is $\frac{2\,c}{1\,pt}$. Multiply, cancel, and simplify:

$3\,pt \times \frac{2\,c}{1\,pt} \rightarrow 3 \times \frac{2\,c}{1} = 6\,c$. The conversion ratio for ounces to cups is $\frac{1\,c}{8\,oz}$. Multiply, cancel,

and simplify: $8\,oz \times \frac{1\,c}{8\,oz} \rightarrow 8 \times \frac{1\,c}{8} = 1\,c$. Joaquin has $6 + 1 = 7$ cups of lemonade.

**Step 3:** The correct answer is **(B)**.

**Step 4:** Confirm that you set up the conversion ratios correctly. Remember that you expect 3 pints to become more than 3 cups and you expect 8 ounces to become less than 8 cups. Checking that your conversions conform to common sense will help confirm that you've set up your arithmetic correctly.

## Conversion Rates in the Metric Measurement System

The metric system is used widely in healthcare. The basic units for the metric system are the gram (for weight), liter (for volume), and meter (for length). Math Chapter 1, Lesson 5: Estimating and Rounding provided information on metric units and conversion between those units. You may want to review the examples in that chapter before moving forward. There, you converted kilograms to grams and millimeters to meters.

## Converting Rates Between Systems

You may have to convert between standard units and metric units. The table shows common conversion ratios.

| Weight | Volume | Length | Temperature |
|---|---|---|---|
| 1 kilogram = 2.2 pounds | 1 liter = 1.06 quarts | 1 inch = 2.54 centimeters | 32° F = 0° C |
| 1 ounce = 28 grams | 1 fluid ounce = 30 milliliters | 1 meter = 39.37 inches | $C = (F - 32) \times \frac{5}{9}$ |
| | 1 teaspoon = 5 milliliters | 1 mile = 1609 meters | $F = C \times \frac{9}{5} + 32$ |
| | 1 gallon = 3.785 liters | 1 meter = 1.094 yards | |

Given the conversion ratio, converting between systems is no different from converting within systems.

Try this one:

How much is 6 kilograms (kg) in pounds (lb.)? Note: 2.2 lb = 1 kg.

- (A)  2.73 lb
- (B)  6 lb
- (C)  13.2 lb
- (D)  15 lb

## Explanation

**Step 1:** The question asks you to convert between two units, kilograms to pounds.

**Step 2:** The conversion ratio is $\dfrac{2.2\ \text{lb}}{1\ \text{kg}}$. Multiple by the conversion ratio: $6\ \text{kg} \times \dfrac{2.2\ \text{lb}}{1\ \text{kg}}$. Cancel the common units: $6 \times \dfrac{2.2\ \text{lb}}{1}$. Simplify: 13.2 lb.

**Step 3:** The correct answer is **(C)**.

**Step 4:** Check your work. Be sure that you set up the conversion ratio correctly. The denominator of the appropriate conversion ratio must have the same unit as the measurement you are converting from. The common units will then cancel, leaving you with the unit you set out to convert to. Here, because the original unit was kilograms, you set up the conversion ratio with kilograms on the bottom.

## Multiple Conversion Ratios

You might encounter a conversion problem that does not give a conversion rate from the given unit to the unit you have to reach. Instead, you might have to work with two rates at once.

For example, you may be asked to convert a length in meters to a length in inches. You may not have the conversion ratio from meters to inches, but you know that 1 meter = 100 centimeters and 1 inch = 2.54 centimeters. From this, you can make the conversion.

Try a question that involves multiple conversion ratios.

Carol is using a pattern that calls for 4 meters of fabric. The store sells fabric by the inch. Approximately how many inches of fabric will Carol need?

- (A)  10 in.
- •(B)  157 in.
- (C)  400 in.
- (D)  1016 in.

$$4\text{m}\ \frac{39.37\text{In}}{1\ meter}$$

## Explanation

**Step 1:** The question asks you convert to from meters to inches. You do not have a direct conversion ratio but can convert in two steps.

**Step 2:** The conversion ratios are $\dfrac{100\text{ cm}}{1\text{ m}}$ and $\dfrac{1\text{ in.}}{2.54\text{ cm}}$. The units meters and centimeters will cancel out, leaving inches as the final measurement in the calculation. Multiply the amount of fabric by the conversion ratios: $4\text{ m} \times \dfrac{100\text{ cm}}{1\text{ m}} \times \dfrac{1\text{ in.}}{2.54\text{ cm}}$. Cancel the common units: $4 \times \dfrac{100}{1} \times \dfrac{1\text{ in.}}{2.54}$. Simplify: ~157 in. The answer choices are pretty far apart, so if you remember that a meter is just a little longer than a yard and there are 36 inches in a yard, you can use this information to estimate the answer. If there were 4 yd instead of 4 m, you'd have $4\text{ yd} \times \dfrac{36\text{ in.}}{1\text{ yd}} = 144\text{ in.}$ Only one choice is a little more than that.

**Step 3:** The correct answer is **(B)**.

**Step 4:** Check your work. Be sure that you set up the conversion ratio correctly. The common units will cancel, leaving you with the unit you set out to convert to.

## KEY IDEAS

- Use dimensional analysis to convert among and between units of a given measurement system.
- Multiply a quantity by its conversion ratio to convert units.
- Use two or more steps to convert units if a direct conversion ratio is not available.

# Converting Measurements Practice Questions

1. What is the approximate volume of 15 fluid ounces (fl oz) of liquid in liters (L)? (1 fl oz = 30 mL and 1 L = 1000 mL)

   (A)  0.045 L
   (B)  0.05 L
   (C)  0.45 L
   (D)  0.5 L

2. Mike's cat weighs 3.3 kilograms (kg). Note that a kg = 2.2 pounds (lb) and 1 lb = 16 ounces (oz). About how many ounces does Mike's cat weigh?

   (A)  10 oz
   (B)  25 oz
   (C)  56 oz
   (D)  116 oz

3. A dosage of 2 teaspoons (t) per day of cough medicine has been prescribed. A measuring device marked in milliliters (ml) is being used. Note that 1 t = 5 mL and 1000 mL = 1 L. How many liters (L) should be ordered if the cough medicine is prescribed for 14 days?

   (A)  0.01 L
   (B)  0.04 L
   (C)  0.14 L
   (D)  1.4 L

**Review your work using the explanations in Part Six of this book.**

# Review and Reflect

Think about the questions you answered in these lessons.

- Were you able to approach each question systematically, using the Kaplan Method for Mathematics?
- Did you feel confident that you understood what the question was asking you to do?
- How well were you able to apply arithmetic and algebra rules to solving problems?
- Were there times when you could have solved more efficiently using critical thinking and estimation, rather than calculation?
- Did you confirm your answer for every question, checking that it made sense and that you had not made any arithmetic or algebra errors?
- If you missed any questions, do you understand why you got the incorrect answer? Could you do the question again now and get it right?

Use your thoughts about these questions to guide how you continue to prepare for the TEAS. If you feel you need more review and practice with arithmetic and algebra, you should study this chapter some more before taking the online Practice Test that comes with this book. Also, consider building your mastery and your confidence further by using **Kaplan's ATI TEAS® Qbank**, which contains over 500 practice questions.

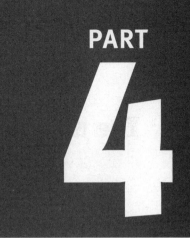

# Science

Nursing and health science program professionals need to understand and be able to use knowledge about the human body as well as other scientific subjects. In your career, you will apply scientific knowledge frequently, and you will need to keep up-to-date on the latest published research to provide your clients with the best possible care. The TEAS *Science* content area tests your understanding of the parts and function of each organ system of the human body, and it asks questions about biology and chemistry. The TEAS also tests your ability to use scientific measurements and tools and to evaluate scientific research.

**Questions by Content Area**

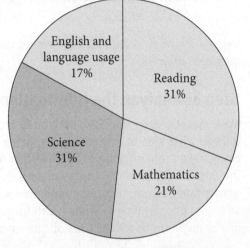

## The TEAS Science Content Area

Of the 170 items on the TEAS, 53 will be in the *Science* content area, and you will have 63 minutes to answer them. Thus, you will have just over a minute (63 minutes ÷ 53 questions ≈ 1 minute 10 seconds) per question.

Of the 53 *Science* questions, 47 will be scored and 6 will be unscored. You won't know which questions are unscored, so do your best on every question.

The 47 scored *Science* questions come from three sub-content areas:

| Sub-content areas | # of Questions |
| --- | --- |
| Human anatomy and physiology | 32 |
| Life and physical sciences | 8 |
| Scientific reasoning | 7 |

To help you prepare for these questions, this part of your book is divided into three chapters:

- Chapter 1: Human Anatomy and Physiology
- Chapter 2: Biology and Chemistry
- Chapter 3: Scientific Procedures and Reasoning

# The Kaplan Method for Science

**Step 1:** Analyze the information provided.

**Step 2:** Recall the relevant facts.

**Step 3:** Predict the answer.

**Step 4:** Evaluate the answer choices.

Using a methodical approach to *Science* questions will help you organize the relevant facts and eliminate incorrect answers.

## Step 1: Analyze the information provided.

Many questions on the TEAS ask you to recall science facts. In these cases, key terms are provided that tell you what area of science you are being tested on and which fact(s) you need to supply. If you are being asked to evaluate an experiment or draw a conclusion based on data or an experimental process, the data will be provided or the process described. This information, which may be in the question itself or in a table, figure, or other information supplied above the question, will be key to answering correctly, so invest enough time to study it carefully. In all cases, a glance at the answer choices may also provide useful guidance about the area of science being tested or the specificity of the answer sought.

## Step 2: Recall the relevant facts.

The TEAS tests many topics in science. Therefore, each time you start a new question, give yourself the time it takes to orient yourself to the question's particular focus. Is it about the endocrine system? Heredity? The experimental method? Call to mind what you know about the topic.

If additional information is provided in the question or above it, then research it. It will either provide the answer to the question or facts you can use to deduce the answer. Read carefully! It would be a shame to know the material but miss the question because you, for example, misread the axis of a graph or named the independent variable instead of the dependent variable.

## Step 3: Predict the answer.

By having the correct answer firmly in mind before you look at the answer choices, you will not choose an incorrect answer that looks similar or one that is a related concept but not the exact concept you need. Sometimes you may not know the science fact the question is asking for. Even in these cases, you can mentally review what you do remember about the topic. This will prepare you to eliminate clear wrong answers and increase your chance of getting the question right.

## Step 4: Evaluate the answer choices.

Choose the answer choice that matches your prediction. If you were unable to make a prediction, eliminate those answer choices that relate to a different organ system or concept. This allows you to make a strategic guess among the remaining choices.

# CHAPTER ONE

# HUMAN ANATOMY AND PHYSIOLOGY

## LEARNING OBJECTIVES

- Identify and describe the parts of the cell and the organization of the human body
- Identify components and features of the following organ systems and describe their function: skeletal, neuromuscular, cardiovascular, respiratory, gastrointestinal, genitourinary, endocrine, reproductive, immune, and integumentary

Of the 47 scored *Science* questions, 32 (68%) will be in the sub-content area of *Human anatomy and physiology*. The TEAS tests your comprehension of the parts and function of human organ systems and your ability to apply this knowledge.

This chapter addresses these topics in 11 lessons:

**Lesson 1:** Human Anatomy and Physiology: An Overview

**Lesson 2:** The Skeletal System

**Lesson 3:** The Neuromuscular System

**Lesson 4:** The Cardiovascular System

**Lesson 5:** The Respiratory System

**Lesson 6:** The Gastrointestinal System

**Lesson 7:** The Genitourinary System

**Lesson 8:** The Endocrine System

**Lesson 9:** The Reproductive System

**Lesson 10:** The Immune System

**Lesson 11:** The Integumentary System

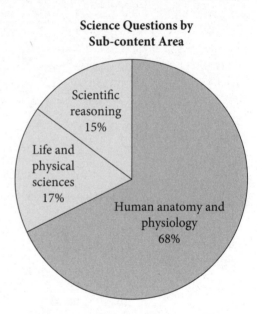

**Science Questions by Sub-content Area**

Scientific reasoning 15%

Life and physical sciences 17%

Human anatomy and physiology 68%

# LESSON 1

# Human Anatomy and Physiology: An Overview

## LEARNING OBJECTIVES

- Identify and describe the functions of different cell parts
- Describe the organization of the body into tissues, organs, and organ systems
- Recognize anatomical positions, planes, and directions

## Components of a Cell

Human cells are **eukaryotic**, meaning that they have a nucleus and membrane-bound **organelles** and are surrounded by a semipermeable **plasma membrane**. This membrane controls the movement of solutes into and out of the cell. The **nucleus** houses the cell's DNA and is surrounded by a double membrane. It is the site of DNA replication and RNA transcription. Outside the nucleus is the **cytoplasm**, an aqueous mixture of proteins and other biological molecules, which surrounds the other organelles. Each organelle has a specific cellular function, so the organelles can be thought of as miniature organs within the cell. The main organelles are summarized by function in the table.

| Function | Organelle | Description |
|---|---|---|
| protein synthesis | **ribosomes** | Either free-floating in the cytoplasm or associated with the endoplasmic reticulum. They are composed of both ribosomal RNA and protein and translate messenger RNA into cellular proteins. |
| protein translation | **rough ER** | Contiguous with the nuclear membrane. It is studded with ribosomes and is the site of translation for membrane-bound or secreted proteins. Rough ER is also the site of protein folding and modification. |
| protein sorting and modification | **Golgi apparatus** | The site of sorting and packaging of proteins. This can be thought of as the cell's "post office." Proteins also undergo posttranslational modification as they transit through the Golgi apparatus. |
| ribosome assembly | **nucleolus** | Substructure of the nucleus. The nucleolus transcribes ribosomal RNA and combines ribosomal proteins to create the large and small ribosomal subunits. |
| waste breakdown | **lysosome** | Acidic compartments that contain hydrolytic enzymes and responsible for breaking down cellular waste. Lysosomes also play a role in the cellular defense against pathogens and apoptosis. |

| Function | Organelle | Description |
|---|---|---|
| energy production | **mitochondria** | Main powerhouse of the cell, producing ATP through aerobic respiration. Mitochondria have a double membrane, a small circular genome, and their own ribosomes. |
| cell organization | **centrosome** | Organizes the microtubules of the cell. The centrioles, a substructure in the centrosome, assemble the mitotic spindle during cell division. |
| detoxification and lipid synthesis | **smooth ER** | The smooth ER is contiguous with the nuclear membrane and produces lipids, phospholipids, and steroids. It also detoxifies metabolic by-products as well as alcohol and drugs. In muscle cells, it functions as a storage site for calcium. |
| locomotion | **cilia** | Celia are cellular protrusions that can beat to enable movement or serve to increase cell surface area to maximize absorption. |

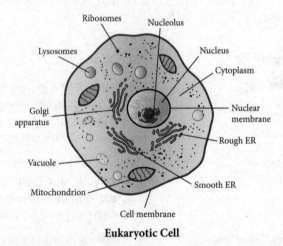

**Eukaryotic Cell**

Different cell types have different organelle compositions to better suit their individual functions. For example, muscle cells that require calcium for contraction have larger amounts of specialized smooth ER, which stores and releases calcium; they also have increased numbers of mitochondria to produce the ATP needed to sustain muscle contraction. Red blood cells lack all membrane-bound organelles so that they can hold large amounts of the oxygen-carrying protein hemoglobin.

Here is how an expert would answer a question about the organelles.

| Question | Analysis |
|---|---|
| An inhibitor targeting the electron transport chain involved in ATP production would most likely target which organelle? | **Step 1:** This question is asking about the specific functions of the organelles. While you may not know specifically what the electron transport system is, the question stem states that it is involved in ATP production. |
| | **Steps 2 and 3:** Recall that the mitochondria of cells are responsible for ATP production. Predict mitochondria. |
| (A)  Ribosomes | **Step 4:** Ribosomes are responsible for protein production. Eliminate. |
| (B)  Golgi apparatus | The Golgi apparatus is responsible for protein modification and packaging. Eliminate. |
| (C)  Mitochondria | Correct. The mitochondria are the main powerhouses of the cell and produce ATP. |
| (D)  Centrosomes | The centrosomes are responsible for microtubule organization. Eliminate. |

## Tissues

Cells working together to perform a specific function form a **tissue**. There are four main tissue types found in the body.

| Tissue Type | Description |
|---|---|
| **epithelial** | Epithelium serves two functions. It can provide covering (such as skin tissue) or produce secretions (such as glandular tissue). Epithelial tissue commonly exists in sheets and does not have its own blood supply. Subsequently, epithelium is dependent on diffusion from nearby capillaries for food and oxygen. |
| **connective** | Connective tissue is found throughout the body; it serves to connect and support different structures of the body. Connective tissue commonly has its own blood supply. The various types of connective tissue include bone, cartilage, adipose (fat), and blood vessel. |
| **muscular** | Muscle tissue is dedicated to producing movement. There are three types of muscle tissue: skeletal, cardiac, and smooth. |
| **nervous** | Nervous tissue provides the structure for the brain, spinal cord, and nerves. Nerves are made up of specialized cells called neurons that send electrical impulses throughout the body. |

# Organs and Organ Systems

An **organ** is a structure composed of multiple tissue types working together to perform a specific function; for example, the lungs oxygenate blood, and the kidneys filter blood. Organs can be further grouped together into **organ systems**, in which multiple organs work together to perform a larger function. There are 10 main organ systems in the body: respiratory, digestive, immune, endocrine, circulatory, urinary, reproductive, muscular, nervous, and skeletal systems. A summary of their function is provided in the table.

| Organ System | Components | Function |
| --- | --- | --- |
| **respiratory** | nose, throat, and lungs | Takes in oxygen and releases carbon dioxide. |
| **digestive** | mouth, esophagus, stomach, small and large intestine | Breaks down foods into nutrients that can be absorbed. |
| **immune** | spleen, bone marrow, lymph nodes | Protects the body from foreign pathogens. |
| **endocrine** | hypothalamus, pituitary, adrenal glands, thyroid, testes, ovaries, pancreas | Produces and secretes hormones to control bodily processes, including glucose regulation, sleep cycles, and gametogenesis. |
| **urinary** | kidneys, ureters, bladder, urethra | Filters blood and eliminates waste through urine. |
| **reproductive** | Males: testes, penis Females: ovaries, uterus, vagina | Produces gametes and facilitates fertilization. |
| **muscular** | muscle | Enables movement of the body. |
| **nervous** | brain, spinal cord, nerves | Receives and processes stimuli, transmits information, controls bodily functions. |
| **skeletal** | bones | Protects internal organs, creates blood cells, provides a framework for muscle. |
| **circulatory** | heart and blood vessels | Moves blood throughout the body to enable nutrient delivery to and waste removal from tissues. |

# Anatomical Planes and Terminology

**Anatomical planes** divide the body into distinct halves. Resting pose is defined as a human standing with feet parallel and facing forward, with arms at sides, palms facing forward and fingers pointing down. There are three main anatomic planes.

| Plane | Description |
|---|---|
| coronal plane | Runs vertically and separates the body into front and back halves. |
| sagittal plane | Runs vertically and separates the body into left and right halves. Note that the left-right division is in relation to the body, not the view looking at the body from the front. In other words, your right hand is on the right side of your body. |
| transverse plane | Runs horizontally and divides the body into top and bottom halves; also called the *axial plane* or *horizontal plane*. |

**Directional terminology** is used to describe the locations of different parts of the human body. Common terms include those in the table.

| Term | Definition | Example |
|---|---|---|
| superior | The top half of the body along the transverse plane | The head is on the superior axis. |
| inferior | The bottom half of the body along the transverse plane | The foot is on the inferior axis. |
| anterior/ventral | The front part of the body along the coronal plane | The clavicle is on the ventral side of the body. |
| posterior/dorsal | The back part of the body along the coronal plane | The shoulder blades are on the posterior side of the body. |
| medial | Toward the midline of the body along the sagittal plane | The thumb is on the lateral side of the body. |
| lateral | Away from the midline of the body along the sagittal plane | The pinky finger is on the medial side of the body. |
| proximal | Toward the post of origin | The proximal convoluted tubule is closest to the Bowman's capsule. |
| distal | Away from the point of origin | The distal convoluted tubule is farthest away from the Bowman's capsule. |

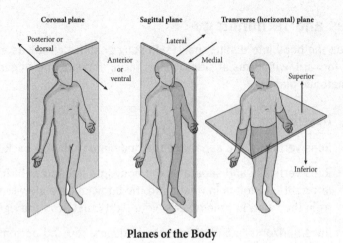

**Planes of the Body**

Directional terms can also be combined to better describe the location of a body part. For example, the nose is both ventral and superior.

Now you try this question on directional terminology.

The collar bone is located on the _____ side of the body.

(A)  superior and dorsal
(B)  superior and ventral
(C)  inferior and dorsal
(D)  inferior and ventral

## Explanation

**Step 1:** This question is asking about the location of the collar bone. Based on the answer options, you need to determine its place relative to the coronal and transverse planes.

**Step 2:** Recall that the coronal plane divides the body into dorsal and ventral halves and the transverse plane divides the body into superior and inferior halves.

**Step 3:** The collar bone is on the ventral side of the coronal plane and the superior side of the transverse plane.

**Step 4:** Answer choice **(B)** matches this prediction.

## KEY IDEAS

- Eukaryotic cells contain membrane-bound organelles, and each organelle performs a specific function or set of functions in the cell.
- Cells are organized into tissues that serve a specific task. Tissues working together for a common function comprise organs. Organ systems are the highest level of organization within the body and are comprised of multiple organs that perform different tasks.
- The body can be subdivided along multiple planes, and specific directional terms can be used to describe the location of different body parts.

# Human Anatomy and Physiology: An Overview Practice Questions

1.  A macrophage, a type of immune cell responsible for phagocytosing and digesting pathogens, is likely to contain more of which of the following organelles?

    (A)  Mitochondria
    (B)  Lysosomes
    (C)  Ribosomes
    (D)  Centrosomes

2.  A buildup of urea, a nitrogenous waste product of protein metabolism, in the body is most likely due to the failure of which organ system?

    (A)  Urinary
    (B)  Endocrine
    (C)  Digestive
    (D)  Immune

3.  The _____ plane runs horizontally through the body and divides it into inferior and superior halves.

    (A)  medial
    (B)  coronal
    (C)  sagittal
    (D)  transverse

**Review your work using the explanations in Part Six of this book.**

# LESSON 2

# The Skeletal System

## LEARNING OBJECTIVES

- Identify specific structures of the skeletal system
- Explain how the muscular system works with the skeletal system to move the body
- Classify different types of joints
- Describe the microscopic and macroscopic structure of bone

The skeletal system has multiple functions in the body including protecting internal organs, facilitating movement, creating new blood cells, and metabolism.

## Parts of the Skeleton

The skeletal system can be broken down into two main divisions: axial and appendicular. The **axial skeleton** consists of the skull, vertebrae, rib cage, and hyoid bone and provides the general scaffold of the body. The **appendicular skeleton** consists of the limb bones, scapula, clavicle, and pelvis and enables movement. The names of the specific bones of the body, as well as their location, are shown here. The TEAS may provide you with a diagram and expect you to be able to identify these bones.

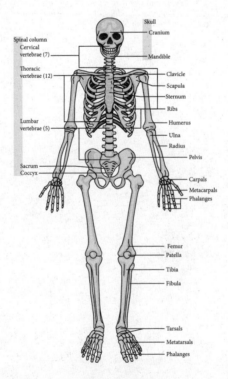

**Human Skeletal System**

There are four main types of bone: long, short, flat, and irregular.

- **Long bones** are hollow, filled with marrow, and longer than they are wide. They function to support the weight of the body and facilitate movement. They are largely part of the appendicular skeleton and include the femur, tibia, fibula, metatarsals, phalanges, humerus, radius, and metacarpals.
- **Short bones** are wider than they are long and provide stability and some movement. They include the carpals and tarsals.
- **Flat bones** provide protection to internal organs and function as areas of attachment for muscles. They include the sternum, ribs, and pelvis.
- **Irregular bones** vary in their structure and shape and thus do not fit into any other category. They include the bones of the vertebral column, the skull, and the knee and elbow.

Bones are connected at joints via **ligaments**. The hyoid bone, which supports the tongue, is the only bone in the body supported solely by muscle. The articulating ends of bone, or points of contact, are covered with **hyaline cartilage** to prevent direct bone contact and cushion the joint. There are three main types of joints:

- **Synovial joints**, including the ball-and-socket, hinge, and pivot joints, are the most common joint in the body and contain lubricating **synovial fluid**. Types of synovial joints include the knee, elbow, hip, and shoulder joints.
- **Fibrous joints** are held together only by ligaments and are not movable. Examples are the joints of the bones in the skull.
- **Cartilaginous joints** occur when two bones meet at a connection made of cartilage and are partially movable, such as joints between vertebrae in the spine.

**Arthritis** develops when cartilage between joints breaks down over time or as the result of joint inflammation. **Rheumatoid arthritis**, an autoimmune disease, is caused by immune cells attacking either the cartilage or joint lining, leading to bone erosion and pain.

Here is how an expert would answer a question about the skeletal system.

| Question | Analysis |
|---|---|
| Which of the following is NOT classified as a synovial joint? | **Step 1:** This question is asking which is *not* synovial, so three answer choices will be synovial, and the correct answer choice will not be. |
| | **Step 2:** Recall that synovial joints are movable joints. Types of synovial joints are the pivot, the ball-and-socket, and the hinge. |
| | **Step 3:** Eliminate answers that fall into these categories. |
| (A) Femur and pelvis | **Step 4:** The femur and pelvis meet at a ball-and-socket joint. Eliminate |
| (B) Skull bones | Correct. The skull bones are not movable and join at fibrous, not synovial joints. |
| (C) Humerus and ulna | The humerus and ulna meet at a hinge joint. Eliminate. |
| (D) Humerus and scapula | The humerus and scapula meet at a ball-and-socket joint. Eliminate. |

The skeletal system also provides a structural framework onto which muscles can attach to move the body. Muscles attach to bone via **tendons.** Tendons are the fibrous connective tissue that attach muscle to bone. At least two muscles attach at the joint of each movable limb and move the limb through antagonistic contraction, in which one muscle contracts and the antagonistic muscle relaxes. The bicep and tricep, for example, are antagonistic muscles. To move the forearm closer to the body, the bicep contracts and the tricep relaxes, but to extend the forearm away from the body, the bicep relaxes and the tricep contracts.

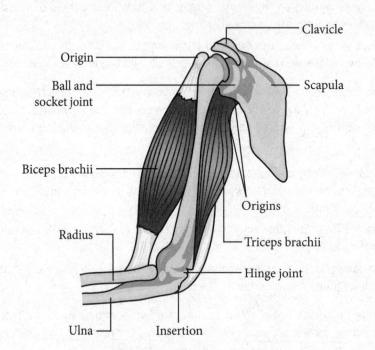

**Antagonistic Muscle Pair: The Biceps and Triceps**

## Macroscopic Structure of Bone

There are two main types of bone tissue: spongy and compact. **Spongy bone**, which is less dense than compact bone and is located in the ends of bones, contains **bone marrow**, the site of red blood cell (erythrocyte) and lymphocyte production. **Compact bone** is much denser; it supports the body and stores calcium.

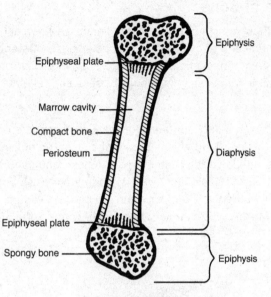

**Basic Structure of Bone**

Long bones are characterized by a cylindrical shaft, called the **diaphysis,** and dilated ends, called the **epiphyses**. The diaphysis is mainly composed of compact bone, which surrounds a hollow cavity containing the bone marrow. The epiphyses are composed of spongy bone surrounding a layer of compact bone. The **epiphyseal plate,** the growth plate, is the site of new bone growth. The **periosteum,** a fibrous sheath, surrounds and protects the bone.

Now you try this question about the skeletal system.

A defect in which of the following parts of bone would be most likely to result in stunted growth?

(A)  Diaphysis
(B)  Epiphysis
(C)  Epiphyseal plate
(D)  Periosteum

## Explanation

**Step 1:** This question is testing your knowledge of the different bone components, specifically the site where bone growth occurs.

**Step 2:** Recall that new bone is made at the epiphyseal plate, or growth plate. A defect in new bone growth would cause stunted growth.

**Step 3:** Predict epiphyseal plate.

**Step 4:** Select answer choice **(C).**

## Microscopic Structure of Bone

Bone is much more dynamic than you might think—approximately 10 percent of the human skeleton is replaced each year through the action of osteoblasts and osteoclasts. **Osteoblasts** build bone, while **osteoclasts** break it down. A great mnemonic is that *blasts build and clasts cleave*. **Osteocytes**, another type of bone cell, are responsible for sensing mechanical stress and regulate both osteoblasts and osteoclasts.

Bone is a vascularized, mineralized matrix containing a calcium phosphate collagen matrix. Bone is synthesized as **osteons**, cylindrical structures comprised of concentric rings of a mineralized matrix known as **lamellae**. **Haversian canals** run down the center of each osteon and contain blood vessels that provide nutrients to the bone cells (the osteoblasts, osteoclasts, and osteocytes). **Volkmann canals** connect the Haversian canals, enabling nutrient exchange between osteons. Cells reside in **lacunae**, spaces found between the lamellae. Microscopic channels, **canaliculi**, connect the lacunae to enable cellular communication.

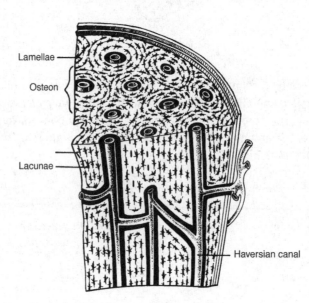

Diseases of the bone include the following:

- **Osteoporosis**, a loss in bone mineral density, is caused by lack of calcium and vitamin D in the body, as well as bone loss that occurs naturally with aging.
- **Osteogenesis imperfecta**, also known as brittle bone disease, is a genetic disease whereby either insufficient or defective collagen is produced, making bones very fragile and easy to break.
- **Osteoarthritis** is a degenerative joint disease characterized by the loss of cushioning cartilage.

Now try this question on the skeletal system.

An overactivation of which of the following bone cells could lead to osteoporosis?

  (A)  Osteon
  (B)  Osteoblast
  (C)  Osteoclast
  (D)  Osteocyte

## Explanation

**Step 1:** The answer choices for this question are all different bone cells, and you are asked which one would most likely contribute to a disease of bone.

**Step 2:** Recall that osteoporosis results from a demineralization of bone. Thus, the function of the cell responsible for osteoporosis must be breaking down bone.

**Step 3:** Predict that osteoclasts "cleave" or break down bone.

**Step 4:** Select answer choice **(C)**.

## KEY IDEAS

- The skeleton can be subdivided into axial and appendicular, and it is comprised of four main types of bone: long, short, flat, and irregular.
- The most common type of joint in the body is the synovial joint; examples are ball-and-socket, hinge, and pivot joints.
- Compact bone is dense and supports the body, while spongy bone contains bone marrow, where certain blood cells are made.
- Bone is a highly dynamic tissue, as it is broken down by osteoclasts and built by osteoblasts.

# Skeletal System Practice Questions

1. Drugs designed to treat osteoporosis would most likely increase the activity of which of the following bone cells?

   (A) ¹Osteoblast
   (B) Osteoclast
   (C) Osteocyte
   (D) Osteon

2. Which of the following bones can be characterized as a long bone?

   (A) Carpal
   (B) ⁴Humerus
   (C) Pelvis
   (D) Vertebra

**Review your work using the explanations in Part Six of this book.**

# LESSON 3

# The Neuromuscular System

## LEARNING OBJECTIVES

- Identify the components of the neuromuscular system and state their role(s)
- Differentiate between the central nervous system and the peripheral nervous system
- Describe the sequence of events that occur before, during, and after muscle contraction

The neuromuscular system consists of the nervous system and muscular system. Working together, these two systems are responsible for coordinating every movement of the body.

## Anatomy of the Nervous System

The **nervous system** allows the body to sense and respond to environmental changes, both those that arise internally as well as those caused by external stimuli. This system consists of two parts: the central nervous system, comprised of the brain and spinal cord, and the peripheral nervous system, consisting of **neurons** (nerve cells) that send and receive signals throughout the body.

The **central nervous system** (CNS) processes information in the brain. The **brain** functions as the control center for the body and occupies the **cranium**, or skull.

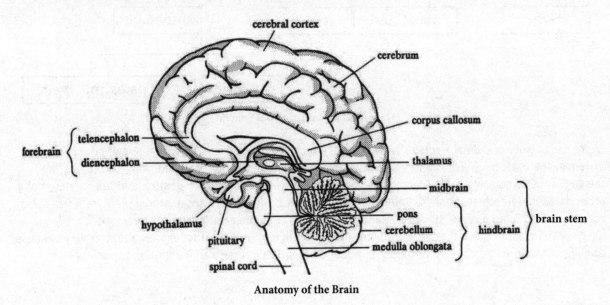

**Anatomy of the Brain**

The largest part of the brain is the **cerebrum**, which is responsible for thought and perception as well as visual and auditory processing. The cerebrum is divided into two halves, connected by nerve fibers that form the **corpus callosum**, which are further subdivided into four lobes: frontal, parietal, occipital, and temporal.

The **brain stem** connects the cerebrum to the spinal cord and controls critical involuntary body functions. Muscle control and balance are coordinated by the **cerebellum,** a dense cluster of neurons located at the base of the brain. The **medulla** regulates breathing, swallowing, and the beating of the heart.

Nerve impulses are transmitted from the extremities of the body to the brain via the **spinal cord,** a cylindrical column of nerves that runs through the center of the spine. **Spinal nerves** contain both sensory fibers and motor fibers. Sensory information such as temperature, pain, or pressure is conveyed to the brain along **afferent (sensory) neurons.** Response commands from the CNS are transmitted back to the musculature along **efferent (motor) neurons.**

The **peripheral nervous system** includes all nerves that exist outside the CNS. It can be further divided into the **somatic nervous system,** which sends and receives signals from skeletal muscle, which is under conscious control, and the **autonomic nervous system,** which regulates body processes that do not require conscious control. These include smooth and cardiac muscle activity and glandular secretions. The **sympathetic** division of the autonomic nervous system controls the body's "fight or flight" response to threat. The **parasympathetic** division returns the body to its resting state. These two systems work in opposition to one another.

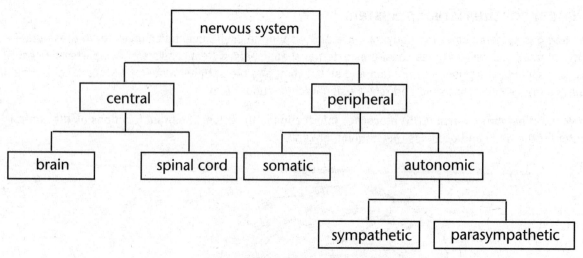

**Organization of the Nervous System**

There are 12 sets of **cranial nerves** that reach the interior of the brain, each with a specific function. For instance, the **optic nerve** transmits visual stimuli from your eye to your brain, allowing you to see, and the **vagus nerve** conveys signals from your abdominal organs, controlling digestion and heart rate among other parasympathetic responses. **Spinal nerves** transmit both sensory and motor signals from the spinal cord to a specific area of the body. The largest spinal nerve is the **sciatic nerve,** which runs from the lower spinal column down the leg. Peripheral nerve damage, or **neuropathy,** can lead to muscle weakness, tingling sensations, numbness, or paralysis depending on the degree and location of the injury.

Here is how an expert would answer a question about the nervous system.

| Question | Analysis |
|---|---|
| The autonomic nervous system would be involved in all of the following EXCEPT | **Step 1:** This question is asking about specific actions of the autonomic nervous system. |
| | **Step 2:** Recall that the autonomic nervous system carries impulses between smooth and cardiac muscle and the central nervous system. Therefore, all actions involving smooth or cardiac muscle will be controlled by the autonomic nervous system. |
| | **Step 3:** Predict that the correct answer to this EXCEPT question will involve skeletal muscle. |
| (A) digesting a meal. | **Step 4:** Digestion is an involuntary process involving the smooth muscle of the stomach and intestines and glandular secretions of the pancreas and gallbladder. Eliminate. |
| (B) exhaling after holding your breath. | Breathing is regulated by the autonomic nervous system, even though temporary voluntary control—such as holding your breath—can be initiated. The smooth muscle of the lungs would be signaled to exhale if receptors recognized a buildup of $CO_2$ in the bloodstream. |
| (C) maintaining blood pressure. | Blood pressure is regulated by the involuntary contraction or dilation of blood vessels, under the control of the autonomic nervous system. |
| (D) jerking away from a painful stimulus. | Reacting to a painful stimulus is a reflex action under involuntary control. However, reflex actions are controlled by skeletal muscle. This is therefore *not* regulated by the autonomic nervous system. Choice **(D)** is correct. |

# Anatomy of the Muscular System

There are three types of muscle in the **muscular system**: skeletal, smooth, and cardiac. Each muscle is an organ containing muscle tissue, connective tissue, nervous tissue, and blood.

**Skeletal muscle** is composed of multiple **fascicles**, bundles of cells surrounded by connective tissue. Each fascicle contains multiple muscle fibers, or cells. These muscle fibers appear striated, or striped, due to the alignment of sarcomeres within each **myofibril**. **Sarcomeres**, which are the contractile unit of the muscle cell, are composed of **actin**, the thin filament protein, and **myosin**.

The largest skeletal muscle in the body is the gluteus maximus, which straightens the leg at the hip and helps keep the body upright. The smallest muscle is the stapedius. This 1 mm long muscle stabilizes the bone in the middle ear and controls the conduction of sound waves into the inner ear.

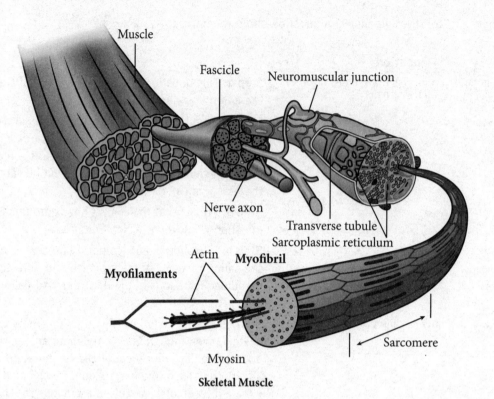

**Skeletal Muscle**

**Smooth muscle** lacks striations and is responsible for involuntary muscular contraction in the walls of hollow visceral organs, like the gastrointestinal tract, and in blood vessels. Actin and myosin are both present, but they are not organized into bundles of sarcomeres. Instead, they are arranged in a diagonal spiral, which causes the muscle to twist, rather than shorten, upon contraction.

**Cardiac muscle** occurs only in the heart. Like smooth muscle, cardiac muscle is also under involuntary contraction. Unlike smooth muscle, cardiac cells are striated and contain myofibrils and **T tubules**. Cardiac muscle is distinguishable from skeletal muscle because it consists of branching chains of striated cells and individual cardiac cells are not regulated by individual neuromuscular junctions.

If muscle is deprived of oxygen for an extended period of time, it will become **ischemic,** meaning the muscle tissue has become damaged or has died as a result of inadequate blood flow. In cardiac muscle, this event is often referred to as a heart attack.

Now try answering this question about the muscular system:

Which of the following neuromuscular processes are involved in chemical digestion?

(A)    Autonomic control by the sciatic nerve
(B)    Somatic control by the vagus nerve
(C)    Smooth muscle contraction in the small intestine
(D)    Skeletal muscle contraction in the stomach

**Explanation**

**Step 1:** This question is asking about the nerves and muscles that control chemical digestion.

**Step 2:** Recall that chemical digestion is an involuntary process that occurs primarily in the stomach and intestines.

**Step 3:** Predict that the correct answer will involve either smooth muscle or autonomic nerves.

**Step 4:** Only answer choice **(C)** matches your prediction. The sciatic nerve controls skeletal muscle. While the vagus nerve is involved in digestion, it is involved in the autonomic nervous system, not the somatic nervous system. The stomach is also comprised of smooth muscle.

# Neural Regulation of Muscle Contraction

Each neuron has a cell body, called the **soma**, multiple branched **dendrites**, and an **axon**. Messages are communicated between the brain and the muscular system by way of electrical signals called **action potentials** that travel along the axon. The process of generating an action potential, called **polarization**, can be triggered when a dendrite receives an impulse from a sensory receptor. Action potentials occur in an "all or none" fashion. Either one is triggered or one isn't.

Most axons are insulated with layers of **myelin**, which helps to increase the speed of the electrical impulse along the nerve cell. Demyelinating disorders, such as **multiple sclerosis**, prevent these impulses from being transmitted effectively and can result in uncoordinated muscle movement.

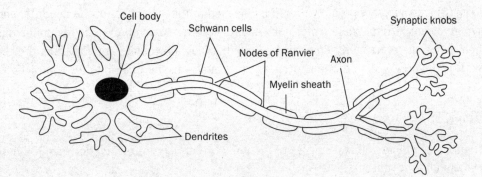

**Anatomy of a Neuron**

The space between the axon of one neuron and the dendrite of another is called the **synapse**. Neurons communicate across the synapse using **neurotransmitters**. At the synapse between a motor neuron and muscle fiber, or the **neuromuscular junction**, the specific neurotransmitter released is called **acetylcholine**, or ACh. In skeletal muscle, acetylcholine triggers the release of $Ca^{2+}$, which causes the actin and myosin to interact. A single motor neuron can communicate to numerous muscle fibers at once, defined as the **motor unit.**

During muscle contraction, the myosin head binds to actin, shortening the sarcomere as the thin filament is pulled over the thick filament. Like action potentials, muscle contraction is triggered in an "all or none" fashion. When contraction is signaled, all fibers of the motor unit contract at full force. The overall force of the muscular contraction varies by how many motor units are contracted simultaneously. Muscles that are not used regularly may **atrophy**; the myofibrils will shrink, resulting in weaker muscular contractions. After prolonged periods of disuse, the nerve supply to atrophied muscle tissue is reduced, and musculature is irreversibly replaced with connective tissue.

**Muscle fatigue** can result when a muscle is exerted strenuously over a long period. This can result from a depletion of ACh at the neuromuscular junction, meaning that contraction can no longer be signaled, or from a buildup of **lactic acid**, which impairs the muscle's ability to contract due to changes in muscle tissue pH. **Muscle strain** occurs when muscle fibers are overstretched or torn.

Now use what you know about muscle contraction to answer the following question:

Muscle contraction will occur only if

(A)   acetylcholine is released by the dendrite.
(B)   an action potential travels down the axon.
(C)   all the motor units are activated.
(D)   the muscle tissue is polarized.

## Explanation

**Step 1:** This question is asking about the process of initiating muscle contraction.

**Step 2:** Recall that muscle contraction begins with the polarization of the dendrite and ends with the binding of actin and myosin.

**Step 3:** Predict that the answer will involve a true statement about the sequence of events in muscle contraction.

**Step 4:** Choice **(B)** matches your prediction. ACh is released at the synapse, not the dendrite, and is only one of many neurotransmitters. While motor units always contract in an all-or-none fashion, a muscle may contract when only some of its motor units are activated; if only a few units are activated, the contraction will be weak. It is the polarization of the neuron, not the muscle tissue, that initiates contraction.

## KEY IDEAS

- Neurons coordinate all movements of the body by carrying messages between the nervous system and the muscular system.
- There are three types of muscle tissue. Skeletal muscle is under voluntary control. Smooth and cardiac muscle are under involuntary control.
- Muscle contraction occurs when an action potential in the neuron triggers the release of neurotransmitter at the synapse. This, in turn, leads to the binding of actin and myosin in the sarcomere.

# Neuromuscular System Practice Questions

1. Signals from touch receptors in the hand are transmitted to the brain via

    (A) an afferent neuron.
    (B) the brain stem.
    (C) an efferent neuron.
    (D) a motor neuron.

2. Damage to the cerebellum would most likely result in

    (A) speech impairment.
    (B) difficulty walking.
    (C) loss of short-term memory.
    (D) life-threatening injury.

3. Which of these statements is correct regarding muscle contraction?

    (A) When a person is at rest, no muscles are contracting.
    (B) Muscle contraction is activated by actin and myelin cross-bridges.
    (C) Sensory neurons stimulate muscle tissue to contract.
    (D) Muscle fibers contract in an all-or-none fashion.

**Review your work using the explanations in Part Six of this book.**

# LESSON 4

# The Cardiovascular System

---

## LEARNING OBJECTIVES

- Identify the components of the cardiovascular system and state their function(s)
- Trace the flow of blood through the cardiovascular system
- Describe how the cardiovascular system is regulated

---

The cardiovascular system supplies oxygen and nutrients to every living cell throughout the body by orchestrating movement of blood and lymph.

## Anatomy of the Cardiovascular System

The cardiovascular system, also called the circulatory system, is composed of the heart, blood vessels, and blood.

The **heart** propels blood through the blood vessels and is the key organ of the circulatory system. There are four muscular chambers of the heart: the right and left atria and the right and left ventricles. The **atria** receive blood returning to the heart from other areas of the body, and the **ventricles** collect and expel blood from the heart. The atria and ventricles are separated by **atrioventricular valves**: the **tricuspid valve** separates the right atrium and right ventricle, and the **mitral valve** (also called **bicuspid**) separates the left atrium and left ventricle. As you learned in Lesson 3, the heart is composed of cardiac muscle tissue.

Blood outside the heart travels through the blood vessels. There are three major types of blood vessels: arteries, capillaries, and veins. **Arteries** are strong, elastic vessels adapted to the high pressure of blood as it leaves the heart. Smaller branches of the arteries (called **arterioles**) supply blood to the **capillaries**, the smallest blood vessels. Capillaries consist of only a single layer of epithelial tissue. This allows substances and gases to be exchanged between the blood and the cells of tissues via **diffusion**. The largest artery in the body is the **aorta**.

Blood returns to the heart from the capillaries via **venules**, which merge to form veins. The walls of **veins** are thinner than those of arteries because veins do not have to carry blood under high pressure. Veins also contain valves to prevent the backflow of blood. The largest vein in the body is the **inferior vena cava**, which brings deoxygenated blood back to the heart. The **pulmonary veins**, which bring blood from the lungs to the heart, are the among the few veins that carry oxygenated blood.

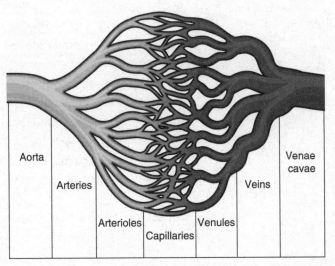

**Blood Vessels**

Blood is an essential bodily fluid that transports oxygen and nutrients to the tissues and removes waste products, including carbon dioxide and ammonia. There are four main components of human blood: red blood cells, white blood cells, platelets, and plasma.

All blood components are suspended in a matrix of **plasma**, the liquid component of blood that accounts for approximately half the blood volume. In addition to the blood cells, plasma contains proteins and electrolytes.

Red blood cells, or **erythrocytes**, account for the second greatest component of blood by volume. The functional unit of an erythrocyte is **hemoglobin**, an iron-containing protein that facilitates gas exchange by binding to oxygen or carbon dioxide. **Anemia** is a condition that occurs when hemoglobin levels are low, either because the body isn't producing enough red blood cells, such as when someone has iron deficiency, or because of another underlying condition that causes the red blood cells to be irregularly shaped, such as the **sickle-cell** trait.

White blood cells, called **leukocytes,** are part of the body's immune response and remove pathogens and foreign material from the blood. There are several different types of white blood cell, each with its own function. **Lymphocytes,** for example, release antibodies in response to disease and harness other immune system responses. White blood cells will be discussed further in Lesson 10: The Immune System.

**Platelets** are cell fragments that prevent bleeding by developing blood clots. They work with coagulating proteins to stick to vessel walls and to each other. Having too few platelets, a condition called **thrombocytopenia**, can result in excessive external bleeding, such as nosebleeds, or in bruising caused by uncontrolled bleeding under the skin.

Here is how an expert would answer a question about the circulatory system.

| Question | Analysis |
|---|---|
| Which of the following blood component levels would be expected to increase in response to a viral infection? | **Step 1:** This question is asking about the role of each blood component. |
| | **Step 2:** Recall that lymphocytes release antibodies as part of the immune response to disease or infection. |

| Question | Analysis |
|---|---|
| | **Step 3:** Predict the correct answer will correctly refer to the lymphocyte. |
| (A) Erythrocytes | **Step 4:** This is a red blood cell, the oxygen-transporting component of blood. Eliminate. |
| (B) Leukocytes | Correct. Leukocytes are white blood cells, of which lymphocytes are one specific type. |
| (C) Plasma | Plasma makes up the majority of the blood volume, which does not change as a result of infection. Eliminate. |
| (D) Platelets | Platelets are the blood-clotting component. Eliminate. |

## Paths of Circulation

The **closed circulatory system** is often described as a double loop because blood flows through the heart twice: once in its oxygenated state on its way to the body and once more when it is deoxygenated and on its way to the lungs. These two pathways are called the systemic circuit and the pulmonary circuit.

The **systemic circuit** carries oxygenated blood away from the left ventricle of the heart and returns deoxygenated blood to right atrium. The systemic circuit includes the aorta and blood vessels leading to the body tissues, as well as all the veins and venae cavae.

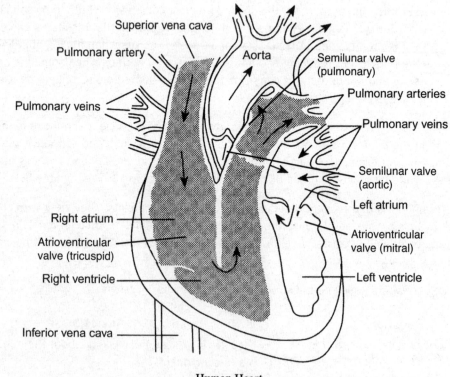

**Human Heart**

The **pulmonary circuit** contains the blood vessels that carry blood to and from the lungs. Deoxygenated blood flows from the right ventricle through the pulmonary arteries to the lungs, where the blood picks up oxygen. It then returns to the left atrium via the pulmonary vein.

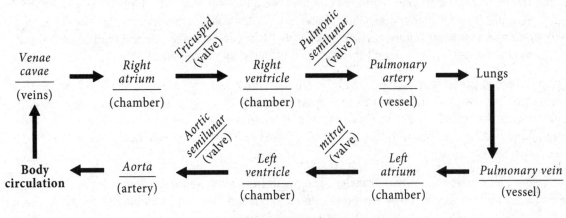

**Double-Loop Circulation**

The open circulatory system, or **lymphatic system**, is a network of capillaries that drain toxins and wastes away from the body tissues into the blood and plays a vital role in monitoring and removing foreign entities in the body. Waste products are absorbed into the **lymph**, a clear plasma-like fluid high in white blood cells, and filtered through one of several **lymph nodes**, which contain high concentrations of lymphocytes. The lymph is eventually drained into the subclavian veins.

Now you try answering a question on circulatory pathways.

> Which of the following statements regarding the pulmonary arteries is correct?
>
> (A) They carry oxygenated blood away from the heart.
> (B) They carry oxygenated blood away from the lungs.
> (C) They carry deoxygenated blood to the heart.
> (D) They carry deoxygenated blood to the lungs.

### Explanation

**Step 1:** This question is asking about properties of the pulmonary arteries, specifically the direction of blood flow and the oxygenation status of the blood.

**Step 2:** Recall that arteries transport blood away from the heart. The pulmonary artery is transporting blood away from the heart to the lungs, so the blood is deoxygenated at this time.

**Step 3:** Predict that the correct answer will be away from the heart in an deoxygenated state.

**Step 4:** Your prediction matches answer **(D)**.

## Cardiovascular Regulation

The **cardiac cycle** describes the period between the start of one heartbeat and the beginning of the next. Unlike skeletal muscle, cardiac muscle does not rely upon neural stimulation to initiate a contraction; cardiac muscle tissue can generate and conduct its own electrical impulses and can contract on its own.

There are two phases to the cardiac cycle: systole (contraction) and diastole (relaxation). During **systole**, contraction forces the blood to move from the chamber either into another heart chamber or into an artery. Atrial systole will move blood into the relaxed ventricles, whereas ventricular systole will pump blood into either the aorta or pulmonary artery, once the pressure of contraction opens the semilunar valves. During **diastole**, the heart muscle relaxes, and the chambers are passively filled with blood. The alternating closures of the atrioventricular and semilunar valve are responsible for the distinct "lub-dub" sound of the heartbeat. **Congestive heart failure** develops when the heart can no longer pump blood effectively, such as when weakened heart valves permit the backflow of blood into the chambers.

A reading of **blood pressure**, the pressure of the blood in the circulatory system, has two numbers (e.g., 120/80) to reflect the different pressures that occur at systole and diastole. Blood pressure is maintained by adjusting cardiac output and vascular resistance. If blood pressure begins to increase, the medulla will signal the heart to beat slower. Likewise, if blood pressure begins to drop, heart rate will increase to adjust.

Chronic high blood pressure, or **hypertension**, can result from multiple factors, including **atherosclerosis** (narrowing of the arteries due to plaque buildup), increased blood viscosity (such as if the blood contains high levels of cholesterol), and heart disease.

## KEY IDEAS

- The heart regulates blood flow through a double-loop system, pumping oxygenated blood to the body tissue and deoxygenated blood to the lungs.
- Blood transports oxygen (via hemoglobin) and nutrients throughout the body by way of the circulatory system.
- Lymph, which moves through the open circulatory system before draining into the veins near the heart, contains infection-fighting white blood cells.

# Cardiovascular System Practice Questions

1. Which of the following valves prevents blood from backflowing between the right atrium and right ventricle?

   (A)  Aortic
   (B)  Bicuspid
   (C)  Mitral
   (D)  Tricuspid

2. Which of the following correctly describes the flow of blood through the double-loop system?

   (A)  Left ventricle - right ventricle - capillaries - pulmonary vein - right atrium
   (B)  Left ventricle - pulmonary vein - lungs - pulmonary artery - right ventricle
   (C)  Left ventricle - aorta - capillaries - vena cava - right ventricle
   (D)  Left ventricle - arteries - veins - right ventricle - right atrium

3. Which of the following blood particles are responsible for blood clotting?

   (A)  Platelets
   (B)  Antibodies
   (C)  Hemoglobin
   (D)  Lymph

**Review your work using the explanations in Part Six of this book.**

# LESSON 5

# The Respiratory System

## LEARNING OBJECTIVES

- Identify the components of the respiratory system
- List the factors that control gas exchange and ventilation rate
- Describe the mechanism of ventilation
- List different conditions that lead to decreased respiratory function

## Components of the Respiratory System

The primary function of the respiratory system is to facilitate gas exchange between the body and external environment and to provide oxygen to the body by working with the cardiovascular system. Oxygen diffuses into the body through the lungs and is disseminated throughout the body by the circulatory system to be used for cellular metabolism. Carbon dioxide, the waste product of cellular metabolism, is returned to the lungs by the circulatory system, and the lungs release it to the environment.

Air first enters the body through the mouth and nasal cavities and passes through the **pharynx**. A flap of cartilage, the **epiglottis**, covers the entrance to the pharynx during swallowing, preventing liquids and food from entering the respiratory tract. Traveling past the epiglottis, air then passes through the **larynx**, also referred to as the voice box, and enters the **trachea**, or windpipe. The trachea splits into two **bronchi** (plural of *bronchus*), which are the main passageways to the left and right lung. As the bronchi move deeper into the lungs, the bronchi split into smaller tubes known as **bronchioles**, which terminate at the **alveoli** (plural of *alveolus*), small sacs only one cell thick. The alveoli are where gas exchange occurs.

This overall pathway of **p**harynx → **l**arynx → **t**rachea → **b**ronchi → **a**lveoli can be remembered using the mnemonic "**p**lease **l**eave **t**he **b**reathing **a**lone."

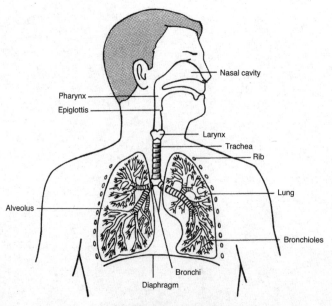

The Respiratory System

Cells lining the respiratory tract secrete mucus and other liquids to both keep the lungs moist and trap inhaled pathogens. One such liquid is **surfactant**, a detergent found bathing the alveoli, which reduces surface tension to prevent lung collapse. Other epithelial cells lining the respiratory tract are covered with short, hairlike **cilia**, which beat rhythmically to keep mucus and other particles flowing across the interior epithelial surface.

Since the heart is located on the left side of the body, the left lung is slightly smaller than the right lung. The right lung has three segments, or lobes, and the left lung has two lobes. Each lobe is covered by a tough, protective double membrane, each part of which is called a **pleura**, with **pleural fluid** between the two *pleurae*. The lungs are therefore described as residing within the pleural cavity.

Here is how an expert would answer a question on the respiratory system.

| Question | Analysis |
| --- | --- |
| Which of the following correctly describes the pathway of air into the lungs? | **Step 1:** This question is asking about the order in which air flows through the parts of the respiratory system. |
| | **Step 2:** Recall the mnemonic for the breathing pathway: **p**lease **l**eave **t**he **b**reathing **a**lone. |
| | **Step 3:** Predict the air travels the path pharynx → larynx → trachea → bronchi → alveoli. |
| (A)  Larynx → pharynx → trachea → bronchi → alveoli | **Step 4:** The pharynx is before the larynx. Eliminate. |
| (B)  Pharynx → larynx → trachea → bronchi → alveoli | Correct. This matches the prediction. |
| (C)  Trachea → pharynx → larynx → bronchi → alveoli | The pharynx comes before the trachea. Eliminate. |
| (D)  Pharynx → larynx → bronchi → trachea → alveoli | The bronchi come after the trachea. Eliminate. |

## Gas Exchange and Regulation of Ventilation

The pulmonary arterioles carry carbon dioxide–rich blood from the right atrium of the heart to the lungs. The blood then enters the capillary beds surrounding the alveoli, where carbon dioxide is exchanged for oxygen. Oxygen-rich blood exits the lungs through the pulmonary venules to be taken back to the left atrium of the heart. From there, the blood flows to the left ventricle, which pumps it into body-wide circulation.

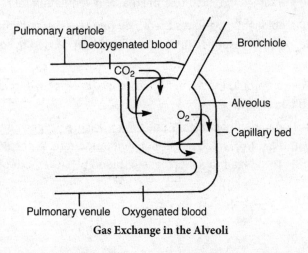

**Gas Exchange in the Alveoli**

The exchange of carbon dioxide for oxygen at the alveoli relies on **simple diffusion**. The **diffusion rate** is directly proportional to the surface area and the concentration gradient and is inversely proportional to the distance between the two gases.

Due to the millions of alveoli in the lung, the surface area for gas exchange is estimated to be between 50 to 75 square meters, or about the size of a tennis court, allowing large amounts of gases to be exchanged quickly. Furthermore, the walls of the alveoli are only one cell thick to minimize distance and maximize diffusion rate.

The diffusion of gases is driven by a concentration gradient. The partial pressure of oxygen is high in the airspace of the lungs and low in the blood, so oxygen will diffuse down its concentration gradient into the blood. The partial pressure of carbon dioxide is higher in the blood than in the airspace in the lungs, so it will diffuse down its concentration gradient out of the blood.

**Ventilation rate** is controlled by the medulla oblongata, located in the brain stem, which monitors blood pH and carbon dioxide concentration in the blood. Carbon dioxide directly affects pH through the bicarbonate blood-buffering system.

$$CO_2 + H_2O \leftrightarrow H_2CO_3 \leftrightarrow H^+ + HCO_3^-$$

Carbon dioxide ($CO_2$) combines with water ($H_2O$) to form carbonic acid ($H_2CO_3$), which can then dissociate into bicarbonate ($HCO_3^-$) and protons ($H^+$). When the concentration of carbon dioxide is high, the equilibrium shifts to the right, favoring protons and bicarbonate. An increase in protons decreases the pH of the blood, causing **acidosis**, and leads to an increase in ventilation rate. When the concentration of carbon dioxide is low, the equilibrium is shifted to the left, favoring carbon dioxide and water, which decreases the concentration of protons and bicarbonate. A decrease in proton concentration increases the pH of the blood, leading to **alkalosis**, and causes a decrease in ventilation rate.

Now try answering this question about the respiratory system.

Which of the following would NOT be expected to cause a decrease in ventilation rate?

- (A) Increase in blood oxygen concentration
- (B) Decrease in blood carbon dioxide concentration
- (C) Increase in blood pH
- (D) Decrease in blood pH

## Explanation

**Step 1:** This question is asking what will *not* lead to a decrease in ventilation rate.

**Step 2:** Recall that the medulla oblongata regulates breathing rate by sensing carbon dioxide levels and pH. Ventilation rate would decrease in response to elevated blood pH caused by low carbon dioxide concentrations in the blood.

**Step 3:** Predict that ventilation rate would increase, not decrease, in response to high carbon dioxide concentration or decreased blood pH.

**Step 4:** Choice **(D)** is correct. The medulla oblongata does not measure oxygen concentration of the blood, so changes in oxygen concentration, (A), would not affect ventilation rate. A decrease in carbon dioxide concentration in the blood, (B), would lead to an increase in blood pH, (C)—both of which would lead to a decrease in ventilation rate.

## Mechanism of Ventilation and Lung Volumes

Humans use **negative pressure breathing**. During inhalation, the diaphragm contracts and flattens, and the intercostal muscles of the ribs contract and push outward, causing the lungs to expand. As the volume of the lungs increases, the pressure inside the lungs drops. Air then flows from outside the body into the lungs down a pressure gradient. During exhalation, the diaphragm and intercostal muscles simultaneously relax, decreasing the volume of the lungs. This decrease in volume increases the pressure in the lungs, forcing air out.

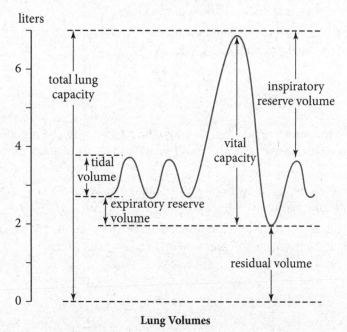

**Lung Volumes**

The **total lung capacity** of an average adult male is approximately 6 liters. This can be further subdivided into the vital capacity and residual volume. **Residual volume** is the amount of air that always resides within the lungs and functions to prevent lung collapse. **Vital capacity** is the total volume of air that can be exchanged through inhalation and exhalation and is composed of the tidal volume, inspiratory reserve volume, and expiratory reserve volume. **Tidal volume** is the amount of air inhaled and exhaled during normal breathing, **inspiratory reserve volume** is the additional volume of air that can be inhaled following normal inhalation, and **expiratory reserve volume** is the additional volume of air that can be exhaled following normal exhalation.

## Factors Impeding Lung Function

Many factors can negatively impact lung function, including genetic disorders, environmental factors, and infection. Genetic diseases arise from mutations in the genome, which can either be spontaneous or inherited from parents. Diseases with a genetic component include the following:

- **Cystic fibrosis** arises due to a mutation of a protein expressed in the respiratory tract, leading to abnormally thick mucus. This leads to difficulty breathing and frequent lung infections.

- **Surfactant insufficiency** results from a mutation in the surfactant proteins, leading to difficulty breathing. This is a common cause of respiratory distress in newborns.

- **Asthma**, which involves environmental triggers as well as a genetic predisposition, is characterized by inflammation and a subsequent narrowing of the airway that makes breathing difficult.

Environmental factors can also affect lung function. Prolonged smoking and chemical exposure can damage the cilia, leading to **emphysema** (breakdown of the alveoli), inflammation, and allergies.

Many pathogens also infect the lungs. Here are a few examples:

- Influenza is caused by a coronavirus. Symptoms include coughing, sneezing, runny nose, and fatigue.
- Tuberculosis is caused by a mycobacterium. Symptoms include coughing up blood and weight loss. If not treated, tuberculosis leads to scarring of the lungs.
- So-called walking pneumonia is caused by infection by mycoplasma bacteria. This leads to mild symptoms including coughing and headaches.

## KEY IDEAS

- Air first enters the respiratory system through the nasal cavity and mouth, then travels through the pharynx, larynx, trachea, and bronchi to reach the alveoli where gas exchange occurs.
- Ventilation rate is controlled by the medulla oblongata, which senses changes in blood carbon dioxide concentration and pH.
- Humans breathe by negative pressure breathing. Muscular contraction increases the volume of the lungs, thus decreasing the pressure and causing air to flow in.

# Respiratory System Practice Questions

1. Which of the following lung volumes is responsible for preventing lung collapse?

   (A)  Tidal volume
   (B)  Residual volume
   (C)  Vital capacity
   (D)  Total lung capacity

2. Which of the following would lead to an increase in ventilation rate?

   (A)  The concentration of oxygen in the blood is decreased.
   (B)  The pH of the blood is increased.
   (C)  The pH of the blood is decreased.
   (D)  The concentration of carbon dioxide in the blood is decreased.

3. Which of the following lung ailments is caused by a mycobacterium infection?

   (A)  Influenza
   (B)  Pnemonia
   (C)  Tuberculosis
   (D)  Asthma

**Review your work using the explanations in Part Six of this book.**

# LESSON 6

# The Gastrointestinal System

## LEARNING OBJECTIVES

- Identify the components of the gastrointestinal system and state their function(s)
- Trace the pathway of food through the gastrointestinal tract
- Describe the role of enzymatic digestion and hormonal regulation in the gastrointestinal system

The **gastrointestinal system,** also called the digestive system or GI system, converts food into nutrients that the body can use. This transformation is accomplished through the processes of digestion and absorption. **Digestion** is the chemical and mechanical breakdown of foods into smaller compounds that can be utilized by the body. After foods have been digested, their nutrients are **absorbed,** or moved into the bloodstream from the intestines.

## The Gastrointestinal Tract

The gastrointestinal system consists of the organs of the **alimentary canal,** the pathway through the body that food travels while being digested and absorbed, as well as the accessory organs that release secretions necessary for digestion to occur.

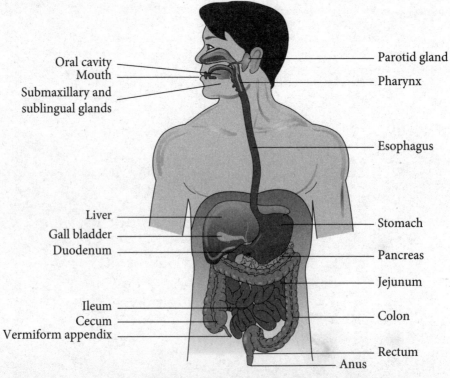

**Components of the Gastrointestinal System**

Food enters the alimentary canal through the mouth, where it is mechanically digested through the chewing process. The **salivary glands** release digestive enzymes that mix with the food to begin chemical digestion and lubricate the mouth. Swallowing is triggered when the chewed food—now referred to as the **bolus**—is sensed by the **pharynx**. The bolus passes through to the **esophagus** and then into the stomach, aided by **peristalsis**, a wavelike contraction of smooth muscle the moves digested material along the digestive tract.

Both chemical and mechanical digestion continue in the **stomach**, a hollow organ separated from the esophagus by the **esophageal sphincter** and from the small intestine by the **pyloric sphincter**. The pH of the stomach is maintained between 1 and 2 by the release of **gastric juice**, which contains hydrochloric acid (HCl) as well as enzymes that begin the chemical digestion of protein.

The contents of the stomach—now called **chyme**—exit the stomach and enter the **small intestine**, where digestion is completed and absorption begins. There are three sections of the small intestine: the duodenum, the jejunum, and the ileum. When chyme enters the intestine, it signals the pancreas and gallbladder to release their digestive secretions into the **duodenum**, the first part of the small intestine. **Bile**, created in the liver and stored in the gallbladder, is secreted into the duodenum through the **common bile duct**. The digestion of protein, carbohydrates, and fats occurs in the duodenum.

As in the esophagus, peristalsis of the smooth muscle moves the chyme through the intestinal tract. The small intestine is lined with **villi** and **microvilli**, finger-like folds in the lining of the intestine that increase surface area to aid absorption. Approximately 90 percent of all nutrients will be absorbed in the **jejunum**, with the exception of Vitamin B$_{12}$, which is only absorbed in the **ileum**. Bile salts and acids are also absorbed in the ileum.

The digested material passes from the ilium through the **cecum**, the pouch at the beginning of the large intestine, into the large intestine. Water, salts, and vitamin K are absorbed in the **colon**, the proximal part of the large intestine. Any remaining waste collects in the **rectum**, the terminal section of the large intestine, to be expelled from the body through the **anus**, regulated by the action of the **anal sphincter**.

Here is how an expert would answer a question about the gastrointestinal system.

| Question | Analysis |
|---|---|
| Which of the following organs is part of the alimentary canal? | **Step 1:** This question is asking about the anatomical components of the alimentary canal. |
| | **Step 2:** Recall that the alimentary canal describes the pathway that food takes through the body. |
| | **Step 3:** Predict that the organ will be in the oral cavity, esophagus, stomach, or intestines. |
| (A) Trachea | **Step 4:** The trachea connects the oral cavity to the lungs. During swallowing, the epiglottis covers the trachea so that food does not enter the trachea. Eliminate. |
| (B) Pharynx | Correct. Stimulation of the pharynx triggers swallowing, and food passes through the pharynx from the mouth to the esophagus. |

| Question | Analysis |
|---|---|
| (C) Larynx | The larynx holds the vocal cords and lies between the trachea and the pharynx. During swallowing, the larynx rises and is covered by the epiglottis so that food does not enter the respiratory tract. |
| (D) Salivary glands | The salivary glands are accessory organs that release digestive enzymes into the oral cavity. Food does not pass through the salivary glands. |

## Digestion and Absorption

Two kinds of digestion work together to convert food and water into usable body nutrients: mechanical digestion and chemical digestion.

**Mechanical digestion** involves the physical breakdown of food into smaller pieces. Chewing, the churning process of the stomach, and the muscular action of peristalsis physically mash food particles apart, creating a greater surface area for chemical digestion to take place.

**Chemical digestion** involves enzymes or acids that break down food at the molecular level. Digestive enzymes are secreted by certain exocrine organs—including the pancreas, liver, and salivary glands—and by specialized cells in the lining of the stomach and intestines.

So they do not digest the cells that synthesize them, enzymes are released in the inactive **zymogen** form and are rendered active only in the presence of other digestive compounds, such as HCl. For example, the chief cells of the stomach synthesize and store pepsinogen, an inactive form of the enzyme that digests protein. In the presence of HCl released in gastric juice, pepsinogen is converted to the active form pepsin. Enzymes that function best in acidic environments (low pH) are most active in the stomach; enzymes that function best in alkaline environments (high pH) are most active in the small intestine.

The TEAS may ask you about the origin and/or function of digestive enzymes, as well as to identify which type(s) of macromolecules are digested in different areas of the alimentary canal. Review the chart to familiarize yourself with the digestive enzymes.

| Secretion | Origin | Function |
|---|---|---|
| Saliva | Salivary glands (mouth) | Lubricates the mouth; contains salivary amylase, which breaks down carbohydrates and starches; contains salivary lipase, which breaks down fats |
| Hydrochloric acid (HCl) | Parietal cells (stomach) | Sterilizes potentially harmful bacteria; causes proteins to denature; converts pepsinogen to pepsin |
| Pepsin(ogen) | Chief cells (stomach) | Digests protein by breaking bonds of amino acids |
| Gastric lipase | Chief cells (stomach) | Digests lipids and fats in the stomach |

| Secretion | Origin | Function |
|---|---|---|
| Mucus | Goblet cells (stomach) | Maintains the mucosal lining of the stomach; protects the stomach walls from the digestive activity of HCl and other gastric enzymes |
| Bile | Liver | Helps neutralizes the acidic chyme as it enters the small intestine; aids in fat digestion and absorption by emulsifying lipid particles |
| Pancreatic bicarbonate | Pancreas | Neutralizes chyme as it enters the duodenum |
| Pancreatic lipase | Pancreas | Digests lipids and fats in the small intestine |
| Trypsin(ogen) (proteases) | Pancreas and small Intestine | Digests proteins in the small intestine |
| Brush border enzymes | Microvilli (small intestine) | Includes lactase and other dissaccharidases that break down lactose and other simple sugars; nucleases that break down nucleic acids; and peptidases that complete protein digestion and convert trypsinogen to trypsin |

Absorption begins in the villi of the small intestine. Most nutrients absorbed in the small intestine move into the capillaries. The capillary network of the digestive tract carries blood to the liver through the **hepatic portal vein**. Digested fats are absorbed into the lymphatic system.

Now try answering this question about digestion:

> Which of the following macromolecule groups is chemically digested for the first time in the stomach?
>
> (A)  Carbohydrates
> (B)  Proteins
> (C)  Lipids
> (D)  Nucleic acids

## Explanation

**Step 1:** This question is asking about the onset of chemical digestion in the stomach.

**Step 2:** Recall that chemical digestion begins in the mouth with salivary lipase and amylase. Lipases digest lipids, and amylases digest carbohydrates. Chemical digestion continues in the stomach with the release of pepsin(ogen), which breaks the bonds of amino acids.

**Step 3:** Predict that the chemical digestion of protein begins in the stomach.

**Step 4:** This prediction matches choice **(B)**, proteins. Nucleic acid digestion begins in the small intestine with the brush border enzymes released by the pancreas.

# Regulation of the GI System

The gastrointestinal system is controlled by the autonomic nervous system and regulated by a series of hormonal feedback loops. The smooth muscle of the GI system is affected by emotions. The sympathetic nervous system, or "fight or flight" response, slows digestion and can cause the bowels to empty in preparation for dealing with a threat; the parasympathetic nervous system, or "rest and digest," increases blood flow to the stomach and intestines.

Digestion is also regulated by the release of hormones into the bloodstream.

| Hormone | Stimulus for Release | Released from | Target | Function |
|---|---|---|---|---|
| Gastrin | Arrival of protein in the stomach | Stomach/Small intestine | Parietal cells of the stomach | Stimulates gastric acid and mucosal secretion; increases motility |
| Ghrelin | Empty stomach | Stomach | Hypothalamus | Induces hunger |
| Leptin | Fat in the bloodstream | Adipose (fat) tissue | Hypothalamus | Reduces hunger by signaling satiety |
| Secretin | Arrival of chyme in the duodenum | Small intestine | Pancreas, stomach, liver | Stimulates pancreas to release bicarbonate; inhibits gastric emptying; increases bile secretion |
| Insulin | Increase in blood glucose levels | Pancreas | Liver, muscle and adipose tissue | Stimulates uptake of glucose for conversion into glycogen; decreases blood glucose levels |
| Glucagon | Low blood glucose levels | Pancreas | Liver | Initiates breakdown of glycogen; increases blood glucose levels |
| Somatostatin | Acid in the stomach | Stomach | Secretory stomach cells | Inhibits gastric secretion and slows digestion |
| Cholecystokinin (CCK) | Fats and amino acids | Small intestine | Gallbladder, pancreas, stomach | Stimulates gallbladder to release bile; stimulates the pancreas to release pancreatic enzymes; inhibits gastric emptying and acid secretion |

## KEY IDEAS

- The gastrointestinal system converts food into usable nutrients through chemical and mechanical digestion.
- Food enters the body through the mouth, passes through the alimentary canal for digestion and absorption, and is eliminated from the body through the anus.
- Enzymes released from accessory organs into the mouth, stomach, and intestines break down macromolecules into smaller units that can be absorbed into the capillaries or lymphatic system.

# Gastrointestinal System Practice Questions

1. Which of the following is absorbed in the colon?

   (A)  Vitamin $B_6$
   (B)  Vitamin C
   (C)  Vitamin D
   (D)  Vitamin K

2. After passing through the pyloric sphincter, a food high in protein would be in which of the following states?

   (A)  Acidic and partially digested
   (B)  Acidic and completely digested
   (C)  Alkaline and partially digested
   (D)  Alkaline and completely digested

3. Which of the following hormones signals satiety?

   (A)  Gastrin
   (B)  Ghrelin
   (C)  Leptin
   (D)  Secretin

**Review your work using the explanations in Part Six of this book.**

# LESSON 7

# The Genitourinary System

## LEARNING OBJECTIVES

- Identify the components of the genitourinary system and state their function(s)
- Describe the role of renal hormones in cardiovascular homeostasis

The **genitourinary system**, the name given to parts of the urinary, renal, and excretory systems, is responsible for removing toxins, waste, and water from the body as well as maintaining the blood pressure and pH.

## Anatomy and Physiology of the Kidney

The genitourinary system is comprised of the kidneys, ureters, urinary bladder, and urethra. The **kidneys** filter blood to remove waste products and maintain fluid balance, and they produce **urine**, a fluid consisting of water, excess electrolytes, and metabolic wastes. Urine travels from the kidneys through the **ureters** to be stored in the **urinary bladder** before being expelled from the body by the **urethra**. In males, the urethra travels through the penis and also carries semen as part of the reproductive system; in females the urethra is shorter and is located above the vaginal opening.

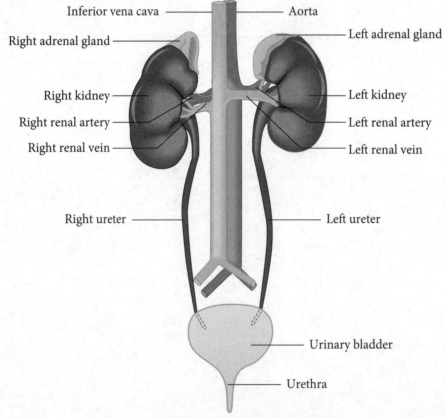

**Anatomic Structures of the Genitourinary System**

## Overview of Kidney Function

The functional unit of the kidney, the **nephron**, is where blood filtration and reabsorption occur. The kidneys receive blood from the left and right **renal arteries**, which carry blood directly from the heart via the abdominal aorta. These arteries branch and feed into the **glomerulus**, a network of capillaries that contains large pores, making it highly permeable to certain ions like sodium and potassium. **Bowman's capsule**, a cup-like end of the nephron, surrounds the glomerulus, and together they make up the **renal corpuscle**, which is the filtration unit of the kidney. The arteriole entering the glomerulus, the **afferent arteriole**, is larger than the arteriole exiting the glomerulus, the **efferent arteriole**. The smaller diameter of the efferent arteriole resists a steady flow of blood, increasing the blood pressure within the glomerulus. This high pressure assists in "pushing" the blood components, with the exception of large proteins and red and white blood cells, out of the blood vessels and into Bowman's capsule.

The filtrate next enters the **renal tubule**, where salts, water, glucose, and amino acids are reabsorbed. The remaining filtrate, which contains significant amounts of **urea** along with excess water and other waste products, then enters the collecting duct, where it can be concentrated and converted into urine.

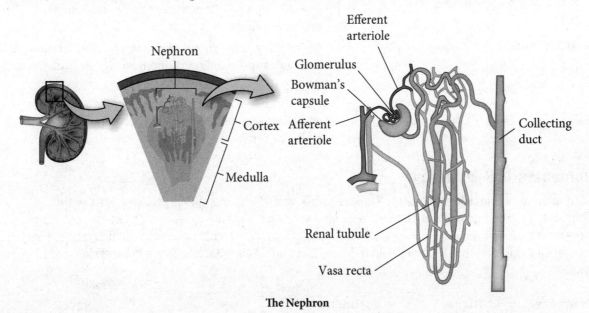

**The Nephron**

The presence of certain solutes in the urine can indicate renal problems or help to diagnosis other conditions. For example, glucose in the urine is a sign of diabetes; dark urine can indicate dehydration; and **hematuria**, blood in the urine, could indicate damage to the urinary tract or kidney itself.

See how an TEAS expert would answer question about the kidney.

| Question | Analysis |
|---|---|
| Which of the following describes the region of the kidney where blood is filtered? | **Step 1:** This question is asking about the anatomical features of the kidney, specifically where filtration takes place. |
| | **Step 2:** Recall that filtration takes place in the glomerulus, a network of capillaries that filters blood into Bowman's capsule, a part of the nephron. |
| | **Step 3:** Predict that the answer will relate to the glomerular region of the nephron. |
| (A) Tubule | **Step 4:** The renal tubule is where reabsorption of water and ions from the filtrate occurs. Eliminate. |
| (B) Pelvis | The renal pelvis is located in the center of the kidney and funnels urine from the collecting duct into the ureter. Eliminate. |
| (C) Corpuscle | Correct. The renal corpuscle is the place of filtration, as it contains the glomerulus and Bowman's capsule. |
| (D) Medulla | The renal medulla houses some parts of the renal tubules as well as the collecting ducts. Reabsorption and blood volume maintenance occur in the renal medulla. Eliminate. |

## Homeostatic Regulation

In addition to filtering out wastes, the kidneys play a vital role in maintaining homeostasis in the circulatory system. The **adrenal glands** are located at the tip of each kidney and secrete several hormones, including those that regulate blood pressure and fluid balance. These hormones react in response to decreased blood pressure to retain fluid balance. The table lists renal hormones that regulate blood pressure.

| Hormone | Trigger | Function | Result |
|---|---|---|---|
| Renin | Decreased blood pressure | Activates angiotensin; increases secretion of ADH and aldosterone | Increases blood pressure |
| Angiotensin | Activated by renin | Constricts arteriolar blood vessels; increases reabsorption of $Na^+$ and $Cl^-$ and water retention in the renal tubules; stimulates ADH secretion | Increases blood pressure |
| Antidiuretic hormone (ADH); also called vasopressin | Decreased blood volume; increased osmolality of blood | Prevents fluid loss to maintain blood volume by increasing reabsorption of water from renal tubules and collecting ducts | Increases blood volume |
| Aldosterone | Decreased blood pressure; increased $K^+$ levels | Increases reabsorption of $Na^+$ from the renal tubules, causing more water to be reabsorbed via osmosis | Increases blood pressure |

Now try answering this question about the kidney:

Which of the following hormones would directly cause urine to become more concentrated?

    (A)  Epinephrine
    (B)  Renin
    (C)  Aldosterone
    (D)  ADH

## Explanation

**Step 1:** This question is asking about one aspect of urine production, namely urine concentration.

**Step 2:** Recall that urine is formed after the filtrate passes through the collecting duct. The amount of water reabsorbed in the collecting duct determines how diluted or concentrated urine will be.

**Step 3:** Predict that the correct hormone will act directly on the collecting duct.

**Step 4:** Answer choice **(D)** matches your prediction. Epinephrine, (A), is produced by the adrenal glands but is responsible for the "fight or flight" response. Renin, (B), helps increase blood pressure by increasing secretion of aldosterone, (C), but neither is directly responsible for urine concentration because it does not act on the collecting duct.

## KEY IDEAS

- The genitourinary system removes waste products and toxins from the body in the form of urine and helps maintain homeostasis of the cardiovascular system.
- Water, salts, and other essential components from the blood are reabsorbed in the nephron, the functional unit of the kidney, while excess water and toxins are filtered out.
- Blood volume and blood pressure are regulated by hormones that act on the kidneys to cause more or less water to be removed from the blood.

# Genitourinary System Practice Questions

1. After passing through the collecting duct, urine flows into which of the following genitourinary structures?

   (A) Bladder
   (B) Nephron
   (C) Ureter
   (D) Urethra

2. Which of the following vessels directs blood into the glomerulus?

   (A) Afferent arteriole
   (B) Bowman's capsule
   (C) Efferent arteriole
   (D) Renal artery

3. Which of the following hormones increase sodium reabsorption in the renal tubule?

   (A) Adrenal and renin
   (B) Aldosterone and epinephrine
   (C) Angiotensin and aldosterone
   (D) Renin and ADH

**Review your work using the explanations in Part Six of this book.**

# LESSON 8

# The Endocrine System

## LEARNING OBJECTIVES

- Describe the mechanism of action and regulation of hormones
- List the various components of the endocrine system and describe the hormones they secrete
- Describe common diseases that arise from the dysregulation of hormones

## Hormone Action and Regulation

The endocrine system consists of multiple organs that secrete **hormones** directly into the bloodstream to control body processes and maintain **homeostasis,** the state in which the body's hormones and nutrient levels are balanced. Hormones then travel through the bloodstream and bind to **receptors** on their target, triggering a response by the target tissue. The two main classes of hormones are steroid and peptide hormones.

- **Peptide hormones** are water soluble and bind to receptors on the surface of target cells. They induce a signaling cascade that leads to a rapid, but short-lived, response.
- **Steroid hormones** are fat soluble and can pass freely through the plasma membrane and bind to receptors inside the cell. They induce changes in cellular gene expression, so their effects are longer lasting.

The body maintains homeostasis through a variety of feedback loops. In **positive feedback,** the response to a deviation will lead to a larger response. These are very rare and often lead to large physiological changes, such as delivery of a baby. Most feedback loops operate under **negative feedback,** a process in which a deviation from normal is detected, a response is made, and the response alleviates need for further action to address the deviation. An example of negative feedback is shown in the figure.

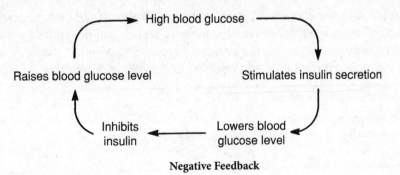

**Negative Feedback**

Here is how an expert would approach a question on feedback loops.

| Question | Analysis |
| --- | --- |
| Which of the following is an example of a negative feedback loop? | **Step 1:** This question is asking for an example of a negative feedback loop. The answers refer to a drop in hormone levels, so you can be more specific with your prediction. |
| | **Step 2:** Recall that in negative feedback, a deviation from homeostasis is detected, a response is made, and the response alleviates the need for further action. |
| | **Step 3:** Predict that a decrease in hormone level will lead to the production of more hormone. Once hormone levels stabilize, no more hormone will be released. |
| (A) A decrease in thyroid hormone levels is detected, and the thyroid produces more hormones. Following the increase in hormone levels, the thyroid produces more hormones. | **Step 4:** A decrease in thyroid hormone would cause more to be released. However, once levels stabilized, the thyroid would release less, not more, hormone. Eliminate. |
| (B) A decrease in thyroid hormone levels is detected, and the thyroid produces less hormones. Following the decrease in hormone levels, the thyroid produces less hormones. | A decrease in thyroid hormone would lead to more, not less, hormone release. Eliminate. |
| (C) A decrease in thyroid hormone levels is detected, and the thyroid produces more hormones. Following the increase in hormone levels, the thyroid produces less hormones. | This is a perfect match for your prediction. Choose choice **(C)**. |
| (D) A decrease in thyroid hormone levels is detected, and the thyroid produces less hormones. Following the increase in hormone levels, the thyroid produces more hormones. | A decrease in thyroid hormone would lead to more, not less, hormone release. Eliminate. |

## The Hypothalamus and Pituitary

The master regulatory gland of the endocrine system is the **hypothalamus**, which is located in the brain under the thalamus. It serves as the link between the nervous system and the endocrine system by releasing hormones that control other endocrine glands in response to different stimuli. The hypothalamus also produces two hormones that are stored and released by the **posterior pituitary**:

- **Oxytocin** stimulates uterine contractions during labor.
- **Vasopressin (antidiuretic hormone)** induces water reabsorption in the kidney. This hormone is discussed in greater detail in Lesson 7: The Genitourinary System.

K

The hypothalamus also releases hormones to induce hormone release from the **anterior pituitary**. The anterior pituitary releases both **direct hormones**, which stimulate a response directly at a target organ, and **tropic hormones**, which induce hormone release by other glands. Following is a summary of the seven hormones released by the anterior pituitary and their functions:

- **Follicle-stimulating hormone (FSH)**: In females, induces the maturation of an ovarian follicle; in males, stimulates spermatogenesis.
- **Luteinizing hormone (LH)**: In females, induces ovulation; in males, stimulates testosterone production.
- **Adrenocorticotropic hormone (ACTH)**: Stimulates the adrenal glands to release hormones.
- **Thyroid-stimulating hormone (TSH)**: Stimulates the thyroid gland to release thyroid hormones.
- **Prolactin**: Induces milk production at the mammary glands in females.
- **Endorphins**: Inhibit the perception of pain.
- **Growth hormone**: Induces growth of the body and increases metabolic rate.

A great mnemonic to remember these hormones is FLAT PEG, where the FLAT hormones are the topic hormones and the PEG hormones are the direct hormones.

## Additional Glands and Hormones and Diseases of the Endocrine System

In addition to the hypothalamus and pituitary gland, many other endocrine glands are either regulated by the hypothalamus or respond directly to physiological changes.

The pineal gland, located in the center of the brain, secretes **melatonin** to regulate sleep cycles. The release of melatonin is governed by light–dark cycles. Melatonin supplements are readily available at drugstores and can be used to induce sleep.

The thyroid and parathyroid are located in the neck and control both metabolism and calcium balance. The parathyroid gland releases **parathyroid hormone** in response to low blood calcium. It induces the breakdown of bone to increase blood calcium levels. The thyroid gland, upon stimulation by TSH, will absorb iodine and produce thyroid hormones. **Thyroid hormones** (T3 and T4) regulate metabolic rate. The thyroid also releases **calcitonin** in response to high blood calcium levels and induces the storage of calcium in bone. It "tones down" blood calcium.

Thyroid diseases include hypothyroidism and hyperthyroidism. **Hypothyroidism** is caused by insufficient thyroid hormone production, and its symptoms include weight gain, fatigue, and cold intolerance. At the other end of the spectrum is **hyperthyroidism**, caused by overproduction of thyroid hormones. Symptoms include weight loss, hyperactivity, and heat intolerance. Additionally, although uncommon in developed countries, insufficient iodine intake can lead to a significant enlargement of the thyroid known as a **goiter**. The widespread availability of iodized salt has greatly reduced the prevalence of goiters.

The pancreas is responsible for regulating blood glucose levels. It releases two main hormones:

- **Insulin** is released in response to high blood glucose. It induces the storage of glucose in glycogen and stimulates glucose uptake by cells.
- **Glucagon** is released in response to low blood glucose. It induces the release of glucose from glycogen stores and gluconeogenesis. A mnemonic for remembering its function is that it is released when the "glucose is gone."

The most common endocrine disease of the pancreas is **diabetes,** caused by insufficient insulin secretion, which leads to abnormally high blood glucose levels. There are two types of diabetes. Type 1 diabetes is caused by damage to the cells that produce insulin and must be treated with administration of exogenous insulin. Type 2 diabetes is caused by insulin resistance: the body still produces insulin, but the cells are unable to respond. Type 2 diabetes can often be managed with diet and lifestyle changes.

The adrenal glands are located just above the kidneys. They are composed of an outer cortex and inner medulla, similar to the kidney. The adrenal medulla secretes **epinephrine,** which induces the "fight or flight" response. The adrenal cortex secretes hormones that regulate salt and sugar balance in the body, including the hormone **aldosterone,** which regulates salt balance and is discussed in greater detail in Lesson 7: The Genitourinary System.

Sex hormones are released by the testes and ovaries. These hormones are steroid hormones and thus have long-lasting effects on the body. **Estrogen** is produced by the ovaries and leads to the development of secondary female sex characteristics. **Progesterone** is also released by the ovaries and maintains the uterine wall. These two hormones are discussed in greater detail in Lesson 9: The Reproductive System in relation to the menstrual cycle. The testes produce **testosterone,** which induces male sexual differentiation in utero and the development of secondary male sex characteristics during puberty.

Now you try a question testing the endocrine system.

Which of the following hormones would be secreted following a drop in blood calcium levels?

(A) Epinephrine
(B) Calcitonin
(C) Parathyroid hormone
(D) Insulin

## Explanation

**Step 1:** This question is asking which hormone is released when blood calcium levels are too low.

**Step 2:** Recall that calcitonin and parathyroid hormone act antagonistically to regulate blood calcium levels. Parathyroid hormone is released when blood calcium is too low, while calcitonin is released when blood calcium is too high.

**Step 3:** Predict that parathyroid hormone would be released due to low blood calcium.

**Step 4:** Choice **(C)** matches this prediction. Epinephrine, (A), is released by the adrenal cortex to initiate the "flight or fight" response. Calcitonin, (B), is released when blood calcium is high, and insulin, (D), regulates blood glucose, not calcium.

## KEY IDEAS

- The endocrine system consists of a number of glands that release hormones into the bloodstream to exert effects on different target tissues.
- Most feedback loops in the body operate under negative feedback, in which the product produced inhibits the release of more product.
- The hypothalamus is the master regulator of the endocrine system and links the nervous system to the endocrine system.

# Endocrine System Practice Questions

1. A client presents with specific overproduction of the hormone aldosterone, which regulates salt balance in the body. This condition can be best explained by a tumor in which of the following endocrine glands?

   (A)  Hypothalamus
   (B)  Anterior pituitary
   (C)  Adrenal cortex
   (D)  Adrenal medulla

2. Which of the following best explains what occurs after a person eats a meal high in refined sugar?

   (A)  Blood glucose rises, triggering a release of insulin and causing blood glucose to increase.
   (B)  Blood glucose drops, triggering a release of glucagon and causing blood glucose to increase.
   (C)  Blood glucose rises, triggering a release of insulin and causing blood glucose to decrease.
   (D)  Blood glucose drops, triggering a release of glucagon and causing blood glucose to decrease.

**Review your work using the explanations in Part Six of this book.**

# LESSON 9

# The Reproductive System

## LEARNING OBJECTIVES

- Identify components of the male and female reproductive systems and their functions
- Describe how the endocrine system regulates the menstrual cycle in females

## Male Reproductive Anatomy

The male reproductive system is responsible for the generation of male gametes, **sperm**. Sperm are generated in the **testes,** which are housed in the **scrotum,** an external pouch that hangs below the penis. The scrotum keeps the temperature of the testes 2–4 degrees Fahrenheit below normal body temperature for sperm production. The scrotum also can be raised or lowered to maintain temperature. The figure highlights some of the components of the male reproductive system.

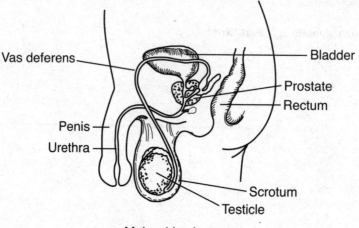

Male: side view

**Male Reproductive System**

Sperm are produced in the **seminiferous tubules** in the testes through the process of **spermatogenesis. Testosterone,** produced by the testes, is responsible for initiating and maintaining sperm production. During spermatogenesis, four haploid sperm cells are produced from one diploid cell through meiotic division, a series of two divisions through which diploid cells produce haploid daughter cells. Sperm are produced continuously in males after the onset of puberty. The sperm cells then travel to the **epididymis,** located just above the seminiferous tubules in the testes, where they gain motility and are stored until ejaculation.

The **vas deferens** carries the sperm from the epididymis to the **ejaculatory duct** during ejaculation. The ejaculatory duct, located just above the prostate gland, is where different glands secrete nutrient-dense fluids that mix with the sperm to produce semen. The **seminal vesicles** secrete a fructose-containing liquid to nourish the sperm, while the **prostate gland** secretes a slightly alkaline fluid that enables the sperm to better survive the acidic female reproductive tract. The **bulbourethral glands** produce a viscous fluid that lubricates the male reproductive tract.

The ejaculatory ducts from the two testes fuse at the **urethra**. Semen travels down the urethra and is ejected from the body through the **penis**. The urethra is also part of the urinary system, as it connects to the bladder.

The pathway through which sperm travel during spermatogenesis through ejaculation can be remembered with the mnemonic SEVEN UP: **S**eminiferous tubules → **E**pididymis → **V**as deferens → **E**jaculatory duct → **N**othing (placeholder) → **U**rethra → **P**enis.

Here is how an expert would approach a question on the reproductive system.

| Question | Analysis |
|---|---|
| The sperm are stored in which of the following sites prior to ejaculation? | **Step 1:** This question is asking where sperm are stored. |
| | **Step 2:** Recall that sperm are produced in the seminiferous tubules and stored in the epididymis prior to ejaculation. |
| | **Step 3:** Predict the correct answer will be epididymis. |
| (A)   Vas deferens | **Step 4:** The vas deferens serves as a conduit for sperm and is not a storage site; eliminate. |
| (B)   Epididymis | Correct. This matches your prediction. |
| (C)   Ejaculatory duct | The ejaculatory duct is where sperm mix with secretions from different glands to form semen; eliminate. |
| (D)   Penis | The penis serves as the final path for sperm to leave the body; eliminate. |

## Female Reproductive Anatomy

The female reproductive system is responsible for the production of female gametes, **ova**, and the incubation of the fetus during pregnancy. The ova are produced in the ovaries through the process of **oogenesis**. During oogenesis, one haploid ovum is produced from one diploid cell along with two polar bodies (dead-end products) through meiotic division, so females have a 1:1 diploid-to-haploid cell ratio whereas males have a 1:4 ratio.

Unlike spermatogenesis, oogenesis is a discontinuous process. Females are born with all the immature ova they will ever have. These immature ova are arrested at the beginning stages of meiotic division. During ovulation, one immature ovum completes the first division and is arrested in the second division. Oogenesis is not completed until after the ovum is fertilized.

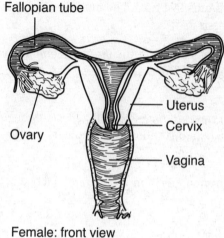

Female: front view

**Female Reproductive System**

During ovulation, the immature ovum is released and travels through the **fallopian tube** to the uterus. If sperm are present, they may fertilize the ovum during its passage through the fallopian tube. If the ovum is fertilized, it will implant in the uterine wall, which is lined with **endometrium**, leading to pregnancy. The endometrium is tissue with many blood vessels that nourishes the developing embryo. It forms the **placenta**, the site of nutrient and waste exchange for the developing fetus. In the absence of pregnancy, the endometrium is shed during **menstruation**.

The uterus connects to the **vagina**, the female reproductive tract, through the **cervix**. During childbirth, the walls of the uterus contract to push the fetus out of the body through the vagina. Additionally, the cervix dilates, increasing in diameter, to allow passage of the fetus.

## The Menstrual Cycle

The female menstrual cycle is approximately 28 days long, though this can vary among individuals. The cycle can be subdivided into two halves: the follicular phase and the luteal phase. In the **follicular phase**, the ovarian follicle matures. Following ovulation, the **luteal phase** begins, during which the ovum awaits fertilization.

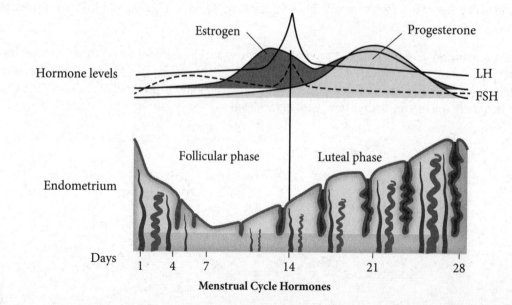

**Menstrual Cycle Hormones**

The cycle starts with menstruation, caused by a drop in hormone levels, which resets the cycle. During the follicular phase, the anterior pituitary releases follicle-stimulating hormone (FSH). FSH acts on the ovaries to induce the release of estrogen. Estrogen leads to the maturation of one **ovarian follicle** and the thickening of the endometrium. Early in the cycle, estrogen inhibits the release of more FSH to prevent the maturation of multiple follicles. However, later in the cycle, estrogen acts in a positive feedback loop to drive more FSH release, culminating in the release of luteinizing hormone (LH). LH induces **ovulation**, during which the ovarian follicle ruptures and releases the egg into a fallopian tube.

Following ovulation, the luteal phase begins. The ruptured follicle develops into the **corpus luteum** and secretes the hormone progesterone to maintain the uterine lining. In the absence of fertilization, the corpus luteum atrophies, causing progesterone levels to drop and triggering menstruation, again resetting the cycle.

Now you try a question on the menstrual cycle.

Which of the following best characterizes the function of estrogen in the menstrual cycle?

(A) Maintains the uterine wall prior to implantation
(B) Induces the rupturing of the ovarian follicle
(C) Induces the thickening of the endometrium
(D) Drives ovulation

## Explanation

**Step 1:** This question is asking for the role of estrogen in the menstrual cycle.

**Step 2:** Recall that estrogen is released from the ovaries in response to the FSH produced by the anterior pituitary. It induces the thickening of the endometrium and development of the ovarian follicle.

**Step 3:** Predict that estrogen will induce follicle development or endometrial thickening.

**Step 4:** Choice **(C)** matches this prediction. Progesterone maintains the uterine wall before implantation, as in choice (A), and LH is responsible for inducing the rupturing of the ovarian follicle, (B), to then drive ovulation, (D).

## KEY IDEAS

- Sperm are produced in the seminiferous tubules of the testes under the control of testosterone.
- During spermatogenesis and ejaculation, the sperm flow through the pathway seminiferous tubules → epididymis → vas deferens → ejaculatory duct → urethra → penis (SEVEN UP).
- Ova are produced in the ovaries and travel through the fallopian tubes, where fertilization occurs, to the uterus, the site of implantation.
- The menstrual cycle is regulated by the hormones FSH, LH, estrogen, and progesterone.

# Reproductive System Practice Questions

1. What hormonal change leads to shedding of the endometrium during menstruation?

    (A)   An increase in LH
    (B)   A decrease in progesterone
    (C)   A decrease in FSH
    (D)   An increase in progesterone

2. Which component of the male reproductive system is also found in females?

    (A)   Vas deferens
    (B)   Epididymis
    (C)   Urethra
    (D)   Cervix

3. In which of the following organs is testosterone primarily made?

    (A)   Testes
    (B)   Uterus
    (C)   Ovaries
    (D)   Penis

**Review your work using the explanations in Part Six of this book.**

# LESSON 10

# The Immune System

## LEARNING OBJECTIVES

- Describe the common barriers to infection
- Identify cellular components of the innate and adaptive arms of the immune system
- List common immune diseases and their causes

The immune system protects our bodies from foreign **pathogens**, or infectious agents. The organs of the immune system include the lymph nodes, thymus, bone marrow, and spleen. All immune cells are born in the bone marrow but can mature in different locations in the body.

The first line of defense against infection is physical barriers, such as the skin, which prevent most pathogens from accessing our bodies. However, when these barriers are breached, immune cells from the innate and adaptive arms target pathogens for destruction. The **innate arm** is quick to respond, but it is not specific to individual pathogens nor does it form memory cells. The **adaptive arm** is slower to activate, but it specifically targets a pathogen and forms memory cells. The figure shows the classification of immune cells into the innate and adaptive arms.

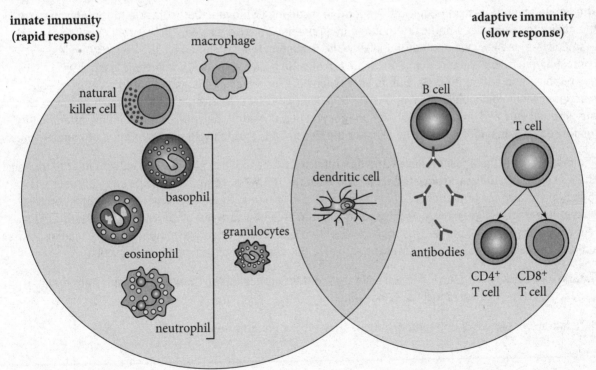

innate immunity
(rapid response)

adaptive immunity
(slow response)

macrophage

natural killer cell

basophil

eosinophil

granulocytes

neutrophil

dendritic cell

B cell

T cell

antibodies

CD4⁺ T cell

CD8⁺ T cell

# Barriers to Infection

Barriers to infection include both physical barriers that block entry of pathogens and proteins that impede pathogen replication. The largest physical barrier is the skin, part of the integumentary system discussed in Lesson 11, which prevents most pathogens from entering the body. The skin also has a moderately acidic pH, between 3 and 5, which discourages replication of most pathogens. The skin is inhabited by **flora**, nonpathogenic microbes that compete for resources and thus prevent pathogen occupancy.

However, the skin does not completely seal the body from the environment, since the body must exchange nutrients and wastes. Other barriers to infection have developed to protect these points of entry, especially the respiratory and digestive systems. The respiratory tract is lined with mucus to trap incoming pathogens. Mucus can be either expelled through coughing, eliminating harmful microbes from the body, or swallowed. Microbes that are swallowed will enter the stomach, where most are killed by the low pH of 2, and survivors must compete for resources with gut flora in the intestines.

In addition to the physical barriers, there are several chemical barriers to infection. Saliva, tears, and mucus all contain the enzyme **lysozyme**, which degrades bacterial cell walls and causes them to lyse, or burst. Cells continuously secrete **antimicrobial peptides** into the bloodstream. These small molecules are broad-spectrum antimicrobials that target and kill many bacterial, viral, and fungal pathogens to prevent infection. If a cell becomes infected, it will secrete **interferon**, a small chemical messenger, to signal to nearby cells the presence of a foreign pathogen and activate innate defenses in those cells.

# Cells of the Innate Immune System

The innate immune system is quick to respond to incoming pathogens but is unable to form **memory**, or the ability to remember a pathogen that has been previously encountered. This system consists of granulocytes, monocytes, and natural killer cells. **Granulocytes** are named for the dense granules, containing reactive oxygen compounds and cytokines, in their cytoplasm and include basophils, eosinophils, and neutrophils. **Basophils** are responsible for releasing histamine and mediating allergic reactions, while **eosinophils** are responsible for killing parasites. **Neutrophils** are the most common of the granulocytes and are responsible for **phagocytosing**, or eating, bacteria and mediating inflammatory responses. **Inflammation** leads to swelling of the tissue and fever, as well as recruitment of immune cells.

The monocytes include macrophages and **dendritic cells**, phagocytic cells that kill extracellular pathogens. They recognize **pathogen-associated molecular patterns (PAMPs)**, common proteins and carbohydrates found on the surface of pathogens that are not specific to one **antigen**, the term for a microbial protein. **Macrophages** also digest dying cells, especially in the spleen where red blood cells die. Dendritic cells, following phagocytosis, present microbial antigens to cells of the adaptive immune system, leading to their activation. Macrophages can also present antigens, but not as effectively as dendritic cells.

**Natural killer (NK) cells** attack and kill cells that contain intracellular pathogens or display abnormal surface antigens. Examples include tumor cells.

Here is how an expert would approach a question on the immune system.

| Question | Analysis |
|---|---|
| Which of the following innate immune cells is most effective at activating the adaptive immune response? | **Step 1:** This question is asking for an innate immune cell that most effectively activates the adaptive immune response. |
| | **Step 2:** Recall that antigen-presenting cells, macrophages and dendritic cells, will phagocytose pathogens and display their antigens to cells of the adaptive immune system. |
| | **Step 3:** Predict that dendritic cells best activate the adaptive immune response. Macrophages also activate it, but do so less effectively. |
| (A)  Neutrophil | **Step 4:** Although neutrophils are phagocytic, they do not display antigens to other cells. Eliminate. |
| (B)  Dendritic cell | Correct. This matches your prediction. |
| (C)  Macrophage | Macrophages are capable of presenting antigens but are not the main cell that does do. Eliminate. |
| (D)  Interferon | Interferon is a protein, not a cell. Eliminate. |

## Cells of the Adaptive Immune System

The adaptive immune system is slower to respond because it must first be activated by antigen presentation by cells of the innate immune system. Once activated, it will specifically target pathogens and host cells displaying the presented antigen. Following clearance of the infection, memory cells are formed, which will activate quickly following a secondary encounter with the same pathogen. The quick activation of memory cells underlies the usefulness of **vaccination**. During vaccination, the immune system is challenged by a weakened pathogen and forms memory cells. These cells will quickly activate and kill the pathogen when exposed a second time, preventing or minimizing infection and the development of symptoms.

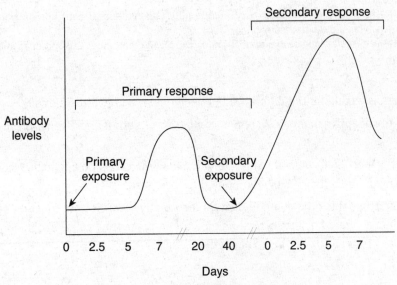

**Activation of the Adaptive Immune System**

The adaptive immune system includes both T and B cells. **T cells** are born in the bone marrow; released into the bloodstream as immune cells; and travel to the **thymus,** a lymphoid organ, for maturation. While in the thymus, T cells can mature into either helper T cells or cytotoxic T cells and then are released to circulate in the blood and lymph systems. **Helper T cells**, following activation by antigen-presenting cells, help to activate other adaptive immune cells such as cytotoxic T and B cells. Helper T cells are targeted and killed by the **human immunodeficiency virus (HIV),** the virus responsible for **acquired immunodeficiency syndrome (AIDS),** leading to a loss of immune function. When a cause of death is written as complications related to AIDS, this indicates that the individual succumbed to infections caused by pathogens that are typically harmless to relatively healthy individuals.

**Cytotoxic T cells,** when activated, will kill a host cell that expresses a foreign antigen. Cytotoxic T cells are antigen specific, meaning that they will only kill a cell that displays the single antigen they were primed to recognize.

**B cells** are both born in and mature in the bone marrow. Following activation, they develop into **plasma cells** and secrete **antibodies,** proteins that specifically bind to viral antigens. A given B cell will only produce one type of antibody. Antibodies will either target pathogens for phagocytosis, coating them to render them noninfectious, or target them for complement-mediated lysis. The **complement system** is composed of multiple proteins that are free-floating in the blood. When coating a pathogen, antibodies recruit these proteins, leading to the formation of a pore in the membrane of the pathogen and causing cell lysis. Antibodies can be acquired either by **active immunity,** through production by plasma cells, or **passive immunity,** through the introduction antibodies from an external source. Common examples of passive immunity include antibody transfer from breastfeeding and therapeutic antibody delivery to people with infections.

Now try a question on your own.

Which of the following correctly identifies the difference between helper and cytotoxic T cells?

(A)  Helper T cells activate antigen-presenting cells, and cytotoxic T cells kill infected cells displaying a particular antigen.

(B)  Helper T cells produce antibodies, and cytotoxic T cells kill infected cells displaying a particular antigen.

(C)  Helper T cells activate cytotoxic T and B cells, and cytotoxic T cells kill infected cells displaying a particular antigen.

(D)  Helper T cells activate cytotoxic T and B cells, and cytotoxic T cells produce antibodies.

## Explanation

**Step 1:** This question is asking for the difference between helper and cytotoxic T cells.

**Step 2:** Recall that the adaptive immune system is composed of both B and T cells. B cells produce antibodies.

**Step 3:** Predict that helper T cells activate other adaptive immune cells and cytotoxic T cells attack cells displaying a particular antigen they have been primed to recognize.

**Step 4:** Choice **(C)** matches this prediction. Choice (A) incorrectly identifies the function of helper T cells because they are activated by, not activators of, antigen-presenting cells. T cells do not produce antibodies, so choices (B) and (D) can be eliminated.

The adaptive immune system is normally **self-tolerant**, in that it does not respond to normal cellular antigens. However in some cases, it targets healthy host cells, leading to **autoimmune disease**. Autoimmune disorders include type 1 diabetes, in which the immune system targets the pancreas, and lupus, in which the immune system targets multiple organs.

## KEY IDEAS

- Barriers to infection include physical barriers and chemical barriers.
- The cellular innate immune system includes cells that recognize common patterns on pathogens and quickly destroy them. However, the innate immune system is not antigen-specific, nor does it form memory cells.
- The cellular adaptive immune system includes cells that target a particular antigen of a pathogen, making them antigen-specific. They are slow to activate during the first exposure to a pathogen, but they form memory cells, which facilitate quicker subsequent responses.
- Depression of immune function leaves the body vulnerable to infection, while overactivation of the immune system leads to the targeting of healthy host cells.

# Immune System Practice Questions

1. Type 1 diabetes is an autoimmune condition caused by the immune system specifically targeting and killing beta cells, which produce insulin in the pancreas, that display a particular antigen. Which of the following best describes the cellular activity responsible for this disease?

   (A) Macrophages phagocytose and kill beta cells that display the antigen.
   (B) Cytotoxic T cells kill beta cells that display the antigen.
   (C) Helper T cells kill beta cells that display the antigen.
   (D) In response to the antigen, neutrophils release interferons that kill beta cells.

2. Which of the following is NOT a component of the innate immune system?

   (A) T cell
   (B) Macrophage
   (C) Dendritic cell
   (D) Neutrophil

3. Which one of the following phagocytoses all kinds of pathogenic cells without specifically targeting them?

   (A) Macrophage
   (B) Helper T cell
   (C) Natural killer cell
   (D) B cell

**Review your work using the explanations in Part Six of this book.**

# LESSON 11

# The Integumentary System

## LEARNING OBJECTIVES

- Identify the structures of the integumentary system and describe their functions
- Describe the role of the integumentary system in thermoregulation

The **integumentary system** is comprised of the largest organ in the human body—the skin—along with hair, nails, and accessory glands. The integumentary system is in constant contact with the external environment and provides protection from and picks up signals about the body's surroundings.

## Anatomy and Physiology of the Integumentary System

The primary organ of the integumentary system is the skin, or **integument**. The skin consists of three principal layers: the epidermis, the dermis, and the hypodermis. The **epidermis** is the outermost layer of the skin. It provides a barrier to infection from environmental pathogens and regulates the amount of water lost to the body's surroundings. The epidermis is constantly being replaced with new skin cells. The **dermis**, or middle layer of the skin, contains nerve endings, hair follicles, sweat and oil glands, and capillaries. The **hypodermis** is the deepest layer of the skin and contains blood vessels and **adipose** (fat) tissues.

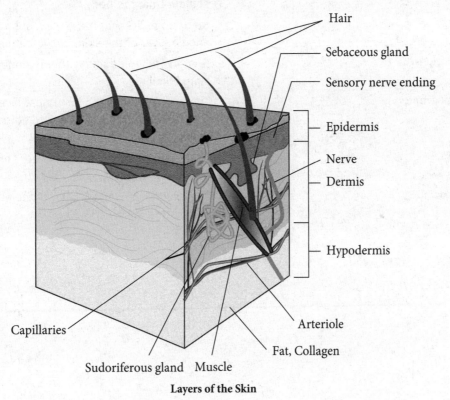

**Layers of the Skin**

Sweat glands, or **sudoriferous glands**, are responsible for the excretion of water and minerals from the body, in particular sodium, chloride, and magnesium. Sweat can also contain trace amounts of urea or other waste products in the blood, like alcohol or lactic acid. There are two types of sweat gland: eccrine and apocine. **Eccrine glands** appear all over the body and are the primary sweat glands of the body; **apocrine glands** are not active until puberty and are found in the armpits, nipples, and groin.

Oil glands, or **sebaceous glands**, secrete sebum, a mixture of fats and proteins that prevents the skin and hair from drying out. Sebaceous glands are found all over the body with the exception of the soles of the feet and palms of the hand.

**Hair follicles** are columns in the skin that have a large concentration of keratin-producing cells. These cells form the hair while adjacent melanin-producing cells give hair its pigmentation. The hairless parts of the body include the soles of the feet, lips, inner labia, and glans penis. Hair protects the body from UV radiation by preventing sunlight from reaching the surface of the skin. Nails, also made of keratin, are formed by keratin-producing cells at the ends of the fingers and toes.

Here is how a TEAS expert would answer a question about the integumentary system.

| Question | Analysis |
|---|---|
| Which of the follow layers of skin contains glands that excrete sodium? | **Step 1:** This question is asking about what anatomical features are found in the layers of the skin. |
| | **Step 2:** Recall that all glands are located in the middle layer of the skin. These include the sudoriferous (sweat) glands, which excrete excess sodium from the body. |
| | **Step 3:** Predict that the correct answer is the middle layer of the skin, or the dermis. |
| (A) Epidermis | **Step 4:** The epidermis is the outermost layer of the skin. Eliminate. |
| (B) Hypodermis | The hypodermis is the innermost layer of the skin and contains blood vessels and adipose tissue. Eliminate. |
| (C) Dermis | Correct. The dermis contains nerve endings, follicles, and glands. |
| (D) Exodermis | The exodermis is not a layer of the human skin. Eliminate. |

# Thermoregulation

The integumentary system plays a vital role in thermal homeostasis, or regulating the body's internal temperature, by controlling how the body interacts with the surrounding environment.

When sensory nerves in the skin indicate that the body is entering a state of **hyperthermia**, meaning that the body temperature is elevated above normal, the integumentary system helps to reduce body temperature through sweat and vasodilation of the blood vessels. The sudoriferous glands deliver water to the skin in the form of sweat, which evaporates from the skin's surface. As the water evaporates, it absorbs and carries away heat with it, cooling the body. Dilated blood vessels in the dermis allow more blood to get near the surface of the skin, carrying excess heat from the body's core. This heat is then released to the external environment as thermal radiation.

The integumentary system also ensures that additional heat is not trapped against the skin's surface. Tiny muscles attached to the hair follicles relax so that the hairs lie flat against the surface. This increases air flow next to the skin and aids in radiative and evaporative heat loss.

When the body enters a state of **hypothermia**, meaning that body temperature drops below normal, the integumentary system prevents heat loss. Blood vessels constrict to reduce the amount of blood flow through the skin, limiting the amount of heat lost to the external environment through radiation. The muscles of the hair follicles contract to lift the hair upright, trapping air against the surface of the skin and helping to insulate the body. This is often referred to as "goose bumps" when the contracted muscles can be seen as bumps beneath the skin.

| Feature | Cooling the Body | Warming the Body |
|---|---|---|
| Blood vessels | Dilate | Constrict |
| Sudoriferous glands | Increase sweating | Cease sweating |
| Hair follicles | Relax | Stand erect |
| | | |

**Thermoregulation by the Integumentary System**

Now try answering this question about the integumentary system.

Which of the following reactions would take place after walking into a very cold room?

(A)   Sebaceous glands would decrease excretion.
(B)   Sudoriforous glands would increase excretion.
(C)   Blood vessels would increase blood flow to the skin.
(D)   Hair follicles would decrease air flow across the skin.

## Explanation

**Step 1:** This question is asking about how the body reacts to a hypothermic environment.

**Step 2:** Recall that when body temperature drops, the skin helps to reduce heat loss by limiting evaporative cooling, reducing blood flow to the surface of the skin, and trapping air against the skin to provide insulation.

**Step 3:** Predict that the correct answer will involve decreased sweating, decreased blood flow, or increased air trapped against the skin.

**Step 4:** Answer choice **(D)** matches the prediction. The muscles of the hair follicles constrict, lifting the hair and trapping air against the skin's surface. This restricts air flow across the surface to limit evaporative cooling. The sebaceous glands, (A), do not assist with thermoregulation, since they produce oil rather than water. Excretion from the sudoriforous glands, or sweat, would decrease rather than increase in this situation, so choice (B) is the opposite of the prediction. Blood vessels would constrict blood flow to the skin's surface, the opposite of what (C) states, making this choice incorrect.

## KEY IDEAS

- The integumentary system is in constant contact with the external environment and thus serves as a protective barrier and as a sensory receptor.
- The integumentary system plays a vital role in regulating body temperature.
- There are three layers to the skin: the epidermis, the dermis, and the hypodermis.

# Integumentary System Practice Questions

1. Hair and nails are comprised of which of the following?

   (A)  Collagen
   (B) ، Keratin
   (C)  Melanin
   (D)  Elastin

2. Which of the following mechanisms does the body use to increase heat loss?

   (A) ، Sweating
   (B)  Vasoconstriction
   (C)  Shivering
   (D)  Panting

3. Which of the following are found in the hypodermis?

   (A)  Apocrine glands
   (B)  Hair follicles
   (C)  Pores
   (D) ، Adipose tissue

**Review your work using the explanations in Part Six of this book.**

# CHAPTER TWO

# BIOLOGY AND CHEMISTRY

## LEARNING OBJECTIVES

- Identify the chemical structure of macromolecules and describe their function in the body
- Explain how chromosomes, genes, and DNA determine the distribution of genotypes and phenotypes in offpsring
- Determine the components and structure of an atom and infer the characteristics of an element based on information from the periodic table
- Classify the physical properties of substances and explain how the physical properties of water and other substances affect their action in the body
- Describe the different states of matter and explain various phase transitions
- Analyze information about chemical reactions, including identifying types of chemical bonds, balancing chemical equations, and interpreting information about pH

Of the 47 scored *Science* questions, 8 (17%) will be in the sub-content area of *Life and physical sciences*. Questions will evaluate your knowledge of the function of macromolecules in the body, heredity and genetics, and various topics in chemistry such as the periodic table, states of matter, and chemical reactions.

This chapter addresses these topics in six lessons:

**Lesson 1:** Macromolecules: Carbohydrates, Proteins, and Lipids

**Lesson 2:** Heredity

**Lesson 3:** Atoms and the Periodic Table

**Lesson 4:** Properties of Substances

**Lesson 5:** States of Matter

**Lesson 6:** Chemical Reactions

**Science Questions by Sub-content Area**

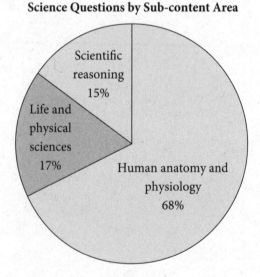

# LESSON 1

# Macromolecules: Carbohydrates, Proteins, and Lipids

## LEARNING OBJECTIVES

- Identify the chemical structure of carbohydrates, lipids, and proteins
- Describe the functions of different macromolecules in the body

Living organisms are made up of four classes of organic **macromolecules**: carbohydrates, lipids, proteins, and nucleic acids. The large molecules are composed of smaller molecules, or **monomers**, that serve as building blocks. Multiple monomers joined together are called **polymers**.

The bonds of polymers are created by **dehydration synthesis**, the removal of a water molecule to create a covalent bond (discussed further in Lesson 6: Chemical Reactions). These bonds can be broken by **hydrolysis**, the addition of a water molecule to split apart the two monomers and release energy.

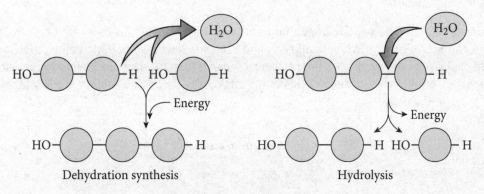

**Dehydration Synthesis and Hydrolysis**

The TEAS may ask you to recognize the monomers, polymers, and bonding patterns of different macromolecules.

## Carbohydrates

**Carbohydrates** are sugars or starches that contain carbon (C), oxygen (O), and hydrogen (H). Carbohydrate monomers, called **monosaccharides**, have the chemical formula $C_nH_{2n}O_n$. Glucose and fructose, for example, both have the chemical formula $C_6H_{12}O_6$, while ribose has the chemical formula $C_5H_{10}O_5$.

When two monosaccharides undergo dehydration synthesis, they form a **disaccharide**. For instance, sugar, or sucrose, is formed from a glucose and a fructose molecule. Mono- and disaccharides are important sources of energy that are found in fruits (sucrose and fructose) and milk products (lactose).

Larger chains of carbohydrates are called **polysaccharides**. Polysaccharides are made of long, repeated strands of monomers that can be linear or branched. Some polysaccharides are composed only of glucose; these include cellulose, starch, and glycogen. **Glycogen** is stored in the liver and muscle tissue as a form of energy. Plants store energy in the form of **starch**, formed from the glucose polymers **amylose** and **amylopectin**, which can be broken down into glucose during the digestive process. Potatoes, grains, rices, and bean products are high in starch. **Cellulose** is a linear polysaccharide that is found in the structural material of plants; the human body lacks the enzyme necessary to break the bonds of of cellulose, so this is not digestible. Instead, cellulose acts as fiber that helps move material through the digestive tract.

Other polysaccharides contain carbohydrate units as well as other compounds. **Chitin** contains glucose and amino acids and forms the exterior skeleton of arthropods. Glycoproteins and glycolipids play important roles in cellular communication.

## Proteins

**Proteins** are found in hair, muscle, bone, and nearly all other tissues and cells. Protein monomers are called **amino acids**. These contain an amino group ($NH_3^+$), a carboxyl group ($COO^-$), hydrogen (H), and a side chain (R group). There are 20 different amino acids, each with different chemical properties due to differences in their R group.

Amino groups are linked by a **peptide bond** that forms with the removal of a water molecule from the carboxyl and amino groups. When multiple amino acids are linked by peptide bonds, they form a **polypeptide chain**, often referred to as the protein's primary structure. The three-dimensional structure of a protein depends on the specific amino acids in the chain; this shape of a protein is a key factor in the role that it plays in the body.

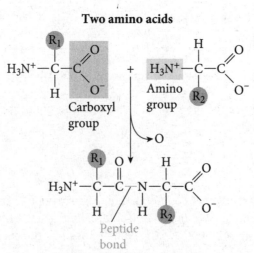

**Amino Acid Structure and Peptide Bond Formation**

**Globular proteins** contain R groups that allow them to be soluble in water. Thus, these proteins can be transported in the blood. The most recognized globular protein is hemoglobin. Globular proteins also serve as cellular messages (e.g., hormones), in the immune system (i.e., immunoglobulins and antibodies), and as enzymes. **Fibrous proteins** do not dissolve in water; these are found in structural compounds like hair and nails (keratin) and connective tissue (collagen).

Membrane proteins that contain both water-soluble and insoluble components are often embedded in cell membranes and serve as receptors for signal transfer between cells and transport ions or other materials across membranes.

**Enzymes** are a special category of proteins that catalyze specific biological reactions. Enzymes speed up the rate of reaction by lowering the **activation energy**, or energy required for the reaction to take place. The shape of an enzyme is specifically suited to bond to one type of substrate at the enzyme's **active site**.

See how a TEAS expert would answer a question about proteins.

| Question | Analysis |
|---|---|
| Which of the following does NOT contain protein? | **Step 1:** This question is asking about the location of protein in different body parts. |
| | **Step 2:** Recall that protein is found in all cell membranes and tissues. |
| | **Step 3:** Predict that the correct answer is *not* part of a cell membrane, a tissue type, or an organ composed of tissues. |
| (A) Cell membrane | **Step 4:** Proteins are embedded within the cell membrane to facilitate transport and cellular communication. Eliminate. |
| (B) Muscle tissue | Muscle tissue, like all tissue, is formed from protein. Actin and myosin are examples of protein filaments found in muscle tissue. Eliminate. |
| (C) Genetic material | Correct. Genetic material, such as DNA or RNA, is formed from nucleic acids. It does *not* contain amino acids. |
| (D) Skeleton | The skeleton is composed of bone tissue, which, like all tissue, contains protein. Eliminate. |

# Lipids

**Lipids**, also commonly called fats, contain long strands of hydrogen (H) and carbon (C) atoms called **hydrocarbon chains**. These chains are **hydrophobic**, meaning they do not dissolve in water, and vary in length. If a hydrocarbon chain ends in a carboxyl group it is called a **fatty acid**. There are three main categories of lipids in the body: triglycerides, phospholipids, and steroids.

**Triglycerides** contain three fatty-acid chains bound to a glycerol molecule. These fatty-acid chains can be **saturated**, meaning that every carbon molecule is bound to two hydrogens, or **unsaturated**, meaning that some carbon molecules in the chain are bound to one hydrogen and double-bonded to the adjacent carbon. Triglycerides are used in the body as a form of long-term energy storage in adipose tissue. Triglycerides also cushion nerves as an important component of the myelin sheath and insulate the body. Fatty acids are consumed in the form of plant oils and animal fats.

**Phospholipids** make up the membrane of every cell. They contain two fatty acids bound to a **hydrophilic**, or water-loving, phosphate group. The phosphate end of a phospholipid will dissolve in water, while the fatty acid end won't.

The third category of lipids is **steroids**. Steroids don't contain fatty acids but are hydrophobic like other lipids. Steroids include cholesterol and sex hormones, like estrogen and testosterone, that are made from cholesterol.

## Nucleic Acids

**Nucleic acids** supply the genetic material for all living cells. The monomer for nucleic acids is called a **nucleotide**. A nucleotide has three parts: a phosphate group, a five-carbon sugar ring, and a nitrogenous base. There are two types of nucleic acids—deoxyribonucleic acid (DNA) and ribonucleic acid (RNA)—each with its own type of nucleotide.

**Deoxyribonucleic acid (DNA)** is found in chromosomes and stores the genetic information of an organism. It has a sugar backbone of deoxyribose and contains the bases adenine, guanine, cytosine, or thyamine (A, G, C, T). **Ribonucleic acid (RNA)** translates the DNA into a form that can be read to create proteins; has a sugar backbone of ribose; and has nucleotides that contain bases adenine, guanine, cytosine, or uracil (A, G, C, U). DNA appears in the body as two chains of nucleotides called a double helix. RNA consists of a single strand.

Nucleotides also function as a source of energy in the form of **ATP (adenosine triphosphate)**.

Now you try answering a question about macromolecules.

> Assuming each macromolecule is of equal weight, which of the following macromolecules would have the greatest number of C-H bonds?
>
> (A) Polypeptide
> (B) Saturated fatty acid
> (C) Polysaccharide
> (D) Unsaturated fatty acid

### Explanation

**Step 1:** This question is asking about C-H bonds.

**Step 2:** Recall that C-H bonds are found in greatest frequency in hydrocarbon chains, which are composed solely of carbon and hydrogen.

**Step 3:** Predict that the answer is a lipid that contains a hydrocarbon chain.

**Step 4:** Choice **(B)** is the answer. Both saturated and unsaturated fatty acids contain hydrocarbon chains, but saturated fatty acids contain the maximum amount of hydrogen atoms. A polypeptide is a protein consisting of amino acids, and a polysaccharide is a carbohydrate.

---

## KEY IDEAS

- Carbohydrates are formed of carbon, hydrogen, and oxygen and play four important roles, providing energy for cells, short-term energy storage, structural support, and cellular communication.
- Proteins are made of amino acids and are found throughout the body.
- Fatty acids are long strands of hydrocarbons and are used for long-term energy storage in the form of triglycerides.
- Nucleic acids are made of nucleotides and are found in genetic material.

# Macromolecules Practice Questions

1. Which of the following is a polysaccharide stored in the liver?

    (A)  Amylose
    (B)  Cellulose
    (C)  Glycerol
    (D)  Glycogen

2. Which of the following nitrogenous bases is found in ribonucleic acid (RNA) but not in deoxyribonucleic acid (DNA)?

    (A)  Guanine
    (B)  Adenine
    (C)  Uracil
    (D)  Thymine

3. Which of the following is a true statement about enzymes?

    (A)  Enzymes are proteins that increase the rate of biological reactions.
    (B)  Enzymes are formed by joining two nitrogenous bases with a peptide bond.
    (C)  Enzymes catalyze reactions by binding to many different types of molecule.
    (D)  Enzymes are fibrous proteins made of amino acids.

**Review your work using the explanations in Part Six of this book.**

# LESSON 2

# Heredity

## LEARNING OBJECTIVES

- Explain the function of chromosomes, genes, and DNA and the relationship and difference between them
- Describe how genetics determine the physical characteristics of an organism
- Distinguish between dominant and recessive traits and between genotype and phenotype
- Use a Punnett square to predict traits of offspring
- Recognize several health problems that are genetically inherited

Even before the science was defined, people recognized that children looked more like their parents than other adults. The passing of traits or characteristics from parents to offspring through the inheritance of genes is called **heredity**.

**DNA** (deoxyribonucleic acid) is a molecule that contains genetic information that determines our physical characteristics or traits. DNA exists in the nucleus of our cells, in rod-shaped structures called **chromosomes**. A **gene**, defined as the unit of inheritance, is a specific section of DNA in a specific location on a chromosome. Genes contain information that codes for proteins, which dictate how a cell functions.

DNA controls the cell's production of proteins. A strand of DNA takes on a characteristic shape, called a double helix, which looks like a ladder that is twisted along its axis. Each rung of the ladder is made of a pair of nitrogen bases. There are four of these bases: adenine (A), guanine (G), thymine (T), and cytosine (C). The four bases pair up in a specific way: A always pairs with T, and C always pairs with G. The sides of the ladder are made of a pentose sugar and phosphate. These items—a pentose sugar, a phosphate group, and the nitrogen base—create a nucleotide. Nucleotides bind together in a specific pattern to form a genetic code that defines the trait and is interpreted by the cell to instruct it how to grow and behave.

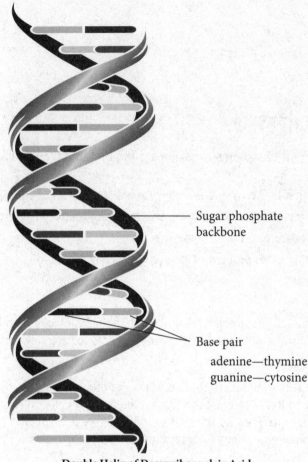

Sugar phosphate
backbone

Base pair
adenine—thymine
guanine—cytosine

**Double Helix of Deoxyribonucleic Acid**

For a protein to be expressed, the DNA must first be **transcribed** to mRNA. This mRNA then leaves the nucleus and is **translated** into protein by ribosomes. Each group of three DNA letters is called a **codon**; each codon codes for an amino acid, and the amino acids are linked together as translation takes place.

## Cell Replication

Most of the body's cells are produced through a process called **mitosis**. Mitosis is a process of cell division that results in two identical daughter cells from a single parent. The number of chromosomes remains the same as the parent, 46. This is a **diploid** cell. During **meiosis**, the original cell divides twice and the four resulting cells each contain a single copy of each chromosome, a **haploid**. In humans, **gametes** (i.e., an ovum and a sperm cell), each of which contains 23 unpaired chromosomes (haploid), unite to produce a zygote, which contains 23 pairs of chromosomes, or 46 chromosomes (diploid).

# Genes and Alleles

**Chromosomes** are compressed bodies of DNA molecules that store codes for the translation of several different kinds of proteins. One chromosome can contain thousands of genes on a single long molecule of DNA.

A gene may come in several variations, known as **alleles**. Alleles specifically code for the traits of an organism. Humans have two copies of every gene (two alleles) for every trait, one inherited from each parent. These alleles may be alike, or may not. If the alleles are alike, that person is **homozygous** for that particular gene. If the alleles are different, the person is **heterozygous** for that particular gene.

When different traits are paired up during the fertilization of an egg, often one allele is **dominant** over the other. A dominant allele hides the expression of the other allele in the phenotype of the offspring. The other allele is called **recessive**. A dominant trait will be expressed even if only one copy (paired with a recessive trait) is present. A recessive trait, on the other hand, is only expressed if the offspring has two copies of the allele. Dominant alleles are typically symbolized with capital letters and recessive alleles with lowercase letters.

If both alleles are the dominant allele, the gene is called homozygous dominant. If both alleles are recessive, the gene is called homozygous recessive. If the organism has different alleles, it is called heterozygous for the gene.

Brown eye color is dominant to blue eye color. If brown eye color is the dominant allele (indicated as B) and blue eye color is the recessive allele (indicated as b), an offspring of parents both heterozygous for the particular gene could have one of three different genotypes (BB, Bb, and bb) when the parents' gametes combine. **Genotype** is the genetic makeup, including both dominant and recessive alleles. The **phenotype** of an offspring is how the genes express themselves in physical characteristics. The table summarizes the possible genotypes, or allele combinations, along with their corresponding phenotype, or visible trait, for this example.

| Genotype | Phenotype | Homozygous or Heterozygous |
|----------|-----------|----------------------------|
| BB | Brown eyes | Homozygous dominant |
| Bb | Brown eyes | Heterozygous |
| bb | Blue eyes | Homozygous recessive |

Different factors can affect phenotype and genotype in offspring. One example is **incomplete dominance**, in which both heterozygous alleles are expressed. The offspring displays a combined phenotype that is distinct from that of either parent. Another factor affecting phenotype and genotype is **codominance**, in which both alleles are independently expressed. For example, a flower with codominant red and white alleles would have red and white patches. However, these same alleles under incomplete dominance would yield a pink flower.

# Punnett Squares

The TEAS may ask for the probability that an offspring of a particular set of parents will have a given trait. For example, brown eye color (B) is dominant over blue eye color (b). To determine the probability that a brown-eyed mother and a brown-eyed father, both with heterozygous genotypes (Bb), will have a blue-eyed child, use a **Punnett square**. Write the genotype of the mother across the top of the grid and that of the father down the left side. Fill the boxes by copying the row and column headers. These squares depict the predicted frequency of all potential genotypes among the offspring each time reproduction occurs.

|   | B | b |
|---|---|---|
| **B** | BB | Bb |
| **b** | Bb | bb |

The probability that these parents will have a child with blue eyes (bb) is 1 out of 4, or 25%.

Here is how an expert would approach a question about predicting the likelihood of an offspring inheriting a particular trait.

| Question | Analysis |
|---|---|
| Dark hair is dominant over red hair. What is the probability that a red-haired mother and a dark-haired father with a heterozygous genotype will have a dark-haired child? | **Step 1:** The question asks about the probability of having a dark-haired child, and dark hair is a dominant trait (D). |
| | **Step 2:** Recall that a dominant trait will be expressed even if only one copy is present. The mother is red haired, which is the recessive phenotype. Therefore, her genotype must be dd. The father is heterozygous, so his genotype is Dd. |
| (A) 25% <br> (B) 50% <br> (C) 75% <br> (D) 100% | **Step 3:** Use a Punnett square to solve the problem. <br><br> |   | d | d | <br> |---|---|---| <br> | **D** | Dd | Dd | <br> | **d** | dd | dd | <br><br> Two of the four genotype combinations in the Punnett square are Dd, so the chance the offspring will have dark hair is 50%. |
| | **Step 4:** The correct answer is choice **(B)**. |

Genetic traits can be classified by whether they are transmitted on autosomal chromosomes (numbers 1–22) or on sex chromosomes (the X most often, as it carries more genes than does the Y). The table identifies characteristics of different inheritance patterns.

| Autosomal Dominant | Autosomal Recessive | X-Linked Dominant | X-Linked Recessive |
|---|---|---|---|
| • Males and females are equally likely to have the trait.<br><br>• Traits do not skip generations.<br><br>• The trait is present if the corresponding gene is present.<br><br>• There is male-to-male and female-to-female transmission. | • Males and females are equally likely to have the trait.<br><br>• Traits often skip generations.<br><br>• Only homozygous recessive individuals have the trait.<br><br>• Traits can appear in siblings without appearing in parents.<br><br>• If a parent has the trait, those offspring who do not have it are heterozygous carriers of the trait. | • All daughters of a male who has the trait will also have the trait.<br><br>• There is no male-to-male transmission.<br><br>• A female who has the trait may or may not pass the affected X chromosome to her son or daughter (unless she has two affected X chromosomes). | • Males are more likely to have the trait because they have only one copy of the X chromosome.<br><br>• Women are affected when they have two copies of the mutant allele.<br><br>• There is no father-to-son transmission, but there is father-to-daughter and mother-to-daughter transmission. |

Marfan's syndrome, which affects the connective tissue, is caused by an autosomal dominant inheritance disease, so only one copy of the trait is necessary for a child to inherit the disorder. On the other hand, cystic fibrosis, which affects the lungs, is caused by a recessive trait that must be inherited from both parents. Other disorders that are caused by genetic traits include some types of cancer, sickle cell anemia, and Huntington's disease.

Now you try a question on inheritance.

Consider two parents who are both heterozygous for sickle cell anemia, a recessive genetic disease. What is the probability that an offspring will have the disorder?

(A) 25%
(B) 50%
(C) 75%
(D) 100%

## Explanation

**Step 1:** The question asks about the probability of an offspring of two parents heterozygous for sickle cell anemia having the disease. If $s$ is used to represent the recessive gene (and $S$ used to represent the gene that does not code for the disease), the parents' genotype is Ss.

**Step 2:** Recall that a recessive trait is expressed only if the offspring has two copies of that allele. The offspring will need two recessive alleles (ss) to express sickle cell anemia.

**Step 3:** Use a Punnett square to solve the problem. It results in three genotypes (SS, Ss, and ss), but only two phenotypes because the dominant trait is expressed in the SS and Ss individuals. The recessive trait shows up in the offspring with a probability of 25%.

|   | S  | s  |
|---|----|----|
| S | SS | Ss |
| s | Ss | ss |

**Step 4:** Choice **(A)**, 25%, is correct. Choice (C) is the probability that the offspring will have at least one dominant allele and thus not have the disease.

## Laws of Mendelian Inheritance

Mendel's Law of Segregation describes the separation of the alleles of the parent genotype in the formation of gametes. There can be a maximum of two different alleles from a single parent; half the gametes get one allele, and the other half get the other allele.

Mendel's Law of Independent Assortment suggests that different genes sort into different gametes, independently of each other. For example, the sorting of alleles for eye color is not affected by the sorting of alleles for earlobe attachment.

Mendel's Law of Dominance states that one factor in a pair of traits dominates the other in inheritance, unless both factors in the pair are recessive.

The first two laws above explain the 3:1 and 9:3:3:1 ratios of phenotypes observed in monohybrid and dihybrid crosses discussed next.

## Monohybrid and Dihybrid Cross

The Punnett square in the previous question depicts a **monohybrid cross**—both parents are heterozygous for the given trait. You can also analyze the inheritance of two genes using a Punnett square. Just account for every combination of the two alleles in each parent's gametes. Try the following question about a **dihybrid cross** between two individuals who are heterozygous for both genes.

Both Tom and Mary Jo are brown eyed, but their baby, John, is blue eyed. Tom and Mary Jo have free earlobes, but John's earlobes are completely attached. Brown eyes (B) are dominant to blue eyes (b), and free earlobes (A) are dominant to attached earlobes (a). What is the probability that John's baby sister will have brown eyes and free earlobes like her parents?

(A) $\frac{1}{16}$

(B) $\frac{3}{16}$

(C) $\frac{7}{16}$

(D) $\frac{9}{16}$

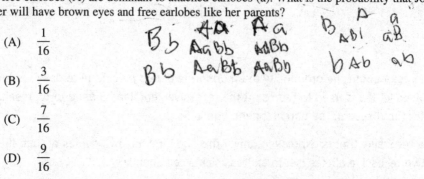

## Explanation

**Step 1:** The question is asking about the inheritance of two traits, eye color and earlobe attachment. You are told that brown eyes and free earlobes are dominant, that both parents have the dominant phenotype for both traits, and that one child has a phenotype of recessive traits (blue eyes, attached earlobes).

**Step 2:** Recall that for an offspring to express a recessive trait, he must have two recessive genes. This means that John inherited a recessive allele from both parents. Since the parents have the dominant phenotype, they must be heterozygous for both traits (BbAa). Make a Punnett square listing all possible combinations for Mary Jo's gametes across the top and for Tom's gametes down the side.

|        | BA    | Ba    | bA    | ba    |
|--------|-------|-------|-------|-------|
| **BA** | *BBAA* | *BBAa* | *BbAA* | *BbAa* |
| **Ba** | *BBAa* | BBaa  | *BbAa* | Bbaa  |
| **bA** | *BbAA* | *BbAa* | bbAA  | bbAa  |
| **ba** | *BbAa* | Bbaa  | bbAa  | bbaa  |

**Step 3:** A child will have the dominant phenotype for both traits if there is at least one B and at least one A in her genotype. Nine of the 16 possible combinations meet this criterion (these are italicized in the square), so the probability that the baby sister will look like her parents in both respects is $\frac{9}{16}$.

**Step 4:** The correct answer choice is **(D)**. Choice (A) is the probability that a child like John, with both recessive traits, is born. Choice (B) is the probability that a child is born with either blue eyes and free earlobes or brown eyes and attached earlobes. Choice (C) is the probability that a child is born with at least one recessive trait. The phenotype ratio of 9:3:3:1 holds for all dihybrid crosses.

## KEY IDEAS

- Different versions of a gene that code for the same trait are alleles. An individual receives one allele from each parent, resulting in a genotype that may be homozygous or heterozygous.
- When one version of the allele is dominant and the other recessive, heterozygotes have the dominant phenotype.
- A Punnett square is used to determine the probability of offspring inheriting specific traits.

# Heredity Practice Questions

1. Dark hair is a dominant trait. If *D* symbolizes the allele for dark hair, which option shows the heterozygous genotype and its matching phenotype?

   (A) genotype: Dd; phenotype: dark hair
   (B) genotype: Dd; phenotype: lighter hair
   (C) genotype: DD; phenotype: dark hair
   (D) genotype: DD; phenotype: lighter hair

2. A student is conducting an experiment to study the trait of fur color in rabbits. Black fur is dominant, and white fur is recessive. She crosses a black male with a white female and is surprised when one of the offspring has white fur. What fact would account for this result?

   (A) The white female is heterozygous.
   (B) The black male is heterozygous.
   (C) The offspring with white fur is heterozygous.
   (D) All of the offspring are homozygous.

3. Which of the following is the result of meiosis beginning with one human cell?

   (A) Two cells, each with 23 chromosomes
   (B) Two cells, each with 46 chromosomes
   (C) Four cells, each with 23 chromosomes
   (D) Four cells, each with 46 chromosomes

**Review your work using the explanations in Part Six of this book.**

# LESSON 3

# Atoms and the Periodic Table

## LEARNING OBJECTIVES

- Describe the basic components and structure of an atom
- Interpret the notation of electron configuration
- Determine the composition of an atom from its atomic number and mass
- Infer characteristics of elements from their position in the periodic table

An **element** is a pure type of matter that cannot be separated into different types of matter by ordinary chemical means. An **atom** is the smallest component of an element that retains the properties of that element. A **molecule** is a group of two or more atoms bonded together. Molecules will be discussed in Lesson 5: States of Matter and Lesson 6: Chemical Reactions.

Atoms are composed of a central **nucleus** and an orbital "cloud" that surrounds the nucleus. **Neutrons** are particles in the nucleus that have no electric charge. **Protons** are positively charged particles in the nucleus. **Electrons** have a negative electric charge. Neutrons and protons have approximately the same mass; the mass of electrons is negligible. Electrons orbit around the nucleus of an atom, and the opposite charges between protons and electrons create an attraction that serves to keep the electrons in the orbital cloud.

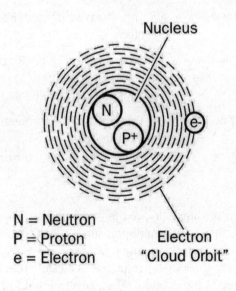

Nucleus

N = Neutron
P = Proton
e = Electron

Electron
"Cloud Orbit"

The number of protons in the nucleus defines an element. Although there is a typical number of neutrons for each element, the number of neutrons in an atom of some elements can vary; these variations in the number of neutrons are termed **isotopes** of the element. Because the numbers of elections and protons remain the same, the different isotopes of an atom have essentially the same properties.

The positive charge of a proton is the same magnitude as the negative charge of an electron, so an atom that contains the same number of each is a **neutral atom.** Atoms that are not electrically balanced because they have either lost or gained electrons are called **ions.** If electrons have been lost, then the ion has a positive charge and is known as a **cation.** If there are extra electrons, then the ion is negatively charged and is an **anion.** For instance, if Mg (magnesium), which has an atomic number of 12, gives up 2 electrons so that its ion has 12 protons and 10 electrons, that ion would now have a $+2$ charge.

Here's how an expert would approach a question on this relationship.

| Question | Analysis |
| --- | --- |
| Which of the atoms described below is an anion? | **Step 1:** The question asks which of the answer choices describes an anion. |
| | **Step 2:** Recall that an anion is negatively charged because it has more electrons than protons. |
| | **Step 3:** Whichever answer choice has more electrons than protons will be correct. |
| (A)  An atom with 9 protons, 10 neutrons, and 10 electrons | **Step 4:** Answer choice **(A)** describes an atom with 10 electrons and 9 protons. This matches the prediction and is correct. |
| (B)  An atom with 9 protons, 10 neutrons, and 9 electrons | This atom is balanced, having 9 of each, so it is a neutral atom. |
| (C)  An atom with 9 protons, 11 neutrons, and 9 electrons | Compared to choice (B), the number of neutrons increases from 10 to 11, but the protons and electrons remain balanced, so this is an isotope of the atom in (B). |
| (D)  An atom with 11 protons, 12 neutrons, and 10 electrons | The protons (11) outnumber the electrons (10), so this is a cation. |

## Electron Configuration

Although electrons move around in the area surrounding the nucleus of an atom, their motion is *not* the same as that of the planets as they orbit around the sun. Each electron can be associated with an **orbital.** However, orbitals are not clearly defined paths. Instead, an orbital describes the probability of the electron's location at any point in time. For instance, a plot of all the orbitals of all electrons of an atom could resemble a cloud, as depicted in the diagram. The electrons could be at any point within this cloud at any time, but there are certain areas where each electron is more likely to be. Each orbital can hold two electrons, which orbit the nucleus in opposite directions; they are said to have opposite spins.

Electron orbitals are grouped into named **subshells**. Each of these subshells has a certain maximum capacity of electrons (based on the number of orbitals per subshell), as shown in this table.

| Subshell Designation | Electron Capacity |
| --- | --- |
| s | 2 |
| p | 6 |
| d | 10 |
| f | 14 |

For example, the s subshell contains only 1 orbital, so it can hold 2 electrons. On the other hand, the d subshell contains 5 orbitals, and since each orbital can hold 2 electrons, the d subshell can hold 10 electrons.

Subshells, in turn, are grouped into numbered **shells**, which describe all the electrons across certain subshells that share the same principle energy level. When a shell reaches its capacity, additional electrons start to fill in the next shell. Each successive shell represents a higher energy level, and as the energy level increases, the electrons are, on average, further away from the nucleus.

All of these conventions lead to a system for describing the **electron configuration** of any element, which describes where all of the electrons for that element reside around the nucleus. For instance, the element chlorine (Cl) has 17 protons and, therefore, 17 electrons in its neutral state. In the first shell, there are 2 electrons in the s subshell. In the second shell, there are 2 electrons in the s subshell and 6 in the p subshell. In the third shell, there are 2 electrons in the s subshell and 5 in the p subshell. The notation for the electron configuration of Cl is thus $1s^2 2s^2 2p^6 3s^2 3p^5$, where the first number is the shell, the letter that follows is the named subshell, and the superscript is the number of electrons in that subshell.

The electrons in the outermost shell are called **valence electrons**. These electrons are crucial to forming bonds with other atoms in chemical reactions, a subject that will be discussed Lesson 6. Most atoms want a valence of 8 electrons, and this tendency to seek that level is known as the **octet rule**. Notable exceptions to this rule are helium, which has a full valence shell of 2 electrons, and hydrogen, which has 1 electron in its valence shell and seeks to have 2. If the outer shell of an atom is almost at its electron capacity, that atom will have a strong attraction for electrons in order to fill that orbital. If the outer orbital is nearly empty, that atom will release electrons relatively easily. If the outer shell is exactly at its full capacity of electrons, the atom will be stable and will not react easily.

Try applying these principles of orbitals to this question.

The element fluorine has the electron configuration $1s^2 2s^2 2p^5$. Which of the following statements is correct based upon that configuration?

(A) Fluorine is very stable and will not react easily with other elements.
(B) Fluorine gives up electrons relatively easily.
(C) Fluorine has a strong affinity for electrons.
(D) Fluorine is a salt.

## Explanation

**Step 1:** The question provides the electron configuration for fluorine and asks what conclusion can be drawn from that information.

**Step 2:** Recall that the last shell is the most critical. Since that shell has a full *s* subshell and a *p* subshell with a capacity of 6 electrons that only is populated with 5, the shell could accommodate just one more electron. As a result, fluorine has a strong affinity for electrons.

**Step 3:** Predict that the correct answer will be related to fluorine's strong affinity for electrons.

**Step 4:** A stable element would have a full outer shell. Eliminate (A). Choice (B) is the opposite of the prediction. Choice **(C)** matches the prediction and is correct. Choice (D) is beyond the scope of the question. For the record, salts contain at least two elements.

## Atomic Numbers and Mass

The **atomic number** of an element is equal to its number of protons (which is also the number of electrons in a neutral atom). The mass of a proton or a neutron is extremely close to 1 **atomic mass unit** (amu). The mass of an electron is only about $\dfrac{1}{1800}$ amu, so a good approximation of the total mass of an atom can be determined by adding up just the numbers of protons and neutrons. If an element has isotopes, the atomic mass shown in the periodic table will be the weighted average of the masses of all the isotopes.

Since the atomic mass is the sum of the number of protons and neutrons, knowing any two of those three numbers will enable you to calculate the third. For instance, the atomic number of carbon is 6, and the mass of its most common isotope is 12. The atomic number of 6 means that carbon has 6 protons. Since the total mass is 12, there must be $(12 - 6) = 6$ neutrons.

## The Periodic Table

An individual element can be identified by its symbol, atomic number, and atomic mass. The descriptive panel for the element chlorine shows one common format for displaying this information. The atomic number, 17, appears above the symbol for this element, Cl. At the bottom, 35.5 is the atomic mass, weighted for the different isotopes of chlorine.

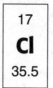

| 17 |
| :---: |
| **Cl** |
| 35.5 |

There are currently 118 known elements. All the elements are shown in the **periodic table**.

| 1 | | | | | | | | | | | | | | | | | 18 |
|---|---|---|---|---|---|---|---|---|---|---|---|---|---|---|---|---|---|
| 1<br>**H**<br>1.0 | | | | | | | | | | | | | | | | | 2<br>**He**<br>4.0 |
| 3<br>**Li**<br>6.9 | 4<br>**Be**<br>9.0 | | | | | | | | | | | 5<br>**B**<br>10.8 | 6<br>**C**<br>12.0 | 7<br>**N**<br>14.0 | 8<br>**O**<br>16.0 | 9<br>**F**<br>19.0 | 10<br>**Ne**<br>20.2 |
| 11<br>**Na**<br>23.0 | 12<br>**Mg**<br>24.3 | | | | | | | | | | | 13<br>**Al**<br>27.0 | 14<br>**Si**<br>28.1 | 15<br>**P**<br>31.0 | 16<br>**S**<br>32.1 | 17<br>**Cl**<br>35.5 | 18<br>**Ar**<br>39.9 |
| 19<br>**K**<br>39.1 | 20<br>**Ca**<br>40.1 | 21<br>**Sc**<br>45.0 | 22<br>**Ti**<br>47.9 | 23<br>**V**<br>50.9 | 24<br>**Cr**<br>52.0 | 25<br>**Mn**<br>54.9 | 26<br>**Fe**<br>55.8 | 27<br>**Co**<br>58.9 | 28<br>**Ni**<br>58.7 | 29<br>**Cu**<br>63.5 | 30<br>**Zn**<br>65.4 | 31<br>**Ga**<br>69.7 | 32<br>**Ge**<br>72.6 | 33<br>**As**<br>74.9 | 34<br>**Se**<br>79.0 | 35<br>**Br**<br>79.9 | 36<br>**Kr**<br>83.8 |
| 37<br>**Rb**<br>85.5 | 38<br>**Sr**<br>87.6 | 39<br>**Y**<br>88.9 | 40<br>**Zr**<br>91.2 | 41<br>**Nb**<br>92.9 | 42<br>**Mo**<br>96.0 | 43<br>**Tc**<br>(98) | 44<br>**Ru**<br>101.0 | 45<br>**Rh**<br>102.9 | 46<br>**Pd**<br>106.4 | 47<br>**Ag**<br>107.9 | 48<br>**Cd**<br>112.4 | 49<br>**In**<br>114.8 | 50<br>**Sn**<br>118.7 | 51<br>**Sb**<br>121.8 | 52<br>**Te**<br>127.6 | 53<br>**I**<br>126.9 | 54<br>**Xe**<br>131.3 |
| 55<br>**Cs**<br>132.9 | 56<br>**Ba**<br>137.3 | * | 72<br>**Hf**<br>178.5 | 73<br>**Ta**<br>180.9 | 74<br>**W**<br>183.8 | 75<br>**Re**<br>186.2 | 76<br>**Os**<br>190.2 | 77<br>**Ir**<br>192.2 | 78<br>**Pt**<br>195.1 | 79<br>**Au**<br>197.0 | 80<br>**Hg**<br>200.6 | 81<br>**Tl**<br>204.4 | 82<br>**Pb**<br>207.2 | 83<br>**Bi**<br>209.0 | 84<br>**Po**<br>(209) | 85<br>**At**<br>(210) | 86<br>**Rn**<br>(222) |
| 87<br>**Fr**<br>(223) | 88<br>**Ra**<br>(226) | † | 104<br>**Rf**<br>(267) | 105<br>**Db**<br>(268) | 106<br>**Sg**<br>(269) | 107<br>**Bh**<br>(270) | 108<br>**Hs**<br>(269) | 109<br>**Mt**<br>(278) | 110<br>**Ds**<br>(281) | 111<br>**Rg**<br>(281) | 112<br>**Cn**<br>(285) | 113<br>**Uut**<br>(286) | 114<br>**Fl**<br>(289) | 115<br>**Uup**<br>(288) | 116<br>**Lv**<br>(293) | 117<br>**Uus**<br>(294) | 118<br>**Uuo**<br>(294) |

| * | 57<br>**La**<br>138.9 | 58<br>**Ce**<br>140.1 | 59<br>**Pr**<br>140.9 | 60<br>**Nd**<br>144.2 | 61<br>**Pm**<br>(145) | 62<br>**Sm**<br>150.4 | 63<br>**Eu**<br>152.0 | 64<br>**Gd**<br>157.3 | 65<br>**Tb**<br>158.9 | 66<br>**Dy**<br>162.5 | 67<br>**Ho**<br>164.9 | 68<br>**Er**<br>167.3 | 69<br>**Tm**<br>168.9 | 70<br>**Yb**<br>173.1 | 71<br>**Lu**<br>175.0 |
|---|---|---|---|---|---|---|---|---|---|---|---|---|---|---|---|
| † | 89<br>**Ac**<br>(227) | 90<br>**Th**<br>232.0 | 91<br>**Pa**<br>231.0 | 92<br>**U**<br>238.0 | 93<br>**Np**<br>(237) | 94<br>**Pu**<br>(244) | 95<br>**Am**<br>(243) | 96<br>**Cm**<br>(247) | 97<br>**Bk**<br>(247) | 98<br>**Cf**<br>(251) | 99<br>**Es**<br>(252) | 100<br>**Fm**<br>(257) | 101<br>**Md**<br>(258) | 102<br>**No**<br>(259) | 103<br>**Lr**<br>(262) |

The elements are arranged in order of increasing atomic number, from left to right and top to bottom. The different rows of elements are called **periods**. These periods are related to the shells of the electrons as described earlier. The highest-numbered shells of each element correspond to the period number. For instance, K (potassium) in the fourth period has an outermost shell consisting of only 1 electron, so its valence configuration is $4s^1$.

The different columns are termed **groups**. All elements in a group need the same number of electrons to complete their outer shell. Therefore, they have similar properties. For example, the elements in the far right column are called **noble gases**. Their outer shells are full and they are odorless, colorless, and inert, meaning they react with other elements only under extreme conditions. As another example, all the elements in the far left column, the alkali **metals**, have one more electron than a noble gas, so that group has just one electron in its valence shell and loses electrons with relative ease. These elements are soft, silvery metals that react strongly with water. The group of elements in the next-to-last column to the right are one electron short of completing a shell and, therefore, have a strong attraction for electrons.

Study how a question about an element in the periodic table can be analyzed and answered.

| Question | Analysis |
|---|---|
| Which of the following can be inferred about the element Br? | **Step 1:** The question asks what can be inferred about bromine. |
| | **Step 2:** Locate the element Br in the periodic table. Its atomic number is 35 and its mass is 79.9 amu. Since Br is just to the left of the noble gases at the far right, which have complete outer shells, you can infer that the elements in group 17 are one electron short of a complete shell. |
| | **Step 3:** Having one electron less than a complete shell means that Br has a strong attraction for electrons. Predict that the correct answer will be based on that fact. |
| (A) Br has a strong affinity for free electrons. | **Step 4:** Choice (A) matches the prediction that Br has "a strong attraction for electrons." |
| (B) Br has more neutrons than protons. | Choice (B) asks about the number of neutrons. Since Br's atomic mass is 79.9, and the number of protons is the same as its atomic number, 35, the average number of neutrons is $79.9 - 35 = 44.9$. This is greater than the number of protons, so (B) is also correct. At this point, you could choose **(D)**, but check out (C) just to confirm. |
| (C) Br has more than one isotope. | Because the atomic number, 79.9, is not a whole number, it must be an average of more than one isotope, so choice (C) is also true. |
| (D) All of the above can be inferred from the information in the periodic table. | Since choices (A), (B) and (C) are all true, the correct answer is **(D)**. |

## KEY IDEAS

- The basic components of atoms are protons, electrons, and neutrons.
- The atomic number of an element is the number of protons of that element.
- The atomic mass of an element is approximately the sum of the number of its protons and the weighted average number of neutrons in its isotopes.
- The group of an element in the periodic table is a key determinant of an element's properties.

# Atoms and the Periodic Table Practice Questions

1. The element boron (symbol B) is listed in the periodic table as having an atomic number of 5 and a mass of 10.8 amu. Which of the following could be true?

   (A) Eighty percent of boron isotopes have 6 neutrons.
   (B) Boron never contains more neutrons than protons.
   (C) The mass shown in the periodic table is incorrect; atomic mass can only be a whole number.
   (D) Boron contains partial neutrons.

2. An element's chemical characteristics are most strongly influenced by

   (A) the amount of the element.
   (B) its physical appearance.
   (C) its group in the periodic table.
   (D) its period in the periodic table.

**Review your work using the explanations in Part Six of this book.**

# LESSON 4

# Properties of Substances

---

## LEARNING OBJECTIVES

- Differentiate between physical and chemical properties
- Classify physical properties as intensive or extensive
- Calculate the density of a substance
- Predict and apply special properties of water resulting from its polar nature
- Predict how molecules in solution diffuse or osmose in different body processes

---

Physical matter that has uniform properties is called a **substance**. A **mixture** is matter that is composed of more than one substance. The TEAS tests specific properties of substances that you should know. Water in particular has unique properties and is extremely important to human physiology.

Since substances are matter, they have **physical properties** that can be readily observed, such as color, shape, and texture. Other physical properties, such as hardness or tensile strength, can be measured. Physical properties can be evaluated without involving the substance in a chemical reaction.

Substances also have **chemical properties** that affect how they interact with other materials. Chemical properties are greatly affected by the valence electron configuration, as outlined in Lesson 3: Atoms and the Periodic Table. These properties can only be observed in the context of chemical reactions, which result in a change from one substance into a different one. For instance, when iron rusts, it combines with oxygen and becomes a new substance, iron oxide. Some chemical properties will be discussed in Lesson 6: Chemical Reactions.

## Physical Properties

Some physical properties depend upon the amount of matter being measured; these are called **extensive properties**. Common extensive properties are mass and volume. Physical properties that do *not* depend upon the amount of a substance are categorized as **intensive properties**. One of the most common intensive properties is **density**. Density is defined as $\dfrac{\text{mass}}{\text{volume}}$.

Study how an expert would answer a question about density.

| Question | Analysis |
| --- | --- |
| A rectangular block of a certain substance is 4 cm wide, 5 cm long, and 2 cm high. The block has a mass of 30 grams. What is the density of this substance? | **Step 1:** The question provides the dimensions of a block of matter and its mass and asks for the density of that substance. The volume of the block is $4 \text{ cm} \times 5 \text{ cm} \times 2 \text{ cm} = 40 \text{ cm}^3$ (cc). The mass is given as 30 g. |
| | **Step 2:** Recall that density is mass divided by volume. |
| | **Step 3:** Calculate density: $$\frac{30 \text{ g}}{40 \text{ cc}} = \frac{0.75 \text{ g}}{1 \text{ cc}}.$$ |
| (A) 0.75 g/cc | **Step 4:** Answer choice **(A)** is correct. |
| (B) 1.33 cc/g | This is the inverse of the correct answer. |
| (C) 7.5 g/cc | This choice misplaces the decimal point. |
| (D) 40 cc | This is the volume, not the density. |

Although the mass and volume of the block in the previous question are measurable extensive properties, density is an intensive property. A different-sized block would have had different volumes and masses, but the density would have still been 0.75 g/cc.

**Melting point,** the temperature at which a substance changes from a solid to a liquid, and **boiling point,** the temperature at which a substance changes from a liquid to a gas, are both common intensive properties. Solid, liquid, and gas are all **states** of matter, a subject that will be covered in more depth in Lesson 5: States of Matter.

Another intensive property is **specific heat capacity**; this is the amount of energy needed to change the temperature of 1 g of a substance by 1°C. **Malleability** describes the ability of a material to be manipulated into different shapes. Other examples of intensive properties include electrical conductivity, hardness, and tensile strength.

Try applying these concepts to this question about physical properties.

The students in a science class conducted an experiment to see whether several samples of different materials were attracted by a magnet. Which of the following type of property were they identifying with their experiment?

(A) Intensive physical property
(B) Extensive physical property
(C) Chemical property
(D) Reactivity property

### Explanation

**Step 1:** The question describes an experiment in which various materials were tested for magnetism. Your task is to identify what type of property this is.

**Step 2:** Recall that characteristics that can be observed without involving a chemical reaction are physical properties and that intensive properties do not rely on the quantity of the substance.

**Step 3:** Since the students were merely observing whether the samples were attracted by a magnet and didn't test the size of the sample, predict that the answer will relate to an intensive physical property.

**Step 4:** The prediction matches choice **(A)**. Since choice (B) mentions extensive, it is incorrect. The experiment did not measure chemical properties or a chemical reaction, so eliminate choice (C). Reactivity, (D), is an example of a chemical property.

## Water

Water, which makes up about 60 percent of an adult human body, is vital to human life because it is needed for many bodily functions. Water is a major component of blood, and it has the important functions of carrying nutrients and oxygen to cells and carrying waste products away from cells. Without water, the body could not properly digest food or regulate body temperature.

As shown in the diagram, a molecule of water is composed of two hydrogen atoms bonded to one oxygen atom at an angle slightly greater than 90°. Each hydrogen atom has a slight positive electrical charge, and the oxygen atom has a slight negative charge. Because of this imbalance, such molecules are termed **polar molecules**. This polarity is responsible for many of the properties of water that make it so uniquely useful.

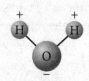

Because polar molecules are attracted to each other, water is **cohesive**; that is, it holds together very well. As a result, water flows well through very small conduits such as capillaries and doesn't require much energy to be pumped from one place to another. Its melting point, boiling point, and specific heat capacity are also much higher than those of substances that have a similar composition due to its cohesive properties.

**Adhesion** is another property that results from water's polar nature. Just as water molecules are attracted to each other, so are the polar molecules or ions of other substances in water attracted to water molecules. Water is nicknamed the "universal solvent" because so many other substances will dissolve in water. **Aqueous solutions** can consist of solids, liquids, or gases dissolved in water.

See how a TEAS expert answers this question about water.

| Question | Analysis |
|---|---|
| Why is water capable of maintaining relatively large amounts of table salt (NaCl) in solution? | **Step 1**: The question asks why water has the capacity to dissolve high concentrations of NaCl in solution. |
| | **Step 2**: Recall that the polar molecules of water will adhere to polar molecules or ions of another substance that is dissolved in water. |
| | **Step 3**: Predict that the correct answer will relate the property of adhesion to solubility. |
| (A)  Salt is lightweight. | **Step 4**: Solubility is due to adhesion, not the weight of what is being dissolved. Eliminate. |
| (B)  NaCl easily separates into $Na^+$ and $Cl^-$ ions. | This agrees with the prediction. The $Na^+$ ions are attracted to the slight negative charge of the oxygen, and the $Cl^-$ ions are attracted to the slight positive charge of the hydrogen. Choice **(B)** is correct. |
| (C)  Heat is created when NaCl dissolves in water. | This is incorrect because no chemical reaction occurs that would generate heat. NaCl merely becomes ionized. |
| (D)  NaCl is a nonpolar molecule when dissolved. | This is opposite of the prediction. |

# Diffusion and Osmosis

When one substance is dissolved into another, the result is a **solution**. Unlike a mixture, a solution has consistent properties. The substance into which another is dissolved is called the **solvent**; the substance that is being dissolved is the **solute**.

In chemistry, **diffusion** is the tendency of substances to move from areas of higher concentration of solute to areas of lower concentration. As a result, substances in solutions will eventually become evenly distributed. The process of diffusion can occur across thin, semipermeable membranes because individual molecules are small enough to pass through. Many life processes rely on the diffusion of solutes. For instance, oxygen molecules diffuse through the very thin membranes of capillaries from the blood into cells with depleted oxygen concentrations.

**Osmosis** is a particular type of diffusion in which an imbalance of concentrations is corrected by the migration of the solvent, rather than the solute. This is accomplished by movement of the solvent from the region with the lower concentration of solute to the region of higher concentration. As a result, the concentrations achieve equilibrium. Osmosis is a process utilized by the kidneys to maintain proper water balance in the body.

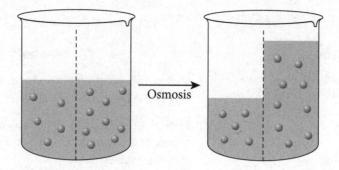

Now apply what you have learned to answer this question.

In the alveolar capillaries, blood returning from the body transfers carbon dioxide to the air in the lungs by _____ and receives oxygen by _____. Which of the following answer choices correctly completes the sentence?

(A)  osmosis; osmosis
(B)  osmosis; diffusion
(C)  diffusion; osmosis
(D)  diffusion; diffusion

## Explanation

**Step 1:** The question asks about the processes by which carbon dioxide is released from blood to the lungs and oxygen is transferred from the lungs into the blood.

**Step 2:** Recall that diffusion is the movement of substances from higher to lower concentrations. If the movement is that of the solvent, the diffusion is categorized as osmosis. In this situation, carbon dioxide is a solute in the blood, and oxygen becomes a solute in the blood.

**Step 3:** Since the two substances being transferred are both solutes, predict that both processes occur via diffusion.

**Step 4:** Answer choice **(D)** matches the prediction and is correct.

## KEY IDEAS

- Physical properties of substances can be visually observed or measured using instruments and are either intensive or extensive. Chemical properties relate to how a substance behaves in chemical reactions.
- Diffusion is the tendency of solute molecules to move from areas of higher concentration to areas of lower concentration. Osmosis is the tendency of solvent molecules to move from areas of lower concentration to areas of higher concentration.
- The special properties of water are mainly due to the polar nature of its molecules.

# Properties of Substances Practice Questions

1.  Ricardo pours sand into water and shakes the container. The sand stays suspended in the water for a while but eventually settles at the bottom of the container. Ricardo created a

    (A)  mixture.
    (B)  substance.
    (C)  solution.
    (D)  solute.

2.  Brandon wants to determine the density of a certain liquid. He selects an empty 50 mL container that has a mass of 30 g. Brandon then pours the liquid into the container, but he only has enough to fill the container to 80 percent of capacity. The mass of the container plus the liquid is 74 g. What is the density of the liquid?

    (A)  0.88 g/mL
    (B)  1.00 g/mL
    (C)  1.10 g/mL
    (D)  1.28 g/mL

3.  When Lucretia spilled some gasoline into a puddle of water, she noticed that the gasoline did not mix with the water. Instead, the gasoline formed a colorful slick on top of the puddle. Which of the following statements explains what she observed?

    (A)  Gasoline has a lower boiling point than water.
    (B)  Gasoline is made up primarily of nonpolar molecules.
    (C)  Gasoline is made up of hydrocarbons with polar molecules.
    (D)  Water is sometimes called the "universal solvent."

**Review your work using the explanations in Part Six of this book.**

# LESSON 5

# States of Matter

> ## LEARNING OBJECTIVES
>
> - Understand the different states of matter and how molecules move in each state
> - Describe how matter undergoes phase transitions
> - Identify the ways in which a substance changes from one state of matter to another

Matter is described as anything that has mass and takes up space, and the four most common states of matter are solid, liquid, gas, and plasma. Because the human body is composed of solids, liquids, and gases, the TEAS will primarily test your understanding of these states.

The states of all substances that make up the body and of many of those in the surrounding environment can have a dramatic impact on a person's health. For example, providing the right concentration of oxygen gas to a client on a respirator could improve that person's brain function. Additionally, certain medications are better absorbed by the digestive system in liquid form rather than as a solid pill. Overall, the more you understand the characteristics of the different states of matter and how substances transition between them, the better able you will be to care for your clients.

## States of Matter

All matter is made up of atoms, which can bond together to form molecules or compounds through **intramolecular forces**. Although the atoms and molecules that make up matter are in constant motion, they are simultaneously ordered and held together by **intermolecular forces** of attraction. Despite the name, this intermolecular attraction can affect both molecular substances (e.g., $H_2O$ or $N_2$) and those comprised of single atoms (e.g., Ar or Hg). To simplify, we will discuss particle behavior more generally in this lesson, since the topics discussed here apply to both kinds of substances. For every substance, the strength of the intermolecular forces between its particles plays an important role in determining its state of matter.

A **solid** has the most highly ordered particles of any state of matter due to the strong attractions between its particles. Because of these strong forces, even though the particles that make up a solid are in constant motion, they typically vibrate together with little change in their relative distance from one another. For this reason, solids typically have fixed shapes and volumes. The most highly ordered type of matter is called a **crystal**.

In a **liquid,** the forces between the particles are strong enough to keep them together but weak enough to allow the particles to move around one another fluidly. Thus, liquids change shape to fit any container or surface. Because the average distance between the particles in liquid remains fairly constant, this state of matter has a defined volume.

The forces that keep particles of **gas** together range from negligible to nonexistent, depending on the type of gas. Gas particles move apart easily and disperse to fill any available space, meaning that gases do not have a fixed volume. The volume of a gas at any given time depends on the amount of pressure that is being exerted on its particles to keep them together. Gases, therefore, can be easily compressed or compacted, while solids and liquids cannot.

The following chart illustrates the primary characteristics of the three most commonly recognized states of matter.

| State of Matter | Fixed Shape | Fixed Volume | Easily Compressible? |
|---|---|---|---|
| Solid | Yes | Yes | No |
| Liquid | No | Yes | No |
| Gas | No | No | Yes |

Here is how a test expert would answer a question about the different states of matter.

| Question | Analysis |
|---|---|
| Suppose scientists have invented a new substance that can be compressed to fit into smaller containers or expanded to fill large spaces. In what state of matter must this new substance exist? | **Step 1:** This question is asking for a state of matter that has certain characteristics. |
| | **Step 2:** Recall that gas is the only state of matter that does not have a fixed volume, which means it can be easily compressed or expanded. |
| | **Step 3:** Predict that the new substance is a gas. |
| (A)  Solid | **Step 4:** The strongly bound particles in a solid give that substance a defined shape and a consistent volume. Eliminate. |
| (B)  Liquid | The particles in a liquid are loosely bound but still maintain a consistent volume. Eliminate. |
| (C)  Gas | Correct. This matches the prediction. |
| (D)  Crystal | Crystals are solids with the most highly ordered and closely bound particles. They must have a defined volume. Eliminate. |

## Phase Transitions

Most substances can exist in each of the three main states of matter. The substance that best illustrates this point is water, which is the only substance on Earth that occurs naturally as a solid (ice), liquid (water), and gas (steam or vapor). Water, like all other substances, does not have to stay in one state but can move from one state to another as conditions change. The change of a substance from one state to another is called a **phase transition**, where *phase* is a term with a similar meaning to *state*. A phase transition occurs when there is a change in environmental conditions, the two most important being temperature and pressure. For example, when the temperature is increased above 0°C under normal atmospheric pressure conditions, an ice cube (water in its solid state) will melt (transition to its liquid state). These transitions occur as changes in temperature and pressure affect molecular movement.

The kinetic molecular theory holds that molecular motion slows down as heat is removed and speeds up as heat is added. For example, at absolute zero, which is 0 K or −273°C, the motion of particles slows to almost (though not quite) a standstill. This near lack of movement is synonymous with a lack of heat. When heat is applied to a substance, the forces that attract the now more active particles to one another are less able to hold them in place, and the particles tend to spread out and move more freely and rapidly. This increased movement also leads to a more disordered arrangement of the particles.

Similarly, outside pressure, such as atmospheric pressure, can play a role in the movement and organization of particles. For example, intense pressure works to pack particles more tightly together and restrict their movement, which corresponds with a higher degree of order. Conversely, a release of pressure allows particles to move apart more easily and become more chaotic, or disordered, in their motion. The figure demonstrates how particles in a solid, liquid, and gas behave when heat is removed or added to each. The solid state is the most highly ordered, while the gaseous state is the most highly disordered.

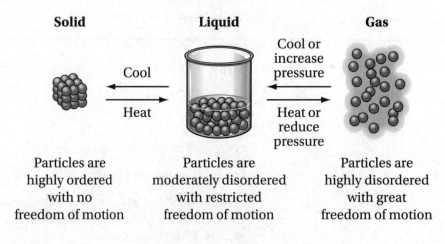

**Solid** — Particles are highly ordered with no freedom of motion

Cool ← / Heat →

**Liquid** — Particles are moderately disordered with restricted freedom of motion

Cool or increase pressure ← / Heat or reduce pressure →

**Gas** — Particles are highly disordered with great freedom of motion

## Types of Changes Between States of Matter

The phase transitions of water provide a helpful illustration of the different ways in which a substance changes from one state into another. As discussed earlier, one of the key factors of this change is the addition or subtraction of heat energy. When pure, liquid water is cooled to 0°C, it turns into solid ice through the process of **freezing**. Through the process of **melting**, ice can turn into liquid water if heat is applied, speeding up its molecular motion and allowing greater fluidity of its particles.

When liquid water is heated to its **boiling point**, it turns into a type of gas called steam. **Evaporation**, or the transition of a liquid into a gas called **vapor**, occurs when heat is transferred primarily to the surface of the liquid. A substance in a gaseous state can change into a liquid state through the process of **condensation**, in which the gas cools, allowing its particles to slow down and gather together at a fixed volume.

Every type of substance needs a certain amount of heat, called **latent heat**, to change from solid to liquid to gas at a constant temperature.

Consider the states of water as an example.

- If ice is below the freezing point, heat must be added to increase its temperature to 0°C, at which point it begins to change into liquid water. As more heat is added, the temperature of the ice stays the same until it has all turned to water. The amount of energy needed to melt the ice after it has reached the melting point is called the **latent heat of fusion**.

- If the temperature of the water continues to rise, it eventually reaches its boiling point. Once the water is boiling, its temperature remains the same until all of the water turns to steam. The amount of energy needed to boil all of the water into steam is called the **latent heat of vaporization**.

- Once all water has turned into steam, any added heat will increase the temperature of the steam.

The diagram illustrates that the temperature of a substance remains constant during phase transitions despite the steady addition of heat.

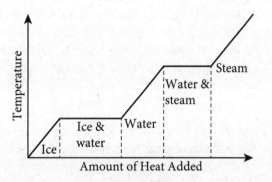

**Latent Heat Diagram**

Latent heat is measured in **calories**. To calculate the amount of heat in calories that is needed to complete a phase change in a substance, use the following formula:

$$H = mL,$$

where $H$ is the change in heat in calories (cal), $m$ is the mass of the substance in grams (g), and $L$ is the latent heat of the substance in calories per gram (cal/g).

Note that if the change in heat energy is positive, the substance is likely to be turning from either a solid to a liquid or a liquid to a gas. If the change in heat is negative, the substance is losing heat energy and likely changing from either a gas to a liquid or a liquid to a solid. Keep in mind that when the processes of vaporization or fusion are reversed, the same amount of latent heat is released during these changes as was needed to bring them about.

Try this question about energy and phase change.

> Mercury is a liquid at room temperature. It has a boiling point of approximately 357°C and a latent heat of 70 cal/g. How much heat is required to completely vaporize a 200 g sample of mercury that has been heated to 357°C?
>
> (A)  1020 calories
> (B)  13,643 calories
> (C)  14,000 calories
> (D)  14,357 calories

## Explanation

**Step 1:** The question asks for the amount of heat necessary to turn 200 g of mercury at 357°C into a gas. You are told that 357°C is mercury's boiling point and its latent heat is 70 cal/g.

**Step 2:** Recall the formula for calculating the change in heat of a substance undergoing phase change: $H = mL$.

**Step 3:** In this case, no heat is needed to bring the mercury to the point where it begins phase change because it is already at the boiling point. Thus, $H = 200\ g \times 70\ cal/g = 14{,}000$ calories.

**Step 4:** Choice **(C)** is correct.

While all substances can undergo phase transitions between different states of matter, they do so at different temperatures. Each substance has its own freezing and boiling points, which are themselves affected by changes in pressure. The less pressure on a substance, the lower the temperature at which the substance will transition from solid to liquid and then liquid to gas. For example, water has a lower boiling point at higher altitudes where there is decreased atmospheric pressure. Conversely, the more pressure on a substance, the more readily that substance will turn from a gas into a liquid and from a liquid into a solid.

The impact of changes in temperature and pressure on a substance's state of matter can be graphed in a **phase diagram**. The point at which environmental temperature and pressure reach an equilibrium such that the solid, liquid, and gas of the substance can all exist at the same time is called the **triple point** on a phase diagram. That point at which temperature and pressure both reach levels at which the liquid and gas phases of a substance have the same density and become indistinguishable is called the **critical point**.

Matter may undergo two other types of phase transitions: sublimation and deposition. In both of these processes, the liquid stage of phase transition is skipped. During **sublimation**, a solid that is at a temperature and pressure below its triple point turns directly into a gas when enough heat energy is applied. You can see this occur with solid carbon dioxide, also known as "dry ice," which sublimates at room temperature. When exposed to the air, solid dry ice quickly absorbs surrounding energy and transitions to gas form without melting first. During the process of **deposition**, the opposite happens: a gas that is at a temperature and pressure below its triple point turns immediately into a solid when heat energy is removed, such as when water vapor in the air freezes directly into snow.

The phase diagram illustrates the phase transitions of a particular substance.

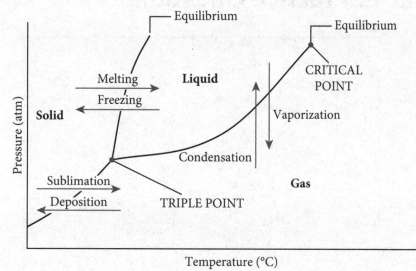

Now try this question on your own about the phase transitions of matter.

Erica left a full glass of water on her windowsill in direct sunlight. When she observed the glass several days later, she noticed that it was only half full. The water that disappeared from Erica's glass likely underwent which type of phase transition?

(A)  Condensation
(B)  Boiling
(C)  Evaporation
(D)  Sublimation

## Explanation

**Step 1:** This question asks you to consider a scenario and determine which phase transition has likely occurred given the circumstances.

**Step 2:** Recall that a liquid can transform into either a solid or a gas. Since the water has disappeared and there is no suggestion that any of the water turned to ice inside the glass, the water likely changed into a gas. Water can complete a phase transition to gas through either boiling or evaporation.

**Step 3:** Predict that evaporation is the correct answer because the direct sunlight would likely not boil off the water but rather only heat the water's surface.

**Step 4:** Answer choice **(C)** matches the prediction and is correct.

## KEY IDEAS

- The three primary states of matter that impact the human body are solid, liquid, and gas, and each is characterized by the way in which particles move in that state.
- Substances undergo phase transitions due to changes in temperature and pressure.
- Substances change states in various ways: melting, sublimation, boiling, freezing, condensation, and deposition.

# States of Matter Practice Questions

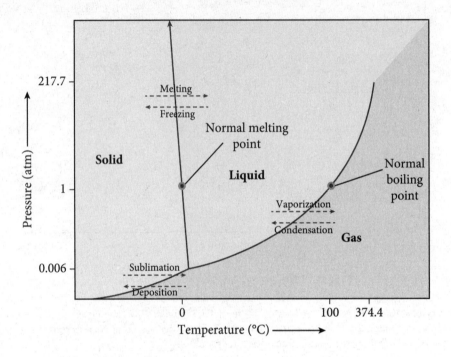

1. The above graph is a phase diagram for water. According to the graph, what environmental conditions allow for deposition?

   (A) High pressure and increasing temperature
   (B) High pressure and decreasing temperature
   (C) Low pressure and increasing temperature
   (D) ¹ Low pressure and decreasing temperature

2. Hydrogen has a boiling point of −253°C. Its latent heat is 108 cal/g. What will be the heat energy change in a 10 g sample of hydrogen at −253°C as it transitions from liquid to a gas?

   (A) −27,320 calories
   (B) −1080 calories
   (C) 1080 calories
   (D) 27,320 calories

3. At what point can a substance exist as a solid, liquid, and gas simultaneously?

   (A) Boiling point
   (B) Freezing point
   (C) Triple point
   (D) Critical point

**Review your work using the explanations in Part Six of this book.**

# LESSON 6

# Chemical Reactions

---

### LEARNING OBJECTIVES

- Identify types of chemical bonds
- Balance chemical equations
- Determine whether a substance is acidic or alkaline from its pH value

---

## Molecules and Bonds

In Lesson 3: Atoms and the Periodic Table, the concept of valence electrons was explained. This lesson will demonstrate how valence electrons are important in chemical reactions. Recall that elements are composed of unique atoms and that molecules are made up of two or more atoms that are bonded together.

The atoms of the elements in the rightmost groups of the periodic table (**non-metal** groups 5, 6, and 7, just to the left of the noble gases), have incomplete outer shells and therefore a strong affinity to acquire electrons. (You can refresh your memory of the periodic table by referring to the complete table in Lesson 3: Atoms and the Periodic Table.) If such an atom were to encounter an atom of an element from the left side of the periodic table (a **metal**), which easily gives up electrons under the right conditions, the first atom would acquire an electron from the second one. This transfer of electrons would create an **ionic bond**. An ionic bond results when one or more atoms gives up one or more electrons, becoming positively charged, and one or more atoms accepts an additional electron or electrons, becoming negatively charged. Since opposite electric charges attract, the new positively and negatively charged ions are bonded together.

Sometimes atoms bond to form molecules by sharing rather than giving up electrons. Oxygen offers one example of this phenomenon. An oxygen atom has 6 electrons in its valence shell, so it would "like" to acquire 2 more. Although oxygen is an element, its natural form is as a molecule made up of two oxygen atoms. This is written as $O_2$; subscripts are used to identify the number of each type of atom in a molecule if there are more than one. Since oxygen atoms want to acquire rather than give up electrons, each atom "shares" 2 of its electrons with the other for a total of 4 shared electrons. This **covalent bond** is illustrated in the figure.

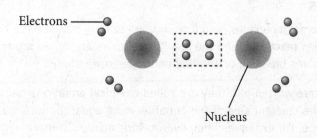

Electrons

Nucleus

Substances that are made up of molecules containing atoms of different elements are called **compounds**. Oxygen, and other elements that have formed molecules without a second element, are not compounds.

There are several common substances that you are likely to encounter on the TEAS. Oxygen ($O_2$) is, of course, vital to human life, as is water ($H_2O$). Sodium chloride (NaCl) and potassium chloride (KCl) are found in the human body, as are the **organic molecules** glucose ($C_6H_{12}O_6$) and ethanol ($C_2H_6O$). All organic molecules contain carbon and hydrogen and are normally present in living things. The macromolecules discussed in Lesson 1 of this chapter are all organic molecules, and most contain elements besides carbon and hydrogen as well.

Study how an expert would answer a question about bonds.

| Question | Analysis |
|---|---|
| Which of the following substances contains an ionic bond? | **Step 1:** The question asks which of the molecules in the answer choices contains an ionic bond. |
|  | **Step 2:** Recall that sharing electrons creates a covalent bond, while a transfer of one or more electrons creates an ionic bond. |
|  | **Step 3:** The correct answer will be composed of elements from both the left (metal) and right (non-metal) side of the periodic table. |
| (A)  C | **Step 4:** Choice (A) is incorrect because a single atom of carbon cannot form a bond by itself. |
| (B)  $N_2$ | Nitrogen (N), like all diatomic gases, shares its electrons in a covalent manner to form a molecule consisting of two identical atoms. Choice (B) is incorrect. |
| (C)  NaCl | Since sodium (Na) gives up electrons easily and Chlorine (Cl) has a strong affinity for them, these atoms form an ionic bond, and choice **(C)** is correct. |
| (D)  $CO_2$ | Carbon and oxygen are both non-metals interested in filling their valence shell, so neither will cede an electron to the other. Therefore, their bond must be covalent, and (D) is incorrect. |

## Chemical Reactions

In a chemical reaction, atoms, molecules, and ions interact to form new substances. The inputs to a chemical reaction are called **reactants**, and the resulting outputs are called **products**. Much of what occurs in chemical reactions involves breaking or creating bonds between atoms.

When chemical reactions are written out, they are called **chemical equations** because the total quantity of each kind of atom on the reactant side of the equation must equal the total quantity of the same kind of atom on the product side. For example, when hydrochloric acid (HCl) reacts with zinc (Zn) to form zinc chloride ($ZnCl_2$) and hydrogen gas ($H_2$), the equation is written $Zn + 2\,HCl \rightarrow ZnCl_2 + H_2$. An arrow is used rather than an equal sign to show the direction in which the reaction proceeds. Notice that the reactants include two of the HCl in order to balance the equation; both the reactants and products have two atoms of H, two atoms of Cl, and one atom of Zn.

There are five basic types of chemical reactions. The example given in the preceding paragraph is a **single displacement reaction** (or, alternatively, a **substitution reaction**) because the Zn displaced the H that was originally paired with Cl.

Another type is the **double displacement reaction**. Here is an example: $Pb(NO_3)_2 + 2\,K \rightarrow Pb_2 + 2\,KNO_3$. You can see that the lead (Pb) and potassium (K) switched places with each other. Notice that the grouping $NO_3$ was treated as if it were a single entity, with the subscript 2 on the reactant side denoting two complete sets of the $NO_3$ grouping, and that it remained intact throughout the reaction. $NO_3$ is a **molecular ion** (alternatively a **polyatomic ion**) that acts in many ways just like an ion of a single atom.

A **decomposition reaction** occurs when a reactant molecule is broken down into its component parts. For instance, when an electric current is passed through water, some water will decompose into hydrogen and oxygen: $2\,H_2O \rightarrow 2\,H_2 + O_2$. The opposite of a decomposition reaction is a **synthesis reaction**, also called a **direct combination reaction**. For example, $2\,H_2 + O_2 \rightarrow 2\,H_2O$.

Another basic reaction is **combustion**. While you may think of combustion as burning, in chemical terms, combustion can be more broadly categorized as an **oxidation reaction** (a reaction involving a combination with oxygen). For instance, when iron rusts, it is becoming iron oxide: $4\,Fe + 3\,O_2 \rightarrow 2\,Fe_2O_3$.

See how an expert would answer the following question.

| Question | Analysis |
|---|---|
| What is the missing coefficient needed to balance this double displacement reaction? <br><br> $4\,FeS + \underline{\quad}\,O_2 \rightarrow 2\,Fe_2O_3 + 4\,SO_2$ | **Step 1:** The question shows a chemical equation with a missing coefficient for one of the reactants and asks for the value that will balance the equation. |
| | **Step 2:** Recall that the numbers of each of the reactant atoms must equal the numbers of the products. |
| | **Step 3:** The missing coefficient determines the amount of O in the reactants. Since in the products, there are 2 complete sets of $Fe_2O_3$ and each has 3 atoms of O, that is a total of 6 O atoms. Similarly, the 4 $SO_2$ contains 8 atoms of O. Thus there is a total of 6 + 8 = 14 O atoms within the products, and this must also be the number in the reactants. Because the missing coefficient is for $O_2$, 7 units are needed. |
| (A)  2 | **Step 4:** Incorrect. |
| (B)  5 | Incorrect. |
| (C)  7 | Correct. |
| (D)  14 | Incorrect. Choice (D) is a trap answer you might choose if you overlook the subscript for oxygen. |

The rate at which a chemical reaction proceeds can be influenced by many factors, including temperature, pressure, and the concentrations of the reactants. Some reactions, such as when coal is burned, give off heat; such reactions are **exothermic**. Other reactions, such as when nitrogen and oxygen react to form nitric oxide, consume heat; these are **endothermic**. Applying more heat, usually by raising the temperature, will generally decrease the rate at which an exothermic reaction proceeds but increase the rate at which an endothermic reaction proceeds. Increasing the air pressure (when there are gaseous reactants) or increasing the concentration of reactants (such as those dissolved in solution) are both ways to increase the chances for successful contact between different reactant particles, and therefore these are also ways to increase reaction rate.

For some reactions, a **catalyst** can speed up the rate by providing a "shortcut" that lowers the amount of energy required for the reaction to occur. The catalyst itself is unchanged by the reaction and does not get used up. Enzymes are biological catalysts that speed up reactions in the human body, such as the metabolism of glucose.

## Acids and Bases

The characteristics of acids and bases relate to the hydrogen ion ($H^+$) and the hydroxide ion ($OH^-$). Acidic solutions have an overabundance of $H^+$ ions, and alkaline (basic) substances have an excess $OH^-$ ions. The quantitative measure of these is **pH**, which is a logarithmic representation of the concentration of $H^+$ ions. The scale of pH ranges from 0 to 14, where 0 is greatest **acidity** and 14 the highest **alkalinity** (also called **basicity**). Pure water is neutral because the $H^+$ ions and $OH^-$ ions are in balance and it has the middle pH of 7.

When acids and bases are mixed together in water, they form a salt (and some more water as well.) Conversely, most salts will dissolve in water and become ionized. For instance, if hydrochloric acid and sodium hydroxide were combined in a solution, the reaction would be $HCl + NaOH \rightarrow NaCl + H_2O$. However, the sodium chloride (NaCl), being a highly soluble salt, would exist in solution in the form of $Na^+$ and $Cl^-$ ions. Sodium chloride and potassium chloride are both salts that are essential to humans.

Try applying what you have learned to the following question:

> Some $Ca(OH)_2$ is dissolved in water. Which of the following could be the pH of the solution?
>
> (A)  0
> (B)  4
> (C)  7
> (D)  8

### Explanation

**Step 1:** The question asks for a possible pH of a solution of $Ca(OH)_2$ in water.

**Step 2:** Recall that pH is related to the balance of hydrogen and hydroxide ion concentrations. Any measure below 7 represents an excess of $H^+$ ions, and any measure above 7 represents an excess of $OH^-$ ions.

**Step 3:** Ca(OH)$_2$ will separate into Ca$^+$ and OH$^-$ ions in water. Because of the subscript 2, there will be twice as many OH$^-$ ions as Ca$^+$ ions. Predict that the pH will be a number greater than 7.

**Step 4:** The correct answer is **(D)**, the only choice greater than 7.

## KEY IDEAS

- Bonds can be either ionic or covalent.
- The total quantity of each type of atom in a chemical reaction equation must be equal on the reactant and product sides.
- There are five basic types of chemical reactions.
- The speed at which a reaction takes place can be altered by changing temperature, concentration, or pressure or by introducing a catalyst.
- Acidity and alkalinity are measured by the pH scale.

# Chemical Reactions Practice Questions

1. Which of the following chemical equations describes a reaction that has a metal and an acid as the reactants and a salt and a gas as the products?

   (A) $Zn + 2 HCl \rightarrow ZnCl_2 + H_2$

   (B) $ZnCl_2 + H_2 \rightarrow Zn + 2 HCl$

   (C) $2 Al(NO_3)_3 + 3 MgS \rightarrow 3 Mg(NO_3)_2 + Al_2S_3$

   (D) $Li + NaCl \rightarrow Na + LiCl$

2. When $MgCO_3$ is dissolved in water, it separates into $Mg^{2+}$ and $CO_3^{2-}$ ions. What type of bond exists between carbon (C) and oxygen (O)?

   (A) Neutron
   (B) Ionic
   (C) Proton
   (D) Covalent

3. Which of the following is NOT an organic substance?

   (A) $C_6H_{12}O_6$
   (B) $MgSO_4$
   (C) $C_2H_6O$
   (D) $C_{12}H_{22}O_{11}$

**Review your work using the explanations in Part Six of this book.**

# CHAPTER THREE

# SCIENTIFIC PROCEDURES AND REASONING

## LEARNING OBJECTIVES

- Use the appropriate metric unit and the appropriate tool to make measurements and be able to determine or infer cause-and-effect relationships based on measurements
- Analyze experimental designs and data to differentiate among different kinds of variables and between research and null hypotheses and to evaluate the validity of results and conclusions

Of the 47 scored *Science* questions, 7 (15%) will be in the sub-content area of *Scientific reasoning*. With these questions, the TEAS assesses your understanding of scientific measurement and the way in which the scientific method explores relationships among variables, as well as your ability to evaluate scientific research.

This chapter addresses these skills in two lessons:

**Lesson 1:** Scientific Measurements and Relationships

**Lesson 2:** Designing and Evaluating an Experiment

**Science Questions by Sub-content Area**

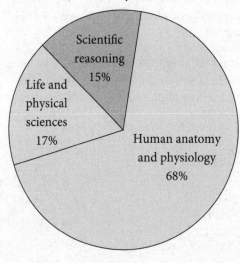

# LESSON 1

# Scientific Measurements and Relationships

## LEARNING OBJECTIVES

- Understand how the metric system functions
- Measure, record, and diagram data using the appropriate tool and metric unit
- Identify cause-and-effect relationships

## The Metric System

The **metric system** is used throughout the world for measurement. In the United States, it is mainly used in scientific and technical applications (including medicine). The TEAS will ask questions about measuring, recording, and diagramming volume, mass, and length using the metric system.

You might see reference to the **SI system**, which refers to the International System of Units. The SI system includes both metric and nonmetric units. The SI base unit for mass is the gram, for length the meter, and for volume the liter. (The SI system is also used to measure time, using seconds as a base. Kelvin, amperes, candela, and mole are other SI base units.) Prefixes are used to increase or decrease the size of a base unit.

The metric system is decimal based, meaning divided into units of 10 (or powers of 10), so converting units is simply a question of moving the decimal point the appropriate number of places to the left or right. (See Mathematics, Chapter 1, Lesson 5: Estimating and Rounding for a conversion chart.)

The most common prefixes are these:

| Prefix | Meaning |
| --- | --- |
| micro- | one-millionth |
| milli- | one-thousandth |
| centi- | one-hundredth |
| deci- | one-tenth |
| deca- | ten |
| hecto- | one hundred |
| kilo- | one thousand |
| mega- | one million |

Hence, a milliliter is one-thousandth of a liter. A hectometer is 100 meters. By custom, some of these prefixes (*deca*, for example) are less commonly used than others.

It's important to know which unit should be used to measure specific things. A person's height is expressed in centimeters, for example, while distances between cities are expressed in kilometers. Thus, the distance between San Jose, California, and San Jose, Costa Rica, is written as 6093 kilometers (km). Small distances, such as the thickness of a mechanical pencil lead, are more likely to be measured in millimeters (mm).

Similarly, small quantities of liquids, such as your toothpaste and shampoo, are expressed in milliliters (mL). Larger volumes of liquids, whether gasoline in a fuel tank or water in a bathtub, are typically measured in liters. A very large amount of liquid, say the water behind a dam, could be measured in megaliters (ML). Small mass amounts, like medicine doses, might be expressed in milligrams (mg). Larger masses—the weight of a human, for example—are more likely to be expressed in kilograms (kg).

## Measuring Tools

In scientific contexts, different tools have different functions, depending on ease of use and accuracy.

Some tools, such as measuring tapes, are commonly used in both scientific and nonscientific applications. Others are typically confined to scientific use. The **graduated cylinder**, for example, is a narrow vessel used to quickly measure liquid volume. Despite its widespread use in science, it is less accurate than other tools. Large volumes of liquids can be more accurately measured using a **volumetric flask**, while smaller volumes are measured precisely using a **volumetric pipette**.

The dimensions of solids can be measured by various tools, including measuring tapes, meter sticks, rulers, or **measuring wheels**. Length, width, and height can then be used to calculate volume.

Mass can be measured on a balance. The **electronic balance** is commonly found in science labs because it is easy to use. You might also come across a **triple beam balance** in a lab at some point.

## Relationships and Causality

**Causality** is the relationship between two events or states such that one brings about the other, with one variable being the cause and the other the effect. For example, think of the relationship between a certain medication and a client's condition. If a medication dosage is increased and the client feels sleepier, this might mean the medication is causing the sleepiness.

Note that just because two things happen consecutively, or even at the same time, does not mean one thing caused the other. Nonetheless, sometimes causation can be established. Some causal relationships are very obvious and easy to determine: if you walk for 1 hour at 3 miles per hour, you will have traveled 3 miles. Others can only be verified by multiple studies. Extensive research has made it clear, for example, that smoking contributes to adverse health conditions such as high blood pressure, vascular disease, some cancers, and emphysema.

Follow along as a TEAS expert tackles a question on scientific measurement.

> *Deinocheirus* is a genus of large ornithomimosaur, or ostrich dinosaur, that lived in the Late Cretaceous epoch, around 70 million years ago. The species name *Deinocheirus mirificus* is Greek for "horrible hand," and this creature's arms were the largest of any bipedal dinosaur.

| Question | Analysis |
|---|---|
| Which would be the appropriate unit to express the length of the arm bones of a *Deinocheirus mirificus*? | **Step 1:** The question asks about the most appropriate unit of measure for the length of the arm bones of a certain dinosaur. |
| | **Step 2:** You are provided with suggestions about the dinosaur's size. Note that *D. mirificus* is called a "large ornithomimosaur," its genus name means "horrible hand," and its arms were the largest of any bipedal dinosaur. |
| | **Step 3:** Use your knowledge of the relative sizes of metric units of measure to select the most appropriate one. Consider which unit you would choose to measure the height of a large animal, for example. |
| (A)  Millimeter | **Step 4:** A millimeter is very small and thus would be cumbersome in this situation. |
| (B)  Centimeter | Although larger than millimeters, centimeters are also too small a unit of measure to express a rough length. |
| (C)  Meter | Correct. A meter would be an appropriate unit to measure *D. mirificus*'s arm bones. |
| (D)  Kilometer | Kilometers are used for great distances, between landmarks or cities for example, and would be inappropriate here. |

Now it's your turn. Try this question about causation.

Color blindness is a hereditary condition present at birth. The human eye normally has three types of cone cells, and each type senses either red, green, or blue light. A person sees color when the cone cells sense different amounts of these kinds of light. Inherited color blindness happens when an individual lacks or has a malfunction in one of these cone cell types. He or she might not see one of the basic colors, see a different shade of that color, or even see a different color entirely. Thus, faulty red cones means that an individual will be unable to see colors containing red clearly.

A person with malfunctioning blue-sensing cone cells would most likely have difficulty distinguishing which of these colors?

    (A)   Pink
    (B)   Turquoise
    (C)   Brown
    (D)   Olive

## Explanation

**Step 1:** The question asks about the likely effect of malfunctioning blue-sensing cone cells on vision.

**Step 2:** The passage explains that the human eye has cone cells dedicated to seeing one of red, blue, or green light. Missing or malfunctioning cell cones can cause difficulty in perceiving one of these basic colors.

**Step 3:** Predict that this person will have difficulty seeing colors containing blue. Look for a choice that names a shade of blue or a color containing blue.

**Step 4:** Turquoise is a shade of green-blue, so a person with blue color blindness would have difficulty perceiving the color correctly. Therefore, **(B)** is the correct choice. Pink, (A), a pale red, and olive, (D), a dark green, should pose no problems for this individual. Brown, (C), is formed by the combination of red and green and likewise would be perceived correctly, provided there were no other issues.

## KEY IDEAS

- Conversions and calculations in the metric system involve multiplying or dividing by powers of ten, as indicated by the prefixes of the units.
- Different units of measure are appropriate for quantities of different sizes.
- Causality can be determined or inferred by considering the relative sizes or amounts of things in combination with changes over time.

# Scientific Measurements and Relationships Practice Questions

1. A student has a brass cube with the following marking: 300 cg. What is another way to express the weight of the cube?

   (A)   3 milligrams
   (B)   3 centimeters
   (C)   ‹ 3 grams
   (D)   3 decagrams

2. Alcohol is classified as a depressant. Consuming alcohol slows down the central nervous system, which decreases motor coordination, reaction time, and intellectual performance. Blood alcohol content (BAC) measures the ratio of alcohol in the blood. For example, a BAC of .10 means 1 part alcohol for every 1000 parts of blood.

The following chart shows how alcohol affects the body at different BAC levels.

| BAC | Effects on Feeling, Behavior, and Function |
| --- | --- |
| 0.02–0.04 | Few obvious effects; slight intensification of mood |
| 0.05–0.06 | Feeling of relaxation and mild sedation; slight decrease in reaction time and in fine muscle coordination |
| 0.07–0.09 | Impaired motor coordination, hearing, and vision; feeling of elation or depression |
| 0.10–0.12 | Difficulty with coordination and balance; distinct impairment of mental faculties and judgment |
| 0.13–0.15 | Major impairment of mental and physical control, including slurred speech, blurred vision, and lack of motor skills |
| 0.16–0.25 | Loss of motor control; mental confusion |
| 0.26+ | Severe intoxication; potential loss of consciousness |

Which of the following describes the likely behavior of a person who consumes two alcoholic drinks, resulting in a BAC of .08?

   (A)   She will experience no changes in her behavior.
   (B)   She will have some difficulty seeing or hearing, even though she might be in a good mood.
   (C)⸱   She will have some difficulty with walking, although she will think she is fine.
   (D)   She will appear confused about her surroundings and her ability to function.

3. Which of the following tools would measure the volume of an object roughly the size of a tennis shoe most accurately?

   (A) ‹ Measuring tape
   (B)   Electronic balance
   (C)   Triple-beam balance
   (D)   Volumetric pipette

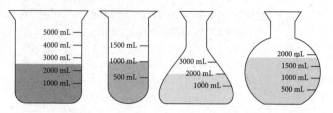

4. Which vessel contains the most liquid?

   (A)   Beaker
   (B)   Test tube
   (C)   Graduated cylinder
   (D)   Globe

**Review your work using the explanations in Part Six of this book.**

# LESSON 2

# Designing and Evaluating an Experiment

## LEARNING OBJECTIVES

- Differentiate among dependent, independent, and controlled variables
- Design experiments to test hypotheses and draw conclusions that are strongly supported by experimental data
- Critique experimental designs

## The Scientific Method

Scientists always take a methodical approach, known as the **scientific method**, to investigate any scientific question. There are five main steps to this method:

1. *Observation:* A scientist notices something that sparks his or her curiosity or identifies a problem that needs to be solved.
2. *Hypothesis:* The scientist formulates a testable statement, called a **hypothesis**, based on his or her original observation.
3. *Experiment:* The scientist tests the hypothesis using a carefully designed procedure, called an **experiment**. In an experiment, measurements and observations are collected.
4. *Data analysis:* The scientist finds out more about what the data mean and determines whether they are reliable.
5. *Conclusion:* The scientist uses the results of the data analysis to determine whether the data support the hypothesis.

To test a hypothesis, a scientist can design an experiment with a **null hypothesis,** which states that there is no causal relationship between the parameter varied and the outcome. For example, if an experimenter's research hypothesis is that drinking during pregnancy leads to fetal alcohol syndrome, the null hypothesis might be that alcohol does *not* lead to the development of fetal alcohol syndrome. To *reject* this null hypothesis, the experimenter must collect experimental data that show a link between drinking during pregnancy and having babies with fetal alcohol syndrome.

## Experimental Design

In designing experiments, it is critical to only vary one experimental parameter at a time so that a direct causal relationship can be established between the varied parameter and the experimental outcome. This varied parameter, or variable, is termed the **independent variable**. The measured parameter would be the **dependent variable**. Graphically, the independent variable is often plotted on the *x*-axis and the dependent variable is plotted on the *y*-axis.

The group in which the independent variable is changed is the **experimental group**. Furthermore, when testing an independent variable, a **control group** must be included: a group identical to the experimental group but without the altered independent variable. All of the variables held constant between the experimental and control groups are termed **controlled variables**.

For example, consider an experiment testing smoking and elevated blood pressure. The presence or absence of smoking would be the independent variable, and blood pressure would be the dependent variable. Two groups would be compared: the experimental group in which individuals are smokers, and a control group similar in every way to the experimental group except that the individuals are nonsmokers.

If this experiment had been run without a control group, anything could be linked to the development of high blood pressure, including diet, lack of exercise, and smoking. By including a control group that is identical in every way to the experimental group except for smoking, if the experimental group shows an increase in blood pressure, the researcher can conclude that the change is due to smoking.

Here is how an expert would approach a question on dependent and independent variables.

| Question | Analysis |
|---|---|
| An experiment is designed to determine the effect of a new drug on controlling blood sugar in people with diabetes. Volunteers of similar ages and diets are enrolled in the study and randomly assigned to two groups: one group receives the drug, and one does not. Following one month of treatment, blood is collected from the subjects to measure blood glucose concentrations. Which of the following parameters is the independent variable? | **Step 1:** This question is presenting you with an experimental design and asking which experimental parameter is the independent variable. |
| | **Step 2:** Recall that the independent variable is the parameter that is changed between the experimental and control groups. The dependent variable is the parameter measured to determine the effect of the independent variable. |
| | **Step 3:** Predict that drug treatment is the independent variable in this experiment. |
| (A) Blood glucose concentration | **Step 4:** Blood glucose was measured in this experiment, so it is the dependent variable and can be eliminated. |
| (B) Drug treatment | Correct. This matches your prediction. |
| (C) Age | Age is held constant between both groups, so this is a control variable. Eliminate. |
| (D) Diet | Diet is held constant between both groups. Eliminate. |

In addition to having the proper controls, it is necessary to have a large sample size. Otherwise small inaccuracies in measurement might skew the data, a phenomenon known as **random error**. If the sample size is too small, random error can lead to unreliable data in which differences between the control and experimental groups are seen, but in actuality do not exist. With a large sample size, random error is minimized, giving much more reliable data.

# Making Strong Conclusions

Drawing strong conclusions depends on gathering reliable data, which must be both reproducible and convincing. When evaluating the reliability of data, consider the following:

- **Bias:** Does the design of an experiment favor one outcome, either intentionally or unintentionally?
- **Control:** Is more than one variable changed at a time?
- **Reproducibility:** Can the results of the experiment be replicated?

If the data are reliable, you can draw some conclusions. However, the conclusions must be based on the experimental evidence; they must be within the scope of what is directly observed in the experiment. Consider the following experiment.

*Example:* A researcher is interested in investigating a new combination drug therapy for treating Alzheimer's disease. She enrolls 200 individuals in the study and randomly assigns them to two groups of 100 subjects. One group is given the combination therapy consisting of drugs X and Y, and the other is given a placebo, or sugar pill, as a control. Members of both groups are instructed to live life as normal and are not told which group they were in. After four months, the researcher finds that the treatment group has experienced improvement in memory while the control group has not. What conclusions can the researcher draw?

Given that there is an observable difference between the two groups, and that drug therapy was the only variable that differed between them, the researcher can conclude that the combination drug therapy improved memory in these study participants. However, the researcher cannot conclude that drug X was responsible for this improvement, as she did not test the drug in the absence of drug Y, or vice versa. The researcher also cannot determine that this combination therapy is the best treatment for Alzheimer's, since she did not compare the treatment to all other available treatments. Conclusions must stay within the scope of the experiment.

Now you try a question that asks you to draw conclusions from experimental data.

A scientist is interested in determining the effect of different wavelengths of light on plant growth. He plants 150 seeds at the start of the experiment and divides them into three groups of 50. Each seed is of the same species and is planted in a separate container in identical soil. One group is grown under red light, another under blue light, and the last under green light. No other wavelengths of light are included. After 30 days, the scientist counts the number of seedlings that germinated and records their heights.

| Lighting | Seeds Germinated | Average Seedling Height |
|----------|------------------|--------------------------|
| Red | 45 | 13 cm |
| Green | 12 | 16 cm |
| Blue | 30 | 14 cm |

Which of the following is the most supported conclusion the experimenter can draw based on the results?

(A) Red light is the most effective lighting source.
(B) Green light inhibits seed germination, but promotes plant growth.
(C) Of the three conditions, red light is optimal for seed germination, but not plant growth.
(D) Blue light is the most effective lighting source.

## Explanation

**Step 1:** This question is asking what conclusions can be drawn based on the experimental results.

**Step 2:** Recall that for a conclusion to be valid, it must be strongly supported by the evidence.

**Step 3:** Based on the experimental data, of the three light sources, red light appears to be optimal for seed germination, while green light appears to be optimal for plant growth. Remember that there are other wavelengths of light that the researcher did not include, so comparisons must be drawn among the three wavelengths studied.

**Step 4:** Based on the data, of the three wavelengths tested, red light appears to be optimal for germination as it has the largest number of germinated seeds. Red light also has the lowest average seedling height, so it is not the best for plant growth. These two conclusions are true based on the experimental data, so choice **(C)** is correct. Because the researcher did not test all wavelengths of light in this experiment, he cannot conclude that one wavelength is the best, only that some are better than others. For this reason, choices (A) and (D) can be eliminated. Furthermore, while 12 was the least number of seeds that germinated in the experiment, nothing in the experiment shows whether this means that germination was inhibited; 12 out of 50 (24%) might be a normal germination rate for this seed, so choice (B) can also be eliminated.

## Critiquing Experimental Design

A failure to control for variables is one of the most common experimental flaws. Many scientists operate under one golden rule: "no control, no experiment." If a control is lacking, a scientist cannot conclusively establish a cause-and-effect relationship between the independent and dependent variables.

> *Example:* A scientist is interested in determining the efficacy of an experimental antiviral drug. She enlists 100 sick volunteers in a study and gives them each three doses of the drug over the course of three days. At the end of the trial, she finds that 100 percent of the study participants show signs of recovery, including a drop in body temperature to normal levels and increased energy. The scientist concludes that the experimental drug leads to increased viral clearance and is better than other drugs currently on the market.

There are several flaws in this experiment. The scientist only has one group of study participants, all of which take the drug. It is thus impossible to determine whether the drug directly led to increased clearance of the virus or study participants simply got better over time. Furthermore, considering that the scientist lacks evidence to show the drug is effective, it is an even bigger stretch to conclude the drug is better than other available therapeutics—no other drugs were included in the study. A conclusion like this goes beyond the scope of the experiment and is not supported by the data.

### KEY IDEAS

- The independent variable differs between experimental and control groups, while controlled variables are held constant between both groups. The variable that is measured is the dependent variable.
- To generate reliable data, a study must be unbiased in the way data are collected, use a large sample size, include adequate controls, and be reproducible.
- Conclusions must be directly supported by the experimental evidence and not go beyond the scope of the study.

# Designing and Evaluating an Experiment Practice Questions

1. A group of researchers is designing a study to test the effect of a specially formulated, vitamin-infused drink on the duration of the common cold in the general population. The researchers recruit 200 participants, 165 women and 35 men. They randomly assign 100 participants to the control group and 100 participants to the treatment group. During the trial, the members of the control group will receive a placebo drink, and the members of the treatment group will receive the vitamin-infused drink. In what way could the design of this experiment be improved?

   (A) Give more participants the vitamin-infused drink.
   (B) Give more participants the placebo drink.
   (C) Recruit more men for the experiment.
   (D) Recruit more women for the experiment.

2. A researcher is designing an experiment to compare a new conductor material to the most commonly used conductor in transistors. Which procedure is likely to lead to the most reliable results?

   (A) Measure the resistance of the new conductor 10 times and compare it to the known resistance of the existing conductor.
   (B) Measure the resistance of the new and old conductors 10 times each under the same conditions and compare the two results.
   (C) Measure the resistance of the new conductor 50 times and compare it to the known resistance of the existing conductor.
   (D) Measure the resistance of the new and old conductors 50 times each under the same conditions and compare the two results.

3. A scientist is interested in studying how caffeine affects heart rate. He gathers a group of 100 college students and randomly assigns them to two groups. One group is given a caffeinated soda and the other is given a caffeine-free soda with the same sugar content. Before starting the experiment, the researcher measures the heart rates of all participants. One hour later, he measures their heart rates again. Which of the following represents the dependent variable in this experiment?

   (A) Caffeine
   (B) Heart rate
   (C) Sugar
   (D) Age

4. The model below shows how a population of the bacterium *Staphylococcus aureus* responds to an increasing concentration of the antibiotic erythromycin.

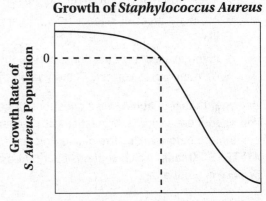

**Effect of Erythromycin on the Growth of *Staphylococcus Aureus***

Which prediction is supported by the model?

   (A) Erythromycin can shrink a population of *Staphylococcus aureus*.
   (B) Erythromycin can shrink a population of any species of bacteria.
   (C) Any antibiotic can shrink a population of *Staphylococcus aureus*.
   (D) Any antibiotic can shrink a population of any species of bacteria.

**Review your work using the explanations in Part Six of this book.**

# Review and Reflect

Think about the questions you answered in these lessons.

- Were you able to approach each question systematically, using the Kaplan Method for Science?
- Did you feel confident that you understood what the question was asking you to do?
- Were you able to recall the facts the question was asking for?
- How well were you able to predict an answer before looking at the answer choices?
- Could you match your prediction to the correct answer?
- Are there areas of science that appear on the TEAS that you don't understand as well as you would like?
- If you missed any questions, do you understand why the answer you chose is incorrect and why the right answer is correct? Could you do the question again now and get it right?

Use your thoughts about these questions to guide how you continue to prepare for the TEAS. If you feel you need more review and practice with human anatomy and physiology, you should study this chapter some more before taking the online Practice Test that comes with this book. Also, consider using **Kaplan's ATI TEAS® Qbank,** which contains over 500 practice questions, to increase your proficiency with the *Science* content area.

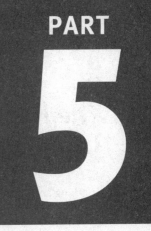

# PART 5

# English and Language Usage

As a nursing or health science student and then later as a healthcare professional, you will be expected to express yourself clearly and correctly in writing. This skill will be important to your ability to communicate with clients and colleagues. You might be adding notes to a client's chart, writing out instructions for a client or colleague, or preparing educational material to distribute to clients or the public. The TEAS *English and language usage* content area tests your ability to use correct spelling, punctuation, and grammar; construct sentences and paragraphs to convey meaning clearly; and use appropriate vocabulary and style to communicate to a given audience.

**Questions by Content Area**

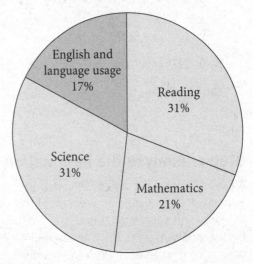

## The TEAS English and Language Usage Content Area

Of the 170 items on the TEAS, 28 will be in the *English and language usage* content area, and you will have 28 minutes to answer them. This means you will have an average of 1 minute per question.

In the *English and language usage* section, 24 of the 28 questions will be scored, and 4 will be unscored. You won't know which questions are unscored, so do your best on every question.

The 24 scored *English and language usage* questions come from three sub-content areas:

| Sub-content areas | # of Questions |
|---|---|
| Conventions of standard English | 9 |
| Knowledge of language | 9 |
| Vocabulary acquisition | 6 |

To help you prepare for these questions, this part of your book is divided into three chapters:

- Chapter 1: Spelling, Punctuation, and Sentence Structure
- Chapter 2: Grammar, Style, and the Writing Process
- Chapter 3: Vocabulary

# The Kaplan Method for English and Language Usage

Thinking through questions step-by-step will help you approach every question with the right rules in mind.

## KAPLAN METHOD FOR ENGLISH AND LANGUAGE USAGE

**Step 1:** Analyze the information provided.

**Step 2:** Predict the answer.

**Step 3:** Evaluate the answer choices.

## Step 1: Analyze the information provided.

Many questions about *English and language usage* will present you with a sentence or short passage and ask you to identify an element of the sentence, complete the sentence correctly, or fix an error. The question will specify what task you are to perform. Read the question and the sentence carefully, paying particular attention to the rule of grammar, spelling, punctuation, or style that you need to apply, as well as context clues in the sentence that point to the meaning of a word or its part of speech, a needed punctuation mark, or whatever you are being asked about.

Not every question is accompanied by a sentence. Some simply ask you to recall facts. In this case, the question still contains key terms that identify which fact you need to apply. The TEAS tests many language arts topics; you might see a question about writing style followed by one about punctuation followed by one about sentence structure. Each time you read a question, give yourself the time it takes for one deep breath to call to mind the particular rules or facts being tested.

## Step 2: Predict the answer.

Before looking at the answer choices, *predict* the answer. You have a much better chance of finding the correct answer if you already have it in mind. Sometimes you may not be able to make a specific prediction. For example, a question might ask you to complete a sentence and there are several ways to complete the sentence correctly. Think of several ways you could complete the sentence and then use this mental checklist as you evaluate the answer choices.

Alternatively, you may have trouble thinking of the exact answer. Say the question asks for the part of a book that lists key terms alphabetically. You may not be able to think of the word *index* right off the bat, but you may know that you find such a list at the back of a book. Even an approximate prediction will allow you to eliminate answer choices you know are not found at the end of a book.

## Step 3: Evaluate the answer choices.

Compare each answer choice to your prediction, eliminating those that are not a match and choosing the one that is a match.

# CHAPTER ONE

# SPELLING, PUNCTUATION, AND SENTENCE STRUCTURE

## LEARNING OBJECTIVES

- Use standard English spelling conventions and common exceptions to these rules to spell words correctly
- Use punctuation correctly according to the standard rules of English
- Construct sentences with various structures and identify parts of speech and the main parts of sentences

Of the 24 scored *English and language usage* questions, 9 (37.5%) will be in the sub-content area of *Conventions of standard English*. The TEAS tests your recognition of and ability to use correct spelling, punctuation, and sentence structure.

This chapter addresses these skills in three lessons:

**Lesson 1:** Spelling

**Lesson 2:** Punctuation

**Lesson 3:** Sentence Structure

**English and Language Usage Questions by Sub-content Area**

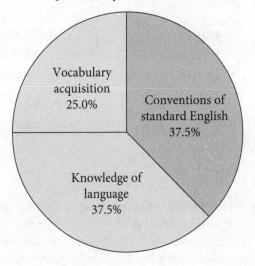

Vocabulary acquisition 25.0%

Conventions of standard English 37.5%

Knowledge of language 37.5%

# LESSON 1

# Spelling

## LEARNING OBJECTIVES

- Spell words using standard English spelling conventions
- Identify common exceptions to standard English spelling conventions
- Recognize common words that have different meanings but are either spelled the same way (homographs) or sound the same (homophones)

English words come from different language families, all of which have rules that govern spelling. As a result, English spelling is notoriously difficult to master because most of its rules have multiple exceptions. Fortunately, the rules can be learned and their exceptions memorized!

## Common Spelling Rules

You may recall learning the rhyme "*i* before *e*, except after *c*," when you were a child. But you may not have learned that there is an easy way to remember additional exceptions to the "*i* before *e*" rule: if it sounds like a long *a* (as in *neighbor* or *weigh*), use *e* before *i*.

| *i* before *e* | "After *c*" and "sounds like *a*" exceptions | Other exceptions |
| --- | --- | --- |
| believe | ceiling | caffeine |
| chief | eight | neither |
| friend | receipt | protein |
| relief | vein | science |
| thief | weigh | weird |

Many spelling errors occur when **suffixes** are added to words incorrectly. It is important to understand the rules and guidelines that dictate whether the endings of a **root word** should change when merged with a suffix; these are the Root Ends and Beginnings of Suffixes (REBS) rules. You may already know some of the REBS rules, but you should memorize any you do not recognize. You should also memorize the most common exceptions to these rules.

| Word that . . . | Rule | Examples | Exceptions |
|---|---|---|---|
| ends in *e* + suffix beginning with a consonant | Keep the *e* if it is silent. | state + ment = statement<br><br>peace + ful = peaceful<br><br>encourage + ment = encouragement | judge + ment = judgment<br><br>awe + ful = awful |
| ends in *e* + suffix beginning with a vowel | Drop the *e* if it is silent. | change + ing = changing<br><br>shove + ing = shoving | Keep the *e* if the word ends in *ce*, *ge*, or *ke* and the suffix is *able* or *ous*.<br><br>change + able = changeable<br><br>outrage + ous = outrageous<br><br>like + able = likeable |
| ends in *y* preceded by a consonant + suffix | Change the *y* to *i* and add the suffix. | carry + er = carrier<br><br>duty + ful = dutiful<br><br>worry + ed = worried | Keep the *y* when adding the suffix *ing*.<br><br>carry + ing = carrying<br><br>rely + ing = relying<br><br>worry + ing = worrying |
| ends in *ay, ey, oy, uy* + any suffix | Keep the *y*. | relay + ed = relayed<br><br>survey + ing = surveying<br><br>destroy + er = destroyer<br><br>buy + er = buyer | |
| ends in a consonant-vowel-consonant and is only one syllable + suffix beginning with a vowel | Double the final consonant and add the suffix. | scrub + ing = scrubbing<br><br>tag + ed = tagged<br><br>run + ing = running<br><br>knit + ed = knitted | Omit the double consonant if the word ends in *w*.<br><br>sew + ing = sewing<br><br>snow + ed = snowed<br><br>blow + ing = blowing |
| ends in a consonant-vowel-consonant but has more than one syllable (and the last syllable is stressed) + suffix beginning with a vowel | Double the final consonant and add the suffix. | control + ing = controlling<br><br>defer + al = deferral<br><br>refer + ed = referred<br><br>occur + ing = occurring | Omit the double consonant if the word ends in *w*.<br><br>renew + ing = renewing |

| Word that . . . | Rule | Examples | Exceptions |
|---|---|---|---|
| ends in *c* + suffix beginning with *e, i,* or *y* | Add a *k* then add the suffix. | panic + ed = panicked<br><br>frolic + ing = frolicking<br><br>garlic + y = garlicky | |

Here is how an expert would answer a TEAS question that tests a spelling rule.

| Question | Analysis |
|---|---|
| Sharla ate a _____ bar on her way to the meeting. | **Step 1:** You need to find the correctly spelled word that fills the blank in the sentence. |
| Which of the following correctly completes the sentence above? | **Step 2:** You cannot predict the word that will fill the blank. However, a glance at the answer choices tells you that spelling rules are involved, so call to mind the rules you know. |
| (A) proteen | **Step 3:** Is this the correct spelling of *protein*? No. |
| (B) protien | Is this the correct spelling of *protein*? No. |
| (C) protein | Is this the correct spelling of *protein*? Yes. This word is an exception to the *i* before *e* rule. |
| (D) protine | This is not the correct spelling of *protein*. |

Now try a question that tests a different rule.

Which of the following is spelled correctly?

    (A)   defered
    (B)   occurred
    (C)   patroled
    (D)   snowwing

## Explanation

**Step 1:** You need to find the correctly spelled word.

**Step 2:** With this type of question, you cannot predict which word will be correctly spelled, but you can call to mind the spelling rules you have memorized. Then evaluate each answer choice and determine which one correctly fills the blank.

**Step 3:** Answer choice **(B)** obeys the REBS rule for doubling the final consonant before adding a suffix: occur + ed = occurred.

## Making Singular Words Plural

Other spelling rules you should be familiar with relate to the formation of plurals. Most of the time, simply adding s to the end of a singular word creates the correct plural form: *peanut* becomes *peanuts*, for example. However, there are rules about when you need to do something different to create a plural. The table lists some of the common rules for forming plurals that you might see tested on the TEAS.

| Word that . . . | Rule | Examples | Exceptions |
|---|---|---|---|
| ends in a consonant other than *s, x, y, z, ch,* or *sh* | Add *s.* | cat/cats<br>dog/dogs<br>owl/owls | |
| ends in *s, x, ch,* or *sh* | Add *es.* | bus/buses<br>box/boxes<br>church/churches<br>wish/wishes | axis/axes<br>ox/oxen<br>appendix/appendixes or appendices |
| ends in *z* | Double the *z* and add *es.* | quiz/quizzes | |
| ends in *y* preceded by a vowel | Add *s.* | holiday/holidays<br>monkey/monkeys | money/monies |
| ends in *y* preceded by a consonant | Change the *y* to *i* and add *es.* | baby/babies<br>story/stories | |
| ends in *f* or *fe* | Change the *f* to *v* and add *es.* | calf/calves<br>leaf/leaves | chief/chiefs<br>proof/proofs |
| ends in a vowel | Add *s.* | coffee/coffees<br>sale/sales<br>taco/tacos | potato/potatoes<br>veto/vetoes |

Learning these rules and the common exceptions will give you an edge on the TEAS *English and language usage* test.

## Homonyms

Words that are spelled the same way but have different meanings are called **homographs**. Those that sound alike but have different spellings and meanings are called **homophones**. Together, homographs and homophones are called **homonyms**. The table lists some homographs, homophones, and other commonly confused words that people often misspell or misuse.

| Word | Meaning | Word in sentence |
|---|---|---|
| accept | to receive willingly | I accept your apology. |
| except | excluding | They were all present except Lara, who stayed home. |
| affect | to impact | The gray weather affects my mood. |
| effect | a result | The drug's effects will wear off soon. |
| content | something contained | The book's content is very disturbing. |
| | at peace or soothed | The baby was content in her mother's arms. |
| close | nearby | His house is close to his birthplace. |
| | to shut | Close the door, please. |
| clothes | apparel | I would like to change clothes first. |
| desert | arid land | I've never been to the desert. |
| | to leave behind | You said you would never desert me. |
| dessert | sweet food served after a meal | A good hostess offers dessert to her guests. |
| fare | money paid for transportation | She paid her subway fare in nickels. |
| fair | just or right | It was only fair that he let you go first. |
| | a festival | After all, it was your first trip to the fair. |
| forth | forward | Go forth and seek adventure! |
| fourth | in the 4th position | Her house is the fourth one on the left. |
| grate | to shred | We will need to grate some cheese before serving the pasta. |
| great | fabulous, fantastic | This will be a great dinner! |
| | of large size | We will eat in the great hall. |
| hole | an opening | This sweater has a hole in it. |
| whole | entire, entirety | I can't believe I ate the whole thing. |
| its | possessive form of the pronoun *it* | The turtle ducked into its shell. |
| it's | contraction of *it is* | It's freezing in here! |
| led | past tense of the verb *lead* | He led the visitors to the cafeteria after the tour. |
| lead | a metal; the material in pencils | My pencil is out of lead. |
| | to guide or bring forward | The captain should lead the charge. |

| Word | Meaning | Word in sentence |
|---|---|---|
| lessen | to reduce or decrease | Hopefully this will lessen the pain a bit. |
| lesson | something you learn or teach | Next time he will have learned his lesson. |
| passed | went by | Have you passed the post office yet? |
| past | opposite of *future* | I lived there in the past but not now. |
| principal | head of a school | The principal will meet with the seniors. |
| | primary, most significant | Cost was the principal reason she cited when explaining the decision. |
| principle | a guiding rule | Failing to act would violate my principles. |
| their | belonging to them | That is their car. |
| there | at that place, opposite of *here* | The car is parked over there. |
| they're | contraction of *they are* | They're going to try to sell it. |
| to | indicates direction | Please go to the store for me. |
| too | also, in addition | Erika will go, too. |
| two | the number 2 | Buy two loaves of bread. |
| weak | the opposite of *strong* | Having the flu has left me feeling weak. |
| week | seven days | I have been sick since last week. |
| your | possessive form of *you* | Don't forget your mittens! |
| you're | contraction of *you are* | You're going to need them on the way home. |

Here is how an expert would answer a question about homonyms.

| Question | Analysis |
|---|---|
| The teacher had prepared his lessons for the week, but on Monday mourning, he was late arriving at school because the bus had passed his house without stopping. | **Step 1:** There are several homophones in this sentence, so these are likely places for an error. |
| Which of the following describes the error in the sentence above? | **Step 2:** Assess the homophones to determine which one is incorrect; *mourning* means sorrow or bereavement and does not work in this sentence. Predict that the correct word here is *morning*, which is a time of day. |

| Question | Analysis |
|---|---|
| (A) The word *lessons* should be *lessens*. | **Step 3**: *Lessons* is the correct word in this sentence. |
| (B) The word *week* should be *weak*. | *Week* is the correct word in this sentence. |
| (C) The word *mourning* should be *morning*. | Correct. This matches your prediction. |
| (D) The word *passed* should be *past*. | *Passed,* the past tense of the verb *pass,* is the correct word for this sentence. |

## KEY IDEAS

- English spelling is governed by rules, but most of these rules have common exceptions.
- Spelling errors commonly occur where word roots meet suffixes, including plurals. Learn the rules and the common exceptions to spot these errors quickly.
- Homophones and homographs are easily confused, so make flashcards with any that give you trouble.

# Spelling Practice Questions

1. Which of the following words is spelled incorrectly?

   (A) Permissible
   (B) Disbelief
   (C) *Wierd
   (D) Judgment

2. Consuming too much salt can be _____ to your health.

   Which of the following correctly completes the sentence above?

   (A) injuryious
   (B) injurieous
   (C) injurrious
   (D) ,injurious

3. The fawn _____ beside the pond, unaware that we were watching.

   Which of the following correctly completes the sentence above?

   (A) *frolicked
   (B) frolicced
   (C) froliced
   (D) frolicted

4. The _____ reason he gave for refusing to wear leather shoes was that doing so violated his _____ as a strict vegetarian.

   Select the pair of homophones that correctly completes the sentence above.

   (A) principle/principals
   (B) ✓principal/principles
   (C) principle/principles
   (D) principal/principals

**Review your work using the explanations in Part Six of this book.**

# LESSON 2

# Punctuation

## LEARNING OBJECTIVES

- Recognize the three sentence punctuation patterns
- Use end punctuation marks and commas to clarify meaning
- Use colons, semicolons, apostrophes, and parentheses correctly within a sentence
- Use direct and indirect quotations according to the standard rules of English

Punctuation is an essential component of written language. These unassuming marks and symbols play a huge role—giving structure and clarity to the ideas expressed in writing and allowing authors to relate meaning, ask questions, identify direct quotations, and emphasize particular ideas or facts.

## Sentence Punctuation Patterns

Punctuation organizes ideas into sentences, which can be characterized as having one of three primary punctuation patterns—simple, complex, or compound.

A **simple sentence** contains only one clause and has a single subject and predicate. The predicate contains the verb and tells us something about the subject.

> *Example:* We divided up the chores.

A **complex sentence** contains both an independent and a dependent, or subordinate, clause. An independent clause has both a subject and a verb and expresses a complete thought. A dependent clause also has a subject and a verb but does not express a complete thought.

> *Example:* Although I ran the marathon last spring, I will not be running it again this year.

A **compound sentence** contains at least two independent clauses, which are connected by either a coordinating conjunction and a comma or a semicolon.

> *Example:* I purchased two tickets to the show, but I am no longer able to attend.

Being able to distinguish the different sentence punctuation patterns is essential to success on the TEAS. The type of sentence pattern determines the type of punctuation required within the sentence.

## End Punctuation Marks

**End punctuation marks** tell the reader the purpose of the sentence. A period indicates a declarative sentence that describes something, states information, or gives a command. A question mark indicates a question. The exclamation point indicates a sentence that expresses strong emotions or excitement.

# Comma Usage

The **comma** is one of the most commonly used punctuation marks. When used correctly, the comma helps the reader understand how ideas in a sentence are connected. There are numerous rules that govern comma usage, and the TEAS may test any of the those listed in the table.

| Comma Usage | |
|---|---|
| **Usage guideline or rule** | **Example** |
| Commas can indicate a pause, such as after introductory information. | *Before the development of Portland cement*, architects rarely used concrete block construction. |
| Commas can present phrases that are not essential to the meaning of the sentence. | Asha, *who is a straight A student*, attends Roosevelt High. |
| Commas are used to show a direct address, or calling a person by name. | *Jake*, please put the roast in the oven. |
| Commas can separate items in a list. | Jodi put *bananas, pears, and oranges* in the fruit salad. |
| Commas divide a series of words, phrases, or clauses. | Today we will *drive to swim practice, stop at the grocery store, and make dinner.* |
| Commas can separate adjectives that both describe a word equally. If you can separate the adjectives with *and*, then a comma is usually appropriate. | Pete visited the *old, crumbling* house one last time.<br><br>Pete visited the *big green* house one last time. (no comma) |
| Commas follow the salutation and the closing in an informal letter or note. | Dear *Jaden*,<br><br>I can't wait to see you.<br><br>*Love*,<br>Mom |
| Do *not* use a comma to set off an essential phrase. Essential phrases often include the word *that*. | Monika ate the cake *that Annie made for her.* |
| Commas are used to separate the elements in dates and place names. | *June 12, 1979*, is my birthday.<br><br>*Detroit, Michigan*, is also known as the Motor City. |

Let's now see how a test expert would tackle a question dealing with commas.

| Question | Analysis |
|---|---|
| Which of the following is a correctly punctuated compound sentence? | **Step 1:** The question asks you to identify a correctly punctuated compound sentence, and the answer choices are four sentences. |
| | **Step 2:** The correct answer will consist of two independent clauses joined by either a comma and coordinating conjunction or a semicolon. |

| Question | Analysis |
|---|---|
| (A) After school lets out the children will go to the park. | **Step 3**: This is a complex sentence, and a comma is missing after "out." Eliminate. |
| (B) All of the children rode their bikes to school, so they will ride to the park as well. | Correct. This sentence has two independent clauses that are correctly connected by a coordinating conjunction and a comma. |
| (C) The weather is warm, they need to drink enough water to stay hydrated. | This sentence has two independent clauses connected by a comma, but the coordinating conjunction is missing. Eliminate. |
| (D) Before they go home for dinner; the children will go down the slide one more time. | This sentence is a complex sentence that incorrectly uses a semicolon in the place of a comma. Eliminate. |

## Colons, Semicolons, Apostrophes, and Parentheses

Familiarize yourself with the rules associated with these punctuation marks.

### Common Punctuation Marks

| Punctuation Mark | Usage | Example |
|---|---|---|
| **colon** | A punctuation mark signaling a list or information that adds to the idea before the colon. Colons may also be used after the salutation in formal letters or memos. | My mother told me to buy the following: a loaf of bread, a container of milk, and a stick of butter. <br><br> To whom it may concern: <br><br> Dear Sir or Madam: |
| **semicolon** | A punctuation mark used to link related independent clauses or a series of items containing commas | The cello player forgot her music; therefore, she had to improvise during her performance. <br><br> For their picnic, Michael purchased apples, bananas, and grapes; Jana bought bread, cheese, and jam; and Julian picked up lemonade and ice tea. |
| **apostrophe** | A punctuation mark used to form possessives and contractions and to pluralize letters, numbers, or other words that have no plural form | Jim's golf clubs, Rosa's house <br><br> Dot your *i*'s and cross your *t*'s! |
| **parentheses** | Punctuation marks used to enclose additional information or explanations that would interrupt the flow of the sentence. | Karyn will (I assume) remember to bring the potato salad. |

Let's see how a test expert would tackle a question testing these punctuation rules.

| Question | Analysis |
|---|---|
| The librarian tried repeatedly to quiet the noisy children, but she was unsuccessful; eventually, she took each childs' book away and escorted the rowdy group to the lobby.<br><br>Which of the following punctuation marks is used incorrectly in the sentence? | **Step 1**: The question asks about punctuation. A sentence is given with two commas, a semicolon, an apostrophe, and an ending period. Examine each in terms of the rules for that mark. |
| | **Step 2**: The word "child" is singular; therefore, the apostrophe should come before the "s" in the possessive form. |
| (A) The comma after the word "children" | **Step 3**: This is a compound sentence, in which the comma correctly comes before the coordinating conjunction that separates the two independent clauses. Eliminate. |
| (B) The semicolon after the word "unsuccessful" | The semicolon correctly separates two independent clauses in this sentence. Eliminate. |
| (C) The comma after the word "eventually" | The comma correctly separates the introductory adverb "eventually" from the rest of the sentence. Eliminate. |
| (D) The apostrophe in the word "childs'" | Correct. The apostrophe should precede the *s*. |

## Punctuation for Quotations

Written dialogue represents the exact language someone has used when speaking. For example, a nurse may need to quote a client's exact words to include on intake or medical reports. When writing a quote, the rules of using **quotation marks** apply.

### Quotation Marks and Dialogue Rules

| Rule | Example |
|---|---|
| Quotation marks must come in pairs. If you open a quotation mark, it must be closed at the end of the quote. | "Always remember to close the quote," the teacher said. |
| Capitalize the first letter of a direct quote if the quote represents a complete sentence. | Danny said, "You never told me it was your birthday!" |
| Do not capitalize the first letter of a direct quote if it is a fragment or incomplete sentence. | Jamie said the new car was "the cat's meow." |
| Do not capitalize the second part of a quote if it is interrupted midsentence. | "I don't know what it was," said Peter, "but it sure was big!" |
| Enclose a comma before closing the quote prior to attribution. | "I've never tried chop suey before," said Katie. |

## Quotation Marks and Dialogue Rules

| Rule | Example |
|---|---|
| A quote within a quote takes single quotation marks. | "And then she said, 'No way!' as she huffed off," Erin told me. |
| Short works such as chapters, songs, poems, and short stories should have their titles enclosed in quotation marks. | We read "Ode on a Grecian Urn" in our English class. |
| The ending punctuation mark for the quote should be enclosed within the quotation marks. Use a comma to transition from quote to attribution. | Jerry said, "All's well that ends well." "She gave me the best present," said Karen. |

Let's see how a test expert would approach the following question.

| Question | Analysis |
|---|---|
| Which of the following sentences correctly punctuates the direct dialogue? | **Step 1:** The question asks about punctuating direct dialogue, and the answer choices are four sentences within quotation marks. Evaluate each sentence in terms of the rules for quotation marks, commas, and capitalization in dialogue. |
| | **Step 2:** Mentally review the applicable rules and prepare to check each answer choice against them. When you see an answer has broken a rule, you can stop reading it and eliminate it. |
| (A) "Whenever the teacher wants the students' attention, she calls out "Silence!" to the class," said the principal. | **Step 3:** This sentence fails to include the comma after the attribution to the teacher, and it uses double quotation marks within the principal's quote. Eliminate. |
| (B) "Whenever the teacher wants the students' attention, she calls out, 'Silence!' to the class," said the principal. | Correct. |
| (C) "Whenever the teacher wants the students' attention, she calls out, "silence!" to the class." Said the principal. | This sentence fails to capitalize the first letter of "silence," it closes the quote with a period rather than a comma, and it has double quotation marks within the principal's quote. Eliminate. |
| (D) "Whenever the teacher wants the students' attention, she calls out 'silence!' to the class," said the principal. | This sentence fails to include the comma after the attribution to the teacher, and it fails to capitalize the first letter of "silence." Eliminate. |

## KEY IDEAS

- Learning the three different sentence punctuation patterns will help you recognize punctuation errors on the TEAS.

- Analyze the content and structure of a sentence to determine which end punctuation is needed and where commas belong.

- Examine the structure of a sentence to determine whether colons, semicolons, apostrophes, and parentheses are either misplaced or incorrectly omitted.

- If a sentence contains a direct quotation, check that it follows standard English rules for capitalization and the placement of quotation marks, commas, and end punctuation.

# Punctuation Practice Questions

1. Which of the following is a correctly punctuated complex sentence?

   (A)  Every weekend in the summer Daniel goes hiking on a mountain trail.
   (B)  Daniel usually hikes alone, however, this time he invited me to join him.
   (C)  Although I am an experienced hiker, I was not prepared for the rocky terrain.
   (D)  I was relieved, when we reached the summit and could stop to enjoy the view.

2. Which of the following examples is a correct method for punctuating this quotation?

   (A)  "We must all do our part" she said, "even when doing so is difficult."
   (B)  "We must all do our part," she said, "even when doing so is difficult."
   (C)  "We must all do our part." She said, "even when doing so is difficult."
   (D)  "We must all do our part," she said. "even when doing so is difficult."

3. Which of the following sentences is correctly punctuated?

   (A)  Because the weather forecast predicted storms we decided to postpone our vacation until next month.
   (B)  Because the weather forecast predicted storms. We decided to postpone our vacation until next month.
   (C)  Because the weather forecast predicted storms; we decided to postpone our vacation until next month.
   (D)  Because the weather forecast predicted storms, we decided to postpone our vacation until next month.

4. Veronica has performed well on every test she has taken this semester_____therefore, she can expect to perform well on the final exam.

   Which of the following punctuation marks best completes the sentence?

   (A)  .
   (B)  ;
   (C)  ,
   (D)  :

**Review your work using the explanations in Part Six of this book.**

# LESSON 3

# Sentence Structure

## LEARNING OBJECTIVES

- Identify the correct use of eight parts of speech
- Construct simple, compound, complex, and compound-complex sentences
- Construct sentences using dependent and independent clauses
- Identify the main parts of sentence structures

## Eight Parts of Speech

The eight parts of speech defined here are the most commonly tested parts of speech on the TEAS.

| noun | a person, place, or thing |
|---|---|
| pronoun | a word (such as *I*, *he*, *she*, *you*, *it*, *we*, or *they*) that is used instead of a noun |
| verb | a word (such as *jump*, *think*, *happen*, or *exist*) that expresses an action or state of being |
| adjective | a word (such as *funny*, *breakable*, or *round*) that describes a noun or a pronoun |
| adverb | a word (such as *quickly*, *cheerfully*, or *very*) used to modify a verb, an adjective, or another adverb |
| preposition | a word expressing a relationship to other words (such as *on* in "the drawing on the page" and *after* in "she arrived after the play") |
| conjunction | a word used to connect independent or dependent clauses (such as *and*, *but*, or *if*) |
| interjection | a word or phrase that expresses sudden or strong feeling (such as *Hooray!* or *Oh!*) |

Here is how an expert would answer a TEAS question about parts of speech.

| Question | Analysis |
|---|---|
| Holland laughed loudly when he heard the joke.<br><br>What are the noun and pronoun pair in the sentence above? | **Step 1:** The question asks you to identify the noun and pronoun in the sentence, and the answer choices list pairs of words from the sentence. |
| | **Step 2:** A noun is a person, place, or thing, and a pronoun is a word used instead of a noun. The noun/pronoun pair in this sentence is "Holland/he." |

| Question | Analysis |
|---|---|
| (A)  Noun: he; pronoun: Holland | **Step 3**: This reverses the noun and pronoun. Eliminate. |
| (B)  Noun: Holland; pronoun: laughed | This gets the noun correct but incorrectly identifies the verb "laughed" as the pronoun. Eliminate. |
| (C)  Noun: he; pronoun: laughed | Here the pronoun is incorrectly identified as the noun, and a verb is used as the pronoun. Eliminate. |
| (D)  Noun: Holland; pronoun: he | Correct. This matches the prediction. |

Now try a question on your own.

> The ballerina danced beautifully despite her broken shoe and torn tutu.
>
> What are the verb and adverb in the sentence above?
>
> (A)  Verb: ballerina; adverb: her
> (B)  Verb: danced; adverb: despite
> (C)  Verb: danced; adverb: beautifully
> (D)  Verb: broken; adverb: shoe

### Explanation

**Step 1:**  The question asks you to identify the verb and adverb in the sentence, and the answer choices list pairs of words from the sentence.

**Step 2:**  A verb is a word that expresses an action or state of being, and an adverb is a word used to modify a verb, adjective, or another adverb. The verb in this sentence is "danced," and the adverb is "beautifully," telling how she danced.

**Step 3:**  Answer choice **(C)** matches the prediction.

## Simple, Compound, Complex, and Compound-Complex Sentences

To be complete, a **simple sentence** must have at least one subject and one verb, and it must express a complete thought. The **subject** is the main noun of the sentence that is doing or being. The verb tells what action the subject is doing. These simple sentences are also called **independent clauses.**

> *Example:* Scarlett attended the training.

 "Scarlett" is the subject, and "attended" is the verb.

Two or more independent clauses can be joined in a **compound sentence.** A compound sentence gives the ideas in the two clauses equal weight. To make a compound sentence, choose a coordinating conjunction (*for, and, nor, but, or, yet, so*) to join the independent clauses and insert a comma before the conjunction. Only these conjunctions can form compound sentences. Use the acronym FANBOYS to help you remember the conjunctions: For, And, Nor, But, Or, Yet, and So.

> *Example:* Scarlett attended the training, so she knows the protocol.

"Scarlett attended the training" is an independent clause, and "she knows the protocol" is also an independent clause. "So" is a coordinating conjunction joining the two clauses.

A **complex sentence** combines an independent clause with a dependent clause. A **dependent clause** has a subject and verb, but it does not express a complete thought. Another term for *dependent clause* is *subordinate clause*. The idea in the dependent clause provides additional information to support the idea in the independent clause.

> *Example:* Scarlett attended the training because it was required.

The independent clause is still "Scarlett attended the training," but now there is a dependent clause, "because it was required." On its own, "Because it was required," would be a sentence fragment instead of a complete sentence.

**Compound-complex sentences** incorporate two independent clauses and one or more dependent clauses. An independent clause contains a subject and verb and expresses a complete thought. A dependent clause contains a subject and verb but does not express a complete thought, so it cannot be a sentence.

> *Example:* Because it was required, Scarlett attended the training, so now she knows the protocol.

Once again, "Scarlett attended the training" is an independent clause, but now it is joined to another independent clause and accompanied by a dependent clause.

Here is how an expert would answer a TEAS question that tests a rule about sentence types.

| Question | Analysis |
|---|---|
| Which of the following is a simple sentence? | **Step 1:** The question asks you to identify a simple sentence, and the answer choices are four sentences. |
| | **Step 2:** A simple sentence contains a subject and a verb and expresses a complete thought. |
| (A)  Driving all the way to the country. | **Step 3:** This is not a complete sentence. It is a sentence fragment. Eliminate. |
| (B)  The car that needed gasoline. | This is also not a complete sentence. Eliminate. |
| (C)  The car needed gasoline because they were driving all the way to the country. | Because two clauses are joined with "because," this is a complex sentence. Eliminate. |
| (D)  The car needs gasoline for the drive to the country. | Correct. This is a simple sentence that uses a subject and a verb and expresses a complete thought. Note that "for" is not used as a coordinating conjunction here because "the drive to the country" is not an independent clause. |

Now you try one.

> Which of the following would NOT complete the sentence correctly with a dependent clause?
>
> She didn't want to drink the coffee, _____.
>
> - (A)  because it was very hot
> - (B)  although she was not in a hurry
> - (C)  and neither did I
> - (D)  since breakfast wasn't ready yet

**Explanation**

**Step 1:** The question asks you to choose the one answer choice that does *not* complete the sentence correctly with a dependent clause, and the answer choices list independent and dependent clauses.

**Step 2:** A dependent clause contains a subject and verb but does not express a complete thought. The correct answer here will *not* be a dependent clause. It may be an independent clause or a fragment (phrase).

**Step 3:** Only answer choice **(C)**, beginning with "and," is not a dependent clause. It expresses a complete thought (*I didn't want to drink the coffee either*) and could stand alone as a sentence. The other answer choices are dependent clauses and could not stand alone.

## Parts of Sentences

Knowing other sentence parts will help you analyze sentence structures that are tested on the TEAS. Here are additional terms that you need to know.

| Part of Sentence | Definition |
| --- | --- |
| subject | the person or thing that is performing the action or being described |
| object | a person or thing that receives the action of the verb |
| indirect object | a person or thing to whom/which or for whom/which something is done |
| predicate | the part of a sentence that expresses what a subject does |
| complement | a word or group of words added to a sentence to make it complete |
| article | a word (such as *a*, *an*, or *the*) used with a noun to limit it or make it clearer |
| modifier | a word (such as an adjective or adverb) or phrase that describes another word or group of words |

*Example:* The girl happily read him the book. It was funny.

In the first sentence, "The girl" is the complete subject, and "happily read him the book" is the complete predicate. "The" is an article, and "happily" is a modifier (an adverb telling how she read). "The book" is the object of her reading, and "him" is the indirect object.

In the second sentence, "It" is the subject, and "was funny" is the complete predicate. "Funny" is a complement because "It was," though consisting of a noun and a verb, would not form a sentence that made sense.

Here is how a test expert would answer a TEAS question that tests the parts of sentence structure.

| Question | Analysis |
| --- | --- |
| She gave me the chocolate.<br><br>Which of the following correctly identifies the direct object and indirect object of the sentence? | **Step 1:** This simple sentence includes the subject "She," the verb "gave," the direct object "chocolate," and the indirect object "me." The question asks about the two kinds of objects. |
| | **Step 2:** The correct answer will identify "chocolate" as the direct object and "me" as the indirect object. |
| (A)   Direct: me; indirect: She | **Step 3:** Incorrectly identifies the indirect object "me" as the direct object and incorrectly identifies the subject "She" as the indirect object. Eliminate. |
| (B)   Direct: She; indirect: me | Incorrectly identifies the subject "She" as the direct object, although it gets the indirect object right. Eliminate. |
| (C)   Direct: chocolate; indirect: me | This matches the prediction. Correct. |
| (D)   Direct: chocolate; indirect: She | Incorrectly identifies the subject "She" as the indirect object. Eliminate. |

## KEY IDEAS

- Knowing the eight parts of speech and the parts of sentences (such as subject, predicate, object, indirect object, complement) is key to analyzing sentence structure.

- An independent clause could stand alone as a simple sentence. A dependent clause cannot stand alone.

- You can distinguish among simple, compound, complex, and compound-complex sentences by whether they include independent and/or dependent clauses and how the clauses are connected.

# Sentence Structure Practice Questions

1. Working hard is important if you want to achieve your goals.

   Which of the following is the subject of the independent clause in the sentence above?

   (A) Working
   (B) important
   (C) you
   (D) goals

2. Bob was generous in his praise of Gil's pleasant nature.

   Which of the following is the pronoun in the sentence above?

   (A) Bob
   (B) generous
   (C) his
   (D) nature

3. Which of the following is an example of a compound-complex sentence?

   (A) Because the book was confusing, Sarah stopped reading it, so now she needs something new to read.
   (B) Sarah stopped reading the most confusing book she had ever encountered.
   (C) Sarah stopped reading the book immediately when it started confusing her.
   (D) Sarah immediately stopped reading the confusing book.

4. He told me a very long and boring story.

   Which of the following is the direct object in the sentence above?

   (A) He
   (B) me
   (C) boring
   (D) story

**Review your work using the explanations in Part Six of this book.**

# CHAPTER TWO

# GRAMMAR, STYLE, AND THE WRITING PROCESS

## LEARNING OBJECTIVES

- Craft sentences using correct grammar and appropriate word choices
- Use the appropriate style for a given writing task and identify the purpose of and intended audience for a piece of writing based on its style
- Use the writing process to produce a well-organized written work that achieves its purpose
- Identify the appropriate use of citations to credit sources

Of the 24 scored *English and language usage* questions, 9 (37.5%) will be in the sub-content area of *Knowledge of language*. With these questions, the TEAS evaluates your ability to use correct grammar and to adopt a style appropriate for the topic and audience, as well as to use the writing process to construct clear, coherent paragraphs.

This chapter addresses these skills in three lessons:

**Lesson 1:** Grammar

**Lesson 2:** Formal and Informal Style

**Lesson 3:** The Writing Process

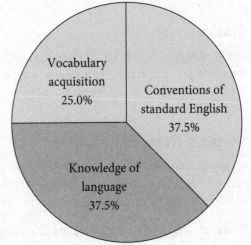

**English and Language Usage Questions by Sub-content Area**

Vocabulary acquisition 25.0%

Conventions of standard English 37.5%

Knowledge of language 37.5%

# LESSON 1

# Grammar

## LEARNING OBJECTIVES

- Craft correct, complete sentences
- Eliminate ambiguous or unnecessary language
- Recognize correct verb usage by using context clues
- Identify appropriate transition words to clarify text

Grammar allows a writer to convey information clearly. The rules of grammar govern topics such as sentence creation, language usage, and flow between ideas; these conventions are accepted as "correct grammar" and are essential to making written communication clear and understandable.

The TEAS tests your ability to recognize both correct and incorrect grammar, including sentence fragments, run-on sentences, and ambiguous language. You may be asked to combine sentences using transition words or to identify synonyms. Refreshing your understanding of these grammar guidelines will help you prepare for the *English and language usage* section.

## Clarity

**Clarity** refers to how clear, or understandable, a text is. Precise, concise language and correct sentence structure present information clearly; vague language, wordiness, and incorrect sentence structure impede clarity and make a text difficult to understand.

## Sentence Fragments

As you learned in Lesson 3 of the previous chapter, a simple sentence has at least one subject and verb and expresses a complete thought. A **sentence fragment** is a combination of words that lacks one or more of these characteristics. Sentence fragments are sometimes called incomplete sentences.

Sentence fragments are often used to provide emphasis when speaking, but they are never correct in written English.

> *Incorrect:* We tried the new restaurant last night. Best tacos ever!

"Best tacos ever!" is a fragment; it does not have a proper subject/verb pairing and does not convey a complete thought. To correct a sentence fragment, fill in the missing piece to make it complete.

> *Correct:* We tried the new restaurant last night. I had the best tacos ever!

## Run-On Sentences

When two or more independent clauses are incorrectly joined, they form a **run-on sentence**. You can correct a run-on by splitting it into separate sentences or by using punctuation and a conjunction to create a compound or complex sentence.

> *Incorrect:* We tried the new restaurant last night and I had the best tacos ever, therefore, you should go there and try them.

> *Correct:* We tried the new restaurant last night, and I had the best tacos ever! You should go there and try them.

## Ambiguity

**Ambiguity** refers to uncertainty of meaning, or a lack of clarity. Ambiguous language is vague and clouds the meaning of a text. To avoid or correct ambiguity, select precise words that paint a clear picture of your intended meaning.

> *Ambiguous:* Our professor is really nice.

> *Unambiguous:* Our professor is upbeat and friendly.

Selecting words to avoid ambiguity also involves considering the **connotation** that matches your intent. Connotation refers to the sense or image associated with a word, such as whether it is positive or negative. *Dog* has a neutral connotation, while *mutt* has a negative connotation. If you wanted to convey a positive image of a dog, you might choose to refer to the animal as *man's best friend*. Choosing words with specific meaning and the proper connotation helps a writer avoid ambiguity.

## Agreement

**Agreement** refers to the appropriate match between a noun and a verb or between a pronoun and its **antecedent** (the noun it represents). A singular noun requires a singular verb and, if paired with a pronoun, requires a singular pronoun. Plural nouns must be paired with plural verbs and/or pronouns.

> *Example:* Ava speaks quickly.

> *Example:* Several boys injured their ankles while at camp.

In the first example, a singular subject, "Ava," is paired with a singular verb, "speaks." In the second example, the plural "boys" is paired with the plural possessive pronoun "their."

Here is how a TEAS expert would tackle a question about clarity.

| Question | Analysis |
|---|---|
| Whether you decide to stay or go. <br><br> Which of the following describes the error above and provides an appropriate correction? | **Step 1:** This is a sentence fragment; it does not have a subject/verb pair and does not convey a complete thought. |
| | **Step 2:** The correct answer will identify that the error is a fragment, and the correction will present a complete sentence. |
| (A)  Run-on sentence; It makes no difference whether you decide to stay or go. | **Step 3:** Incorrect. The error is a sentence fragment, not a run-on sentence. |
| (B)  Run-on sentence; Whether you decide to stay or go, I will support you. | Incorrect. The error is a sentence fragment, not a run-on sentence. |
| (C)  Sentence fragment; Whether you decide to stay or go, I will support you. | Correct. This matches the prediction. |
| (D)  Sentence fragment; Whether you decide on staying or going. | Incorrect. This correctly identifies the error, but the proposed correction remains a sentence fragment. |

Now tackle one on your own.

Gabby wanted to rearrange the office Erika was against the idea and they couldn't agree and finally Erika changed her mind.

Which of the following describes the error above and provides an appropriate correction?

(A)   Run-on sentence; Gabby wanted to rearrange the office, but Erika was against the idea. They couldn't agree until finally Erika changed her mind.

(B)   Run-on sentence; Gabby wanted to rearrange the office, Erika was against the idea, they couldn't agree, finally Erika changed her mind.

(C)   Sentence fragment; Gabby wanted to rearrange the office, but Erika was against the idea. They couldn't agree until finally Erika changed her mind.

(D)   No error; the sentence is correct as written.

## Explanation

**Step 1:** This is a run-on sentence. It contains four independent clauses.

**Step 2:** The correct answer will identify the error as a run-on sentence, and the correction will present correct complete sentences.

**Step 3:** Only answer choice **(A)** correctly identifies the error and provides two correct complete sentences. Choice (B) correctly identifies the error but does not correct it, choice (C) incorrectly identifies the error, and choice (D) neither identifies nor corrects the error.

## Verb Tense

As you learned in the previous lesson, a verb expresses an action or state of being. The **verb tense** expresses the time at which the action or state takes place. Verb tense must be consistent and correct for writing to make sense.

**K**

| Tense | Form | Use | Example |
|---|---|---|---|
| Present | talk/talks | an action, general truth, or state of being | He talks to me every morning. |
| Past | talked | a completed action | He talked to me last night. |
| Future | will talk | an action that has not yet happened | He and I will talk tomorrow. |
| Present progressive | am/is/are talking | an action that is in progress | We are talking right now. |
| Present perfect | have/has talked | an action that began in the past and continued, either for some indefinite period or through the present | He has talked to me every morning this week. |
| Past perfect | had talked | a completed action that took place before a specific time in the past | I had talked to him before he got on the bus. |
| Future perfect | will have talked | an action that will be completed by a specific time in the future | I will have talked to him by lunchtime. |

Verb tense must be used consistently. Sentences may provide clues to indicate the correct tense; time references such as *yesterday* or *tomorrow* and the tense of other verbs make clear which tense is correct.

> Incorrect: The store has offered a discount next week.

> Correct: The store will offer a discount next week

Let's see how an expert would answer a TEAS question that tests verb tense.

| Question | Analysis |
|---|---|
| Which of the following sentences uses correct verb tense? | **Step 1:** This question requires you to assess the answer choices. |
| | **Step 2:** Instead of predicting an answer, read each answer choice and identify the one that includes the correct verb. |
| (A) Before you looked at the answers, be sure to check your work. | **Step 3:** This sentence incorrectly uses a past tense verb, "looked," where a present tense verb would make sense. |
| (B) Before you looked at the answers, be sure you will check your work. | This sentence incorrectly uses a past tense verb, "looked," with a future tense verb, "will check." |
| (C) Before you look at the answers, be sure you will check your work. | This sentence incorrectly uses a future tense verb, "will check." |
| (D) Before you look at the answers, be sure you check your work. | Correct. The present tense verbs "look" and "check" match and make sense in this sentence. |

## Transition Words

**Transition words** provide the framework for a reader to understand a text. They guide the reader from one idea to the next and help provide both clarity and flow. The table lists some types of transitions that occur within texts and some of the more common transition words used to show how ideas are related.

| Transition | Sample Words |
|---|---|
| Cause | because, since, due to |
| Effect | therefore, thus, as a result, consequently |
| Contrast | however, although, despite |
| Example | for example, for instance, such as, to illustrate |
| Sequence or Order | first, second, before, after, then, next, meanwhile |
| Elaboration | additionally, furthermore, moreover |

## KEY IDEAS

- Be able to spot fragments and run-ons and know how to fix these errors.
- Verb tense must match the timing of the information in the sentence.
- Appropriate transition words lead the reader between sentences or paragraphs, as well as from one idea to the next.

# Grammar Practice Questions

1. Before 1906, postcards had space for a message on one side and the recipient's address on the other it was illegal to write a message on the address side.

   Which of the following correctly identifies and corrects the error in grammar or usage in the sentence above?

   (A) Run-on sentence; Before 1906, postcards had space for a message on one side and the recipient's address on the other. It was illegal to write a message on the address side.
   (B) Verb tense error; Before 1906, postcards have had space for a message on one side and the recipient's address on the other, and it has been illegal to write a message on the address side.
   (C) Ambiguity; Before 1906, postcards had space for a short message on one side and the recipient's address on the other side it was illegal to write words on the address side.
   (D) Inappropriate transition word choice; Since 1906, postcards had space for a message on one side and the recipient's address on the other it was illegal to write a message on the address side.

2. Laundry should be separated by colors, despite the chance that vivid items may run while being washed.

   Which of the following describes the error of grammar or usage in the sentence above?

   (A) Sentence fragment
   (B) Verb tense error
   (C) Inappropriate transition word choice
   (D) Run-on sentence

3. Which of the following sentences is an example of correct subject-verb and pronoun-antecedent agreement?

   (A) The client will be late to her appointment.
   (B) Several people has asked about eating before they are admitted to the hospital.
   (C) None of the procedures is covered by Dana's insurance, so she will have to pay for every treatment.
   (D) Find a physician who explains what they are doing during the exam.

4. Which of the following sentences is grammatically incorrect?

   (A) Laundry should be separated by colors due to the chance that vivid items may run while being washed.
   (B) Most people have experienced a sorting error that resulted in discolored laundry coming out of the washer.
   (C) Washing a red shirt with white towels, for example, could result in a load of pink towels!
   (D) Some detergents have prevented colors from bleeding in the wash if you forget to sort by colors.

**Review your work using the explanations in Part Six of this book.**

# LESSON 2

# Formal and Informal Style

## LEARNING OBJECTIVES

- Distinguish between formal and informal writing style
- Choose the writing style that best fits a particular scenario
- Identify a narrator's setting and situation from the language used

Correct grammar is the foundation of strong, clear writing, but good writing must go beyond simply being free from error. Skilled writers adapt their writing style so their communication is both accessible and appropriate for their intended audience.

Different situations call for the use of different styles. As a health care professional, you will need to be able to recognize which writing style is appropriate for a particular situation. Two main types of writing style are formal and informal.

## Formal and Informal Writing Style

For certain kinds of writing, such as business letters, research papers, or scientific reports, a **formal style** of writing is appropriate. This style is more direct, serious, and impersonal than is informal writing, and it generally follows certain conventions or expected formats.

Formal writing tends not to use contractions, abbreviations, **slang**, **clichés**, or **colloquialisms**. However, it may include **jargon**, special terms that are specific to a particular industry, business, or area of study.

Informal writing is more relaxed than formal writing and does not necessarily follow conventions. This type of writing tends to be personal, casual, and conversational in tone. Writers typically use an **informal style** when addressing a familiar audience; crafting a narrative; or discussing a topic that is emotional, lighthearted, or entertaining. Slang, clichés, and other informal expressions that would be out of place in an academic paper or journal article can fit naturally into informal pieces of writing when used correctly.

Recognizing the differences between formal and informal language is a key skill for success on the TEAS, but it is also important to understand that much of the English language can be adapted to either formal or informal contexts. The table lists some types of informal language with examples and shows some formal writing style options for expressing the same idea.

| Types of Informal Language | Examples | Formal Alternatives |
|---|---|---|
| Clichés | raining cats and dogs<br>the time of my life<br>bells and whistles | raining heavily<br>an enjoyable time<br>quality features |
| Colloquialisms | kids<br>guys<br>awesome | children<br>people<br>exciting |
| Slang | have a blast<br>chill out | have fun<br>relax |
| Abbreviations | TV<br>ASAP | television<br>as soon as possible |
| Contractions | can't<br>it's | cannot<br>it is |
| Letter expressions | Hi Joe,<br>Best wishes, | To Whom It May Concern,<br>Sincerely, |

Let's see how a test expert would identify the usage of informal language on the TEAS.

| Question | Analysis |
|---|---|
| Ever since the new disease was discovered, researchers have been working diligently to find a cure, but with so little known about the illness, their early efforts to create a treatment are more a shot in the dark than a targeted approach.<br><br>Which of the following phrases from the sentence above is an example of informal language? | **Step 1:** This question asks you to identify a phrase in the stimulus that can be characterized as informal language. |
| | **Step 2:** Informal language may come in many forms, such as slang, clichés, colloquialisms, contractions, and abbreviations. The correct answer will likely fall into one of these categories. |
| (A)  working diligently | **Step 3:** This phrase is formal. Eliminate. |
| (B)  find a cure | This phrase is neutral. Eliminate. |
| (C)  shot in the dark | Correct. This phrase is a cliché that refers to an effort with little chance of success due to a lack of information. |
| (D)  targeted approach | This phrase is formal. Eliminate. |

# Language Choice

In addition to having the correct style and tone, a piece of writing has to include the right words in order to achieve its intended purpose and reach its target audience.

For example, both an article in a scientific journal and an article about current events in a newspaper require a formal tone, but the language used in each demonstrates that their purposes are very different. A scientific journal article will typically use highly technical language that is directed to scientists with a certain specialty, while an article covering a current event will use direct, clear language that is accessible to the general public.

When determining which writing style and word choice are appropriate for a particular situation, consider the writing medium used and the intended audience of the piece.

Let's see how a test expert would choose the the right language to fit a particular situation on the TEAS.

| Question | Analysis |
|---|---|
| Our newest product line has proven to be a slam dunk; our revenue has skyrocketed in the last quarter, and we expect that these latest gains are just the tip of the iceberg.<br><br>Which of the following revisions of the above sentence would be appropriate for a formal business report? | **Step 1:** This question asks you to choose a revised sentence that has a formal tone appropriate for a business report. |
| | **Step 2:** To create a formal tone, the correct answer must replace all informal phrasing in the stimulus with formal language. The informal phrases include "slam dunk," "skyrocketed," and "tip of the iceberg." The formal language of a business report should be professional, clear, and direct. |
| (A) The performance of our newest product line has thoroughly exceeded our expectations; our revenue has dramatically increased in the last quarter, and we anticipate even more substantial gains in the future. | **Step 3:** Correct. This sentence replaces each informal phrase with a formal phrase that clearly expresses the intended meaning. |
| (B) Our newest product line is growing by leaps and bounds; our revenue has grown significantly in the last quarter, and we expect that the best is yet to be in terms of profitability. | This sentence introduces different informal phrasing, such as "growing by leaps and bounds" and "the best is yet to be." Eliminate. |
| (C) You will not believe how well our new product line is doing; our revenue is on an upswing, and we expect it will keep on climbing down the road. | This sentence is even more informal than the original since it addresses the speaker in second person. It also introduces new clichés, such as "on an upswing," "keep on climbing," and "down the road." Eliminate. |
| (D) The commendable performance of our illustrious new product line has left us flabbergasted; the prodigious revenue growth we have witnessed indicates that our latest venture will continue to produce outstanding results into the foreseeable future. | This sentence eliminates all informal language but replaces it with overly complex phrasing that is inappropriate for a business report. Eliminate. |

# Narrative Settings and Situations

To narrate is to tell a story, and a narrative or story may be categorized as either fiction or nonfiction. Narratives typically have an identifiable setting and tell about how one or more characters interact with their setting and, usually, other characters.

An author helps the reader understand a story's setting and the characters' situation by revealing key information through word choice. For example, a writer might indicate that a narrative is set in a particular time period by referring to a specific historical event as a current event or by using certain slang words from a historical period in dialogue. Similarly, a reader might learn more about the relationship between two characters based on whether the author chooses positive or negative words to describe their interactions.

Let's see how a test expert would use context clues to determine a narrative's setting.

| Question | Analysis |
|---|---|
| A change in the wind told Aida a storm was brewing, and she had barely settled the animals in the barn and lit the oil lamp on her table when the torrential rains came down. <br><br> In which type of narrative setting is the sentence above likely to appear? | **Step 1:** This question asks you to identify the setting of a narrative based on the clues given in the sentence. |
| | **Step 2:** The setting clues in the stimulus are the fact that Aida owns animals and a barn and that she uses an oil lamp in her home. These clues indicate that the character is living in a rural setting without access to electricity. |
| (A)  A contemporary suburban home | **Step 3:** This does not match the prediction. Eliminate. |
| (B)  A modern cottage in the woods | This does not match the prediction. Eliminate. |
| (C)  A rustic farmhouse in the country | Correct. *Rustic* means "simple" or "unsophisticated," which could describe a home that does not have working electricity. The farmhouse and country setting match the prediction. |
| (D)  A secluded hut on a tropical island | This does not match the prediction. Eliminate. |

## KEY IDEAS

- Being able to distinguish formal language from informal language will help you to determine whether a piece of writing has the appropriate style for its purpose and audience.
- Consider the medium and intended audience of a piece of writing to determine what type of language it should include.
- Use content clues to determine the setting and situation of a narrative.

# Formal and Informal Style Practice Questions

1. Multiple studies now indicate that the amount of independent reading a young child engages in directly correlates with that child's future level of academic success.

   Which of the following statements would best adapt the above statement from an article in an academic journal on education into a message that a principal would send to her students' parents?

   (A) Research indicates that promoting a positive attitude toward reading is sure to cultivate lifelong benefits for young readers.
   (B) Giving your young children access to books encourages them to read early and often and prepares them for a lifetime of learning.
   (C) The minds of children are primed to retain a great deal of information from a very early age, and literacy is a key component of optimal retention.
   (D) Reading is an awesome way to help kids become great learners!

2. The client is exhibiting multiple symptoms, including fever, cough, fatigue, and loss of appetite.

   Which of the following is the most likely medium for the sentence above?

   (A) An article in a medical journal
   (B) An advertisement for a new medication
   (C) A research paper on a new medical procedure
   (D) A physician's note on a medical chart

3. Which of the following sentences best indicates that the setting is early colonial America?

   (A) Eli reached the station just in time to see the train pull away, so he settled patiently on a bench to await the next one.
   (B) In the early days of the war, Diana listened to the radio every evening to hear the latest news from the front.
   (C) Anna knew that the long winter days would soon be upon them, so each day she helped her father and mother gather firewood, salt meat, and stow away the few vegetables they were able to grow that first year.
   (D) Sailing around the ancient city, Daniel was struck by the ornate architecture and towering structures that had withstood centuries of changing political and cultural tides.

**Review your work using the explanations in Part Six of this book.**

# LESSON 3

# The Writing Process

## LEARNING OBJECTIVES

- Apply knowledge of the elements of the writing process, including planning, drafting, and revising
- Organize ideas in logically ordered paragraphs
- Identify when a citation is needed and cite sources appropriately

## Elements of the Writing Process

Writing is a highly individual activity, and everyone who undertakes it goes about the task a little differently. However, there are three common phases in the writing process: planning, drafting/writing, and editing.

The first step in the writing process is planning. Some authors make a plan for when and where to write and set up a schedule. For all authors, an important part of planning is determining the **thesis**, or main idea, and their purpose for writing. **Brainstorming**, or thinking of a list of ideas for approaching a task, problem, or project, can help take the process from concept/thesis to written word. Before an author can put pen to paper or fingers to keyboard, she must determine what research is needed to fully explore the topic. In the case of a piece of personal writing, researching may be as simple as taking some time to think. For pieces that require more background or detailed information, the writer may consult a variety of reference sources, many of which will require citations. Finally, before creating a draft, it can be helpful to organize material into a logical framework, or **outline**.

The next phase of the writing process is the actual writing. With a plan and an outline in place, the author can create a first draft. It is important to follow conventions of good writing, such as organizing thoughts in logical paragraphs. Knowing the parts of a paragraph can help a writer communicate ideas effectively.

The last phase of the process is editing and **proofreading**. The author may make changes as significant as restructuring the entire piece or as small as correcting the placement of commas and refining word choice. The writer will fix errors of spelling, grammar, and style. Good writing is easy to understand; the reader should never have to reread a sentence to grasp its relevance or meaning.

Let's see how a test expert would distinguish between parts of the writing process on the TEAS.

| Question | Analysis |
|---|---|
| During the writing process, which of the following tasks would likely take place last? | **Step 1:** The question asks which step would take place last in the writing process. |
| | **Step 2:** The final part of the process for most writers is editing and proofreading. The correct answer will represent this type of task. |
| (A) Writing an outline | **Step 3:** Writing an outline is a part of planning, which is an initial phase. Eliminate. |
| (B) Setting up a daily writing schedule | Setting up a writing schedule is also a part of planning. Eliminate. |
| (C) Checking for typos | Correct. Checking for typos is part of the proofreading process. |
| (D) Reading resource material to gather quotes | Gathering quotes from resource material is part of the planning process. Eliminate. |

## Parts of a Paragraph

An effective **paragraph** includes a group of related sentences. All the sentences should help develop the same main idea so that the paragraph is coherent and the writer's meaning is clear.

The author's main idea should be summarized in the **topic sentence** of a paragraph. The topic sentence often appears at the beginning of the paragraph. A topic sentence must not only state the main idea of the paragraph but identify the point, if any, that the writer will make about the topic. The sentences that follow include **supporting details** that explain and develop the main idea.

In the following paragraph, note that the topic sentence tells the subject of the paragraph (pet ownership) and states the central point the author is making (pet ownership is beneficial to humans and can have positive health effects). The sentences that follow develop the main idea by providing supporting details.

> Pet ownership is beneficial to humans and can have various positive health effects. The human-animal bond positively influences the health and well-being of both people and their pets. Pet ownership has been found to lower blood pressure and decrease mental stress. Dog ownership in particular may reduce risk for cardiovascular disease. In several studies, pet ownership has been linked to healthcare cost savings related to decreased doctor visits.

Here is how a test expert would approach a question about the parts of a passage.

| Question | Analysis |
|---|---|
| Which of the following would be the correct topic sentence for a paragraph? | **Step 1:** The question asks you to find the correct topic sentence for a paragraph. |
| | **Step 2:** A topic sentence summarizes the main idea of a paragraph. Sentences that develop the topic further offer supporting details. |
| (A)  Butterflies and bees are examples of insects. | **Step 3:** This sentence provides examples that further develop the topic. Eliminate. |
| (B)  Some classes of animals include amphibians, reptiles, and mammals. | This sentence gives details that develop the topic. Eliminate. |
| (C)  There is a detailed classification system used to organize different types of animals. | Correct. This sentence summarizes the main idea. |
| (D)  The classification system is separated into kingdom, phylum, class, order, family, genus, and species. | This sentence provides details that develop the topic sentence. Eliminate. |

# Citations

When an author supports his ideas with specific references to other sources, the writing becomes more credible. Information taken directly from research requires citation. A **citation** is a formal acknowledgment of a source that gives credit where credit is due, allows the reader to evaluate the credibility and perspective of the source, and enables readers to find the source to read it themselves if desired. A citation must be used to identify the following:

- The source of a verbatim quote
- The person/people from whom the writer got an idea
- The document from which the writer got information not generally known

The following material does not need a citation:

- Facts that are widely documented as true (e.g., humans first landed on the moon in 1969)
- Ideas that cannot be attributed to a specific person or group (e.g., cholesterol is bad for your health)

In less formal writing, citations may be provided entirely within the text. Sometimes brief citations are provided within the text that point the reader to a complete list of sources. Citations may also be provided in footnotes or endnotes. Here is a less formal example of citation:

> In an August 18, 2010, *US News & World Report* article, Megan Johnson explains that as little as one hour of sleep more or less than usual may bring on a headache.

And here is an example of a more formal citation format that uses a reference list:

> According to an article in *US News & World Report* (Johnson, 2010), participants in a small Turkish study reported fewer and milder migraines following aerobic exericse, such as on a treadmill.

**Reference List**

Johnson, M. (2010, August 18). Headache relief: 6 tricks to ease the pain. *US News & World Report*. Retrieved December 1, 2016, from http://health.usnews.com/health-news/family-health/brain-and-behavior/articles/2010/08/18/headache-relief-6-tricks-to-ease-the-pain

Here is how an expert would answer a TEAS question about citations.

| Question | Analysis |
| --- | --- |
| Which of these situations requires the use of a citation? | **Step 1:** The question asks you to identify a situation in which the writer must include a citation. |
| | **Step 2:** Citations must be used when a source is quoted directly or when another person's ideas are referenced. |
| (A)  The author quotes another author's book. | **Step 3:** Correct. A citation must be used when an author quotes from another source. |
| (B)  The author writes a list of ideas during brainstorming. | A list of the author's own ideas does not require a citation. Eliminate. |
| (C)  The author uses a hypothetical example. | Made-up information does not require a citation. Eliminate. |
| (D)  The author mentions the name of a historical figure. | Simply mentioning an important person does not require citation. Eliminate. |

## KEY IDEAS

- The writing process can generally be categorized into planning, drafting, and revising.
- To communicate information effectively, a paragraph should include a topic sentence followed by supporting details.
- Citations must be used when reference sources are quoted directly, when another person's ideas are used, or when facts are drawn from a specific source.

# The Writing Process Practice Questions

1. Which of the following sentences must be supported by a citation?

   (A) The word *nightmare* is derived from an Old English word for a mythological creature that torments people with scary dreams.
   (B) I had a nightmare about having my wallet stolen on New Year's Eve.
   (C) Nightmares are scary and disturbing, and repeated nightmares can interfere with restful sleep.
   (D) Some people believe that nightmares are caused by eating too late at night.

2. I. Ballet dancers are subject to a number of physical injuries.
   II. Stress fractures and ankle sprains are also very common.
   III. Swelling in the tendons of feet and joints can lead to tendinitis.
   IV. Common injuries result from repetitive movements during many hours of practice.

   How should a writer order these sentences to produce an effective paragraph?

   (A) IV, I, II, III
   (B) II, I, III, IV
   (C) I, IV, III, II
   (D) IV, III, II, I

3. Which of the following is NOT a part of the planning stage of the writing process?

   (A) Thinking of various ideas related to the topic
   (B) Rereading the first draft to find errors and make improvements
   (C) Researching the chosen topic
   (D) Determining what days of the week and time of day writing will occur

4. Which of the following is NOT an example of a topic sentence?

   (A) You can pursue many types of jobs with a business degree.
   (B) To be an effective writer requires regular practice.
   (C) One way to gain more experience in the field is to volunteer.
   (D) The role of a caregiver involves balancing many needs.

**Review your work using the explanations in Part Six of this book.**

# CHAPTER THREE

# VOCABULARY

## LEARNING OBJECTIVE

• Use context clues or word parts to determine the meaning of a word or phrase

Of the 24 scored *English and language usage* questions, 6 (25.0%) will be in the sub-content area of *Vocabulary acquisition*. To answer these questions, you will need to determine the meaning of words and phrases from their parts, such as prefixes and roots, as well as from the context in which they appear.

This chapter addresses this skill in one lesson:

**Lesson 1:** Using the Correct Word

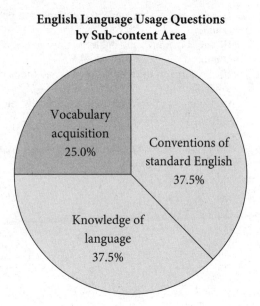

**English Language Usage Questions by Sub-content Area**

# LESSON 1

# Using the Correct Word

## LEARNING OBJECTIVES

- Determine the meaning of a word or phrase by using context clues
- Analyze the parts of a word to determine its meaning

Each word in a sentence plays a particular role, but if a word is unfamiliar or has many possible definitions, its meaning might be difficult to decipher. Earlier in this book, you were introduced to strategies for determining the meaning of a word in the *Reading* content area of the TEAS. The *English and language usage* content area will test the same skill, though it will ask you to apply it in slightly different ways. For some questions, you will need a supporting cast of context clues to help you determine the word's or phrase's meaning. For other questions, you may need to take a word apart in order to discover its definition. Overall, you will not have to determine the exact meaning of a word or phrase to get a question correct. Having a general understanding of a term is enough to make a strong prediction and narrow down the choices to the right answer.

## Context Clues

**Context clues** are the words and phrases in a sentence that help the reader understand unfamiliar terms. There are many types of context clues that can help you infer the meaning of a word.

## Synonyms

When you are unsure of the meaning of a word in a sentence, look for clues that point to a similar idea. Another word or a phrase with a related meaning may appear in the sentence.

> *Example:* The witness intentionally tried to *obfuscate* the facts of the case by confusing the detective with conflicting accounts of the event.

> *Analysis:* The clues "confusing" and "conflicting" point to the meaning of the verb *obfuscate*, which means "to confuse" or "to make unclear."

## Contrast Words

You can determine the meaning of an unfamiliar word by looking for clues that point to a contrasting idea in the sentence.

> *Example:* The team members were surprised by their manager's *churlish* behavior at the meeting, since he was usually polite and pleasant to everyone on the staff.

> *Analysis:* The clues "surprised" and "usually" indicate that the word *churlish* means the opposite of "polite" and "pleasant." *Churlish* is defined as "rude" or "uncivil."

## Tone Words

Positive or negative tone words can provide clues to the meaning of an unfamiliar word in a sentence.

*Example:* The *pernicious* rumor threatened to ruin her reputation.

*Analysis:* The clues "threatened" and "ruin" set a decidedly negative tone for the sentence, which indicates that *pernicious* also has a strongly negative meaning. *Pernicious* is defined as "extremely harmful."

## Words in a Series

When a word appears in a series of similar or related terms, use context clues to determine whether the word's meaning is related to the meanings of the other terms.

*Example:* My grandfather was well-known for his generosity to schools, hospitals, orphanages, and other *philanthropic* organizations.

*Analysis:* The word *philanthropic* appears in a list of organizations that help people in different ways. *Philanthropic* is an adjective that describes a person or act that is "dedicated to the ensuring the welfare of people."

## Cause and Effect

Some context clues help the reader understand the relationship between the ideas in the sentence. Recognizing a cause-and-effect relationship between the unfamiliar word and another portion of the sentence can help you understand the word's meaning.

*Example:* The *incontrovertible* evidence presented at the trial proved the defendant's involvement in the crime.

*Analysis:* This sentence describes a cause-and-effect relationship between the type of evidence presented at the trial and the level of certainty regarding the defendant's participation in the crime. Since the evidence "proved" that the defendant was involved, the term *incontrovertible* must mean "undeniable" or "completely certain."

## General Idea of a Sentence

Context clues can provide information about the general subject matter or situation described in the sentence. These details can help you predict the meaning of an unfamiliar word that appears in that context.

*Example:* The mother *admonished* her daughter for driving recklessly on the icy roads.

*Analysis:* The word *admonished* is used to describe how a mother reacted to her daughter's dangerous driving. Since "reckless driving" is a risky behavior and a mother would likely want her child to drive safely, *admonish* must mean "to scold" or "reprimand."

See how a test expert would use context clues to determine the meaning of unfamiliar words in a sentence.

| Question | Analysis |
|---|---|
| Due to the impending hurricane, we had to abbreviate our vacation and leave three days earlier than expected.<br><br>Which of the following is the meaning of "abbreviate" as used in the sentence above? | **Step 1:** This question asks about the meaning of the word "abbreviate." The sentence offers context clues that point to the word's definition. |
| | **Step 2:** With "Due to," the sentence indicates a cause-and-effect relationship between the storm and the decision to cut the vacation short. Predict that "abbreviate" means to "shorten something." |
| (A)  Reschedule | **Step 3:** This does not match the prediction. Eliminate. |
| (B)  Cancel | This does not match the prediction. Eliminate. |
| (C)  Extend | This is the opposite of the prediction. Eliminate. |
| (D)  Shorten | Correct. The storm forced the speaker to shorten the vacation by three days. |

# Word Parts

Many words are built by combining smaller word parts. By taking an unfamiliar word apart and analyzing the meaning of each of its components, you can often decode the word's general meaning.

## Common Affixes

The smallest meaningful unit of grammar in a language is called a **morpheme**. An **affix** is a morpheme that attaches to the beginning or end of a word **root** to make a new word. Although affixes cannot stand alone, they do have specific meanings and roles. Affixes that change the grammatical function or essential meaning of a word are known as **derivational morphemes**. Affixes that do not change a word's meaning but indicate tense, number, possession, or comparisons are called **inflectional morphemes**. By becoming familiar with the meanings and functions of the most common affixes, you will be able to understand how they shape the definitions of the words they help build.

A **prefix** is a type of affix that is added to the beginning of a word root to create a new word. Some prefixes, such as *in-*, can have several meanings, so you may also need to use context clues in your analysis of a word's general definition. Examine the table to familiarize yourself with some of the most common prefixes.

| Prefix | Meaning | Example |
|--------|---------|---------|
| anti- | against | antisocial |
| auto- | self | autobiography |
| de- | opposite, down | deactivate |
| dis- | not, opposite of | disinterest |
| en- | to cause to be | entangle |
| in- | in, into, toward, near | indoctrinate |
| in- | not | inaccurate |
| inter- | between | interstellar |
| mid- | middle | midline |
| mis- | wrongly | misinterpret |
| non- | not | nonsense |
| pre- | before | prelude |
| re- | again | return |
| sub- | under | submarine |
| trans- | across | transcontinental |
| un- | not | unhappy |

Some prefixes can only attach to words of a particular part of speech. For example, the prefix *mid-* can only be paired with a noun base. Additionally, some prefixes require the use of hyphens when combining them with a word root. The following chart illustrates the conventions for adding a hyphen after a prefix.

| Hyphen Conventions | Examples |
|--------------------|----------|
| Hyphenate a prefix that appears before a proper adjective or noun. | trans-American<br>mid-June |
| Add a hyphen after the prefixes *all-*, *ex-*, and *self-*. | all-access<br>ex-employee<br>self-expression |
| Hyphenate when necessary to add clarity or distinguish between similar words. | re-form (to form again) vs. reform (to improve) |
| Hyphenate to separate a prefix from a number or to make a compound with a single letter. | mid-1900s<br>T-shirt |

Word roots can also combine with suffixes to form new words. A **suffix** is an affix that attaches to the end of a word, and it can change both a word's meaning and its grammatical function or part of speech. The following list outlines some of the most common suffixes in the English language.

| Suffix | Meaning | Example |
| --- | --- | --- |
| -able, -ible | capable of being | passable |
| -acy | state or quality | democracy |
| -ate | become | fixate |
| -ed | past | wanted |
| -en | become | enlighten |
| -er, -or | one who | teacher |
| -ful | full of | joyful |
| -ify, -fy | make or become | magnify |
| -ious, -ous | characterized by | pious |
| -ist | one who | pianist |
| -ize, -ise | become | energize |
| -less | without | wordless |
| -ly | characteristic of | happily |
| -ment | action or resulting state | retirement |
| -ness | state of being | fullness |
| -ology | study of | biology |
| -s, -es | plural | lights |
| -ship | position held, character | friendship |
| -sion, -tion | state of being | tension |
| -y | characterized by | weepy |

## Word Roots

Understanding the meaning of an unfamiliar word's root can help make decoding the word much easier. Many terms in the English language take their roots from Greek and Latin words. For example, the root word *derma-* is from the Greek word for skin, and a doctor who cares for the skin is called a *dermatologist*. The root appears in many other words as well—*epidermis*, *hypodermic*, and *dermatitis*, to name a few. Once you are familiar with the meaning of a root, you can apply that knowledge to decoding several words.

As a healthcare professional, you will especially benefit from becoming familiar with the common roots that appear in medical terminology; however, the TEAS will ask you to determine the meaning of words and their roots that do not have strictly medical usage. The table highlights some common roots that appear in medical terms.

| Root | Meaning | Examples |
|------|---------|----------|
| acous- | hearing | acoustic |
| bronch- | lungs | bronchitis |
| cutane- | skin | subcutaneous |
| glyc- | sugar | hypoglycemic |
| hemo- | blood | hemoglobin |
| nephro- | kidney | nephrologist |
| ocul- | eyes | oculist |
| osteo- | bone | osteoporosis |
| pod- | foot | podiatrist |
| pulmon- | lungs | pulmonary |
| vas- | vein | vascular |

By putting your knowledge of prefixes, roots, and suffixes together, you will be able to decode even the most complex words on the TEAS.

*Example:* neonatologist = neo (*new*) + natal (*born/birth*) + ologist (*one who studies*)

*Analysis:* A neonatologist is one who specializes in the development and health concerns of newborns.

Try a question that asks you to take apart an unfamiliar word to decode its meaning.

Marjorie's primary physician referred her to a hematologist for a second opinion on her condition.

Marjorie likely has a condition related to which of the following?

(A) Hands
(B) Lungs
(C) Blood
(D) Liver

## Explanation

**Step 1:** This question asks for what condition someone would see a hematologist. The answer choices relate to different parts of the body. Taking the word "hematologist" apart into its components will identify this area of expertise.

**Step 2:** The root of "hematologist" is *hemato-*, which has to do with blood. Another word with this root is *hemoglobin*, which is an important part of blood. The suffix *-ologist* indicates one who studies something. Therefore, a "hematologist" is one who studies or specializes in blood conditions.

**Step 3:** Answer choice **(C)** matches the prediction. The other choices all relate to other parts of the body.

## KEY IDEAS

- Analyzing context clues in a sentence can give you enough information to predict the meaning of an unfamiliar word.
- When possible, take a challenging word apart into its prefixes, roots, and suffixes and combine the meaning of each component to infer the word's general meaning.

# Using the Correct Word Practice Questions

1. In which of the following sentences does "check" mean "to restrain or slow down"?

   (A) The voter was unsure of which box to check on the ballot.
   (B) The mechanic has offered to check the car's oil and fluid levels after changing its flat tire.
   (C) The airline required us to check our luggage before we boarded our flight.
   (D) The new budget will help to check government spending in the coming year.

2. Which of the following words means "prior to birth"?

   (A) Antepartum
   (B) Perinatal
   (C) Postpartum
   (D) Neonatal

3. Marco thought that this part of the property would make the perfect plot for his new garden.

   Which of the following is a synonym for "plot" as used in the above sentence?

   (A) Conspiracy
   (B) Scenario
   (C) Patch
   (D) Story

4. The student's failing grade on the test was an aberration in his otherwise perfect academic record.

   Which of the following is the meaning of "aberration" as used in the above sentence?

   (A) Regularity
   (B) Abnormality
   (C) Deceit
   (D) Error

5. Which of the following terms means "an enlarged heart"?

   (A) Auxocardia
   (B) Bronchiolitis
   (C) Osteoporosis
   (D) Tachycardia

6. She chose not to engage in any activities that would put further strain on her injured hand.

   Which of the following is the meaning of the word "engage" as it is used in the sentence above?

   (A) To give attention to something
   (B) To participate in something
   (C) To enter into conflict
   (D) To pledge or promise oneself

**Review your work using the explanations in Part Six of this book.**

# Review and Reflect

Think about the questions you answered in these lessons.

- Were you able to approach each question systematically, using the Kaplan Method for English and Language Usage?

- If one or more sentences were provided, were you able to analyze them efficiently, identifying clues to the correct answer?

- Did you feel confident that you understood what the question was asking you to do?

- How well were you able to predict an answer before looking at the answer choices?

- Could you match your prediction to the correct answer?

- Are there areas of language arts that appear on the TEAS that you don't understand as well as you would like?

- If you missed any questions, do you understand why the answer you chose is incorrect and why the right answer is correct? Could you do the question again now and get it right?

Use your thoughts about these questions to guide how you continue to prepare for the TEAS. If you feel you need more review and practice with spelling, punctuation, and sentence structure, you should study this chapter some more before taking the online Practice Test that comes with this book. Also, consider increasing your knowledge of English and language usage by using **Kaplan's ATI TEAS® Qbank**, which contains over 500 practice questions.

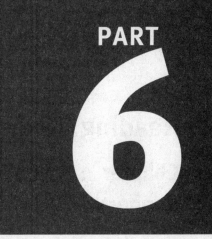

# Answers and Explanations

In this part of your book, you will find answers and explanations for every set of practice questions at the end of the lessons.

Even if you got a question correct, you may still learn something from the explanation. Therefore, review all of the explanations carefully. If you missed a question, first read the explanation to understand why you missed it. Then try that question again in a few days or a week to make sure you still remember how to do it. While reading about how you could have done a question correctly is helpful, actually doing the question correctly is an even more effective way of reinforcing your learning.

As you review, keep track of both your strengths and areas where you would like to improve. Use your performance to determine where you will focus your study time so you can maximize your score on the TEAS.

Good luck!

# Reading: Answers and Explanations

## Chapter 1: Main Ideas and Supporting Details

### Lesson 1: Strategic Reading

#### Questions 1–6: Passage Map

Topic: Urban legends
Scope: What they are
Purpose: Inform
¶ 1: Urban legend = modern folktale, not true
¶ 2: Example—alligators in sewers
¶ 3: Example—kidney removal; ULs sometimes widely believed

1. **(B) urban legends.** The topic, urban legends, is introduced in the first sentence, and the rest of the passage provides more information about them and two examples, making choice **(B)** correct. Choices (A) and (C) are details about urban legends, and choice (D) is a detail from the example showing how they change.

2. **(D) a basis in reality.** This is an EXCEPT detail question, so the correct answer is the one that does *not* characterize successful urban legends. Because you can't find something that isn't there, research the answer choices one by one and eliminate those that are stated in the passage. The author calls urban legends "folktales" and "stories," which means that they are fictional, leaving **(D)** as the correct answer. All other answers are in paragraph 1.

3. **(A) Their themes change with the times.** This question is about a specific claim made in the passage, so it is a detail question. The first sentence of the third paragraph states that urban legends change over time, matching choice **(A)**. Choice (B) is the opposite of what the passage says; most urban legends cannot be verified. Choice (C) is also an opposite, since urban legends have emerged "in modern society." Choice (D) contradicts the information in the last sentence that urban legends are mainly transmitted "through emails and social media."

4. **(C) a new form of folklore.** The author's primary concern is the topic of the passage. The entire passage is about urban legends, so predict that as the topic and match it with answer choice **(C)**. Choices (A) and (B) are details from two legends, and choice (D) refers to a word in the third paragraph, another detail.

5. **(D) aligned with popular beliefs.** The phrase "according to the passage" always signals a detail question, and the answer is directly stated in the passage. In the first paragraph, the author writes that urban legends "persist . . . for the transmission of popular values and beliefs." Another way of saying this is that the legends are compatible, or align with, popular beliefs. Thus, choice **(D)** is correct. Choice (A) is out of scope; though "urban" means "city," the author never says urban legends persist in cities only. Choice (B) is the opposite of the information in the passage, and (C) is extreme in its use of the word "never." Certainly some people believe urban legends or they wouldn't tell them over and over.

6. **(B) All urban legends instill fear in listeners.** Like question 2, this asks for a detail that is not in the passage. Again, research the answer choices and eliminate those that are stated in the passage. Having done this, you are left with choice **(B)**. Choice (A) is in paragraph 2, (C) is in paragraph 3, and (D) is in paragraph 1.

### Lesson 2: Reading for Details

#### Questions 1–2: Passage Map

Topic: Basis of life
Scope: Sun/photosynthesis important to most, but not all life
Purpose: Inform
¶ 1: Life not dependent on sun was considered very rare
¶ 2: Recent discoveries: Whole ecosystems not dependent on sun

1. **(D) Sunlight** The first sentence states that "[m]ost life is fundamentally dependent on organisms that store radiant energy from the Sun." That's a longer way of saying "most life depends ultimately on sunlight." The photosynthetic plants and algae of choice (A) ultimately derive their energy from the sun, while sub-sea ecosystems (B) and chemosynthetic bacteria (C) refer to details that only concern research into deep-sea life.

2. **(A) Both are at the base of their respective food chains.** The first paragraph describes ecosystems that are dependent on photosynthetic organisms, while the second paragraph describes ecosystems that are dependent on chemosynthetic organisms. In both cases, though, the organisms serve similar functions as primary producers at the base of their different food chains. Choice (B) is incorrect because only chemosynthetic organisms are described as dependent on

energy from within the Earth. Choice (C) is incorrect because according to the passage, chemosynthetic organisms get their energy from the Earth, not sunlight. The relative numbers of these organisms, choice (D), is never discussed in the passage.

3. **(B) 2** According to the timeline, only *Queen Nofretete* and *Nike of Samothrace* are dated before the Common Era (BCE). All the other artwork dates have no postscript, which by convention means the dates are of the Common Era.

4. **(A)** *Nike of Samothrace* **and Lindisfarne Gospels** The timeline indicates that the *Nike of Samothrace* and the Lindisfarne Gospels are separated by nine centuries, making **(A)** the correct choice. The artworks in choice (B), *Arnolfini Wedding Portrait* and *Mrs. Siddons,* are also separated by centuries, but the gap is only about 350 years. Both choice (C), *Robie House* and *Girl Before a Mirror,* and choice (D), *The Scream* and *Robie House,* feature artworks separated by only a few decades and can be quickly eliminated.

5. **(D) Gettysburg** The map indicates that the Battle of Gettysburg took place in Pennsylvania. Gettysburg is further north than choice (A), First Battle of Bull Run, Virginia; (B), Antietam, Maryland; and (C), Shiloh, Tennessee.

6. **(C) West Virginia** Referring to the map's legend, you can see that West Virginia was a slave state that remained loyal to the Union. Choice (A), Texas, joined the Confederacy, choice (B), Arizona, was a territory during this period, and choice (D), Ohio, was a free state.

## Lesson 3: Making Inferences

### Questions 1–5: Passage Map

Topic: Arizona Desert products
Scope: Robe and blanket—benefits
Purpose: Sell the products
¶ 1: Have economy + comfort w/AD products
¶ 2: Blanket, robe keep you warm
¶ 3: Easy to maintain & safe

1. **(A) an advertising brochure.** The tone of the passage is very sales-like. You can infer that it is meant to convince a generic person to purchase this product and is not addressed to a specific person, as a personal email, (D), would be. Sales material, like advertising copy from a brochure, is written to tout the benefits of a product, not provide an objective evaluation as a consumer magazine, (B), or government report, (C), would try to do.

2. **(B) consumers who use Arizona Desert products will lower their heating costs.** You are looking for an idea that can be inferred but is not directly stated. Despite the comparison to a toaster, we know this blanket is meant to warm people up, not toast bread. It's the power consumption that is similar (less than 15 cents per day). But although this sounds inexpensive, it doesn't explain how the blanket could pay for itself unless it creates cost savings somewhere else. We can infer, then, that consumers using this blanket will not run their heating as much, and using the blanket will cost less than heating the home. The passage certainly implies that cost is an important consideration for consumers, so choice (D) is not supported.

3. **(B) air conditioners use more energy than fans.** In the first paragraph, the author compares noisy fans and energy-hogging air conditioners. It's implied that each alternative for staying cool has its own drawbacks. From this, you can reasonably infer that an air-conditioning unit is not loud relative to a fan, and a fan is low in its energy usage compared to an air conditioner. Therefore, choice **(B)** is correct. Choice (A) is not supported by the passage. Choice (C) contradicts the implication that the company has been around for some time, having at least one well-established product and one it has just released. Choice (D) might seem reasonable at first glance, but the beginning of the second paragraph implies that people use electric blankets in order to turn down their central heating, not because they don't have any. In fact, in cold parts of the country, central heating is generally not considered optional.

4. **(D) Country of manufacture** The passage's author makes a point of mentioning (C) comfort, (A) the energy usage or energy cost of the blanket and robe relative to regular household heating, and even (B) safety, when noting there is no danger of contact with the chemical fluid. We can infer that the author, who appears to be writing advertising copy, believes these factors to be important to a person making a consumer decision. The author never mentions country of manufacture, so it's also reasonable to infer that he considers this less important than the other three factors.

5 **(C) Choking hazard—do not swallow.** The passage does not say anything about warning labels, but you can infer the answer based on information in the passage concerning safety. The third paragraph states that "you are never exposed to any risk" from the chemical fluid. This strongly implies that the chemical would not be safe if you were to break open the tubes and spill it or drink it. It would be appropriate to note its toxicity on a warning label, (A). You know from the first paragraph that this is an electric blanket (or robe), so a warning not to submerge it in water is reasonable, (B). The warning in the last paragraph to return the blanket right away if it

malfunctions or is damaged and not to replace or repair parts yourself also suggests danger, so this is likely to end up on a warning label (D). Only answer choice (C) is not supported. These products are a blanket and robe large enough to cover an adult. There is no reference to small, detachable parts that a person could conceivably swallow, so there is no evidence of a choking hazard.

# Lesson 4: Understanding Sequences of Events

## Questions 1–4: Passage Map

Topic: Flower arrangement
Scope: How to make it—materials & directions
Purpose: Explain step-by-step

1. **(A) at the 4:00 position** Reread the steps looking for "third-longest stem" or look at your notes. The third-longest stem should be in the 4:00 position, which matches answer choice **(A)**. All other answer choices refer to other elements of the arrangement.

2. **(C) adding water to the dish.** Rereading the steps or using your notes, look for the first step. In the instructions, the key word "first" identifies this step, which is to add water to the dish. Choice (A) is the second step, (B) is the last, and (D) is the third.

3. **(C) pine, chrysanthemum, bamboo, iris** Because the directions state that stems are placed in decreasing order of their length, identify the longest as the first to be placed, which is pine. Now check the answer choices and eliminate any that do not start with pine. Only (A) and (C) are left. The next-longest item is the chrysanthemum, making choice **(C)** correct. All other answers are out of sequence, and choice (B) is completely backward, from shortest to longest.

4. **(A) in any place.** According to the directions, the third-longest stem (that is, the shortest) is the last stem to be placed in a specific position; after that, the florist can arrange any other plant materials in "any position that pleases you."

## Questions 5–8: Passage Map

Topic: GG Bridge
Scope: When built, length, usage
Purpose: Inform

5. **(B) in a car.** According to the passage, pedestrians can cross the bridge only until 6:00 PST, but cars can cross at any time. Thus, a person crossing the bridge at 8:00 PM PST would need to be in a car. Choices (A) and (C) are incorrect because electric scooters and skateboards are never allowed on the bridge, and choice (D) is incorrect because pedestrians cannot walk across the bridge after 6:00 PST.

6. **(D) 1964.** The stimulus states that the Golden Gate bridge lost its title as the longest suspension bridge "when the Verrazano-Narrows bridge was built in New York in 1964," which matches choice **(D)**. All other dates are in the wrong decades.

7. **(D) 200,000** When the bridge opened to pedestrians on May 27, only one person was allowed to cross, but as the passage states, the next day, May 28, 200,000 people walked over the bridge. This matches answer choice **(D)**. Choice (A) gives the number of people who walked the bridge on opening day, choice (B) is the length of the bridge, and choice (C) is the number of vehicles that cross the bridge each day.

8. **(D) under construction.** The stimulus states that the bridge "was started in 1933 and finished in 1937," meaning that in 1936 it must still have been under construction. All other answers are incorrect use of details from the stimulus.

9. **(B) The square numbered 10 is above the square numbered 15.** The question asks you to identify a true statement about the results of arranging numbered shapes according to a set of instructions. Work step-by-step. The first four steps have you create 4 × 4 squares by arranging certain numbered squares from least to greatest in a clockwise direction.

1.

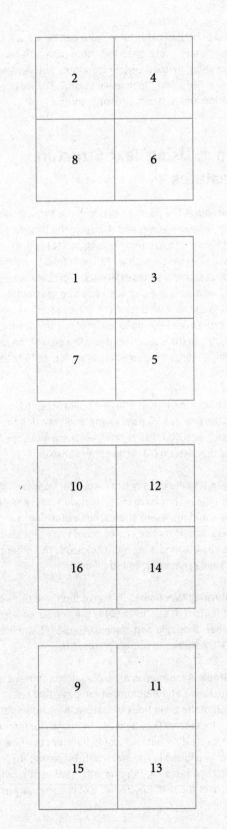

| 2 | 4 |
|---|---|
| 8 | 6 |

2.

| 1 | 3 |
|---|---|
| 7 | 5 |

3.

| 10 | 12 |
|----|----|
| 16 | 14 |

4.

| 9 | 11 |
|----|----|
| 15 | 13 |

While the previous steps had you arrange numbered squares *clockwise* to make 4 × 4 squares, step 5 has you arrange the 4 × 4 squares created in steps 1−4 *counter-clockwise*. So the 4 × 4 square containing the largest single number, 16, is at the upper left. Of the remaining 4 × 4 squares, the one containing the largest number is the one with 15, and it goes below the 4 × 4 square containing 16. The next 4 × 4 square, containing 8, goes to the right of that. And the final 4 × 4 square, whose largest number is 7, goes at the top right.

| 10 | 12 | 1 | 3 |
|----|----|---|---|
| 16 | 14 | 7 | 5 |
| 9  | 11 | 2 | 4 |
| 15 | 13 | 8 | 6 |

# Chapter 2: Passage Structure and Word Choices

## Lesson 1: Understanding the Author's Purpose and Point of View

### Questions 1–4: Passage Map

Topic: US immigrants circa 1900
Scope: Difficulties
Purpose: To explain problems & role of organizations in helping/hurting
¶ 1: Life was hard; some orgs helped
¶ 2: DAR's position & actions; made immigrants "second-class citizens"

1. **(A) It describes the living conditions and political environment for immigrants to America around 1900.** This passage is informative, not persuasive, so (B) and (C) are not correct. The focus of the passage is on describing the conditions of immigrants. It discusses the Daughters of the American Revolution to describe the welcome some immigrants received. Therefore (D) is not correct.

2. **(B) Unsympathetic** The author of the passage used an opinion key word at the end of the first paragraph, describing the organization's approach as "harsher." The answer choice that matches this characterization is **(B)**, while (D), "Warm," expresses the opposite. Choices (A), "Heroic," and (C), "Patriotic," are positive words, while the passage is neutrally factual or slightly negative when referring to the group. The group's name has a patriotic ring, but the question asks for the author's opinion, not the group's opinion of itself.

3. **(D) On the whole, new immigrants to the United States were not treated fairly compared to native-born citizens.** The author uses several opinion key words, such as "trapped in poverty" and "exploited by . . . employers," making choices (A) and (B) incorrect. While choice (C) may seem reasonable, the passage never mentions how life in America compared to life in other countries, so there's no support for the idea that the author would agree with this sentiment. Choice **(D)** is correct. The author states that immigrants were exploited and that laws in some places made them "second-class citizens."

4. **(C) Most immigrants to the United States near the end of the 19th century were poor.** This is the only verifiable, factual statement. Poverty can be objectively defined, such as in terms of household income, so it can be shown whether most immigrants ("most" meaning more than 50%) were poor ("poor" meaning below a certain income). "Anti-American," (A); "unfairly," (B); and "look down upon," (D), are open to interpretation and thus a matter of opinion.

## Lesson 2: Using Text Structure and Features

1. **(C) Procedural** The passage explains the steps involved in submitting, nominating, and choosing the Best Foreign Language Film at the Academy Awards, so **(C)** is the correct answer. Note key words such as "after," "final," and "subsequently" that signal a series of events. A problem and solution are identified only in the last sentence and are not the focus of the paragraph as a whole, so (A) is incorrect. The author does not express an opinion or attempt to convince the reader of something, so (B) is also incorrect. The goal of the passage is not to tell a story with characters and plot, so (D) can be disregarded.

2. **(A) First** After the introductory first sentence, the author describes the process for nominating and choosing the Best Foreign Language Film. The second sentence gives the first step in the process, so **(A)** is the correct answer.

3. **(A) Legend** A map usually has a key that indicates what the symbols on the map refer to in the real world; for example, black lines could represent streets, wide blue lines could represent rivers, and stars and circles could represent towns and cities. The key is called a legend, choice **(A)**. The other choices are not features commonly found on maps.

4. **(D) If Morning Ever Comes** By convention, the titles of novels are italicized, so choice **(D)** is the correct answer. Proper names of people and places, (A) and (C), are not, and neither are the names of literary prizes, (B).

5. **(B) Footnote** A footnote is an explanatory comment or source note found at the bottom of the page that refers to a specific part of the main body of text. Authors often put source citations in footnotes. They also use footnotes for information they deem interesting but that would interrupt the flow of ideas were it included in the main text. Therefore, **(B)** is the correct choice. A heading, (A), and subheading, (C), indicate the structure of the text. Bold print, (D), is commonly used for emphasis.

# Lesson 3: Determining Word Meaning

1. **(A) A kind of priest** "Canon of Rouen" is mentioned as an example of Coutances's "ecclesiastical appointments," so "canon" must be some kind of religious office, **(A)**. Even if you were unfamiliar with the meaning of "ecclesiastical," you could still derive the meaning of "canon" from context. The passage states that although Coutances held political appointments, he also accumulated ecclesiastical ones, so political and ecclesiastical must mean two different things. Thus (B), "diplomat," and (D), "politician," can be eliminated. (C), "a large gun," makes little sense here; a *cannon*, one type of large gun, is a homonym of *canon*, meaning the words sound the same but are spelled differently.

2. **(B) There was so much activity at the center that people resembled bees working in a hive.** The writer is using figurative language to describe the community center during a busy time, which resembled the activity of a beehive, **(B)**. Although baking could be found at the carnival, there is no support for the notion that the author was expecting to find honey in the baked goods, (C). When the author mentions "a jar of honey," he is speaking metaphorically for emphasis. (A) is incorrect because the police closed the street for the children's parade, not to protect them from bee stings. Finally, there is no reason to believe an apiarist, an expert in bees, was present at the carnival, or indeed that any actual bees were there, so (D) can be rejected.

3. **(A) Industriously** Even if you didn't know the meaning of the word "assiduously," you could surmise its meaning from its context. Winston wants to approach his work in a way that his boss would approve of, so he will work hard. **(A)**, "industriously," is the correct choice. The employer would hardly approve of Winston if he worked "carelessly," so (B) is incorrect. Since Winston is working in a certain way for a purpose—to gain approval—choice (C), "needlessly," can be rejected. And finally, since Winston wants credit for his work, (D), "anonymously," is incorrect—he wants to be acknowledged.

4. **(D) The politician thundered.** Choice (A), "The wind whistled," is an example of personification because it gives wind, a nonhuman thing, a human activity, whistling. "The lion roared," (B), is not figurative language, since roaring is what lions do. Choice (C), "The icy road was like a sheet of glass," is a simile because it uses "like" to compare two things, the road and glass. **(D)** is a metaphor because it compares two things, the politician and thunder, without using *like* or *as*.

5. **(C) A biography of a well-regarded writer** Note that this question asks for the *least* useful resource, so you are looking for a choice that would not be helpful in writing an essay. Both a dictionary, (A), and a thesaurus, (B), would be useful when writing, since the former will give you denotative, or literal, meanings of words while the latter will provide synonyms. (D), a poetry collection, could also be useful because it could provide examples of figurative language you could use as inspiration. A biography of a writer, **(C)**, though, would be of little use since it would consist of the writer's life story, which would not help you make word choices.

6. **(C) orated** This question relates to how different words convey different tones. If a person is speaking about a topic of major importance, the verb has to reflect the manner in which one would speak of weighty matters. Of the choices, only **(C)**, "orated" (meaning "delivered a speech, declaimed") has the appropriate degree of seriousness. (A), "chatted," and (B), "gossiped," are too trivial. An individual of authority like a governor should never mumble about important matters (and if she did, the audience would hardly be "attentive"), so (D) is incorrect.

# Chapter 3: Integrating Ideas to Draw Conclusions

## Lesson 1: Comparing and Contrasting Multiple Sources

### Questions 1–2: Passage Map

*Poem*
Topic: Death in battle
Scope: Importance of continuing the fight
Purpose: Urge the living not to "break faith" with the dead—keep up the fight ("Take up our quarrel")

*Letter*
Topic: Battle tomorrow
Scope: Excitement about the battle
Purpose: To describe his enthusiasm ("biggest thing yet," "glad to be going in first wave," "supreme experience")

1. **(C) a glorious death on the battlefield.** Both the poem and the letter, each written about a World War I battle, are concerned with the dead or the possibility of dying and the glory of fighting for a cause. The poem is written from the perspective of soldiers who died in battle and says, "To you from failing hands we throw/The torch; be yours to hold it high." It warns that if the living do not continue the fight, "We shall not sleep." Seeger's letter refers to the possibility of his death ("... if I get through all right. If not, ...."), but adds that "We are to have the honor of marching in the first wave," and "this is the supreme experience." Choice (A) is outside the scope of both sources, and choice (B) omits any reference to dying, placing it outside the scope of the poem. Choice (D) is a misread of the poem, which doesn't make this contrast.

2. **(D) By arguing that fighting for a cause can be worthwhile** The poem and letter speak of both the risk of dying and how taking that risk is worthwhile. Thus, both authors would agree with choice **(D)**. It cannot be assumed that Seeger and McCrae would think the statement is cowardly, as in choice (A), since while Luttrell laments the loss of his friends, he does not express any reluctance to risk his own life. Choice (B) is incorrect because Luttrell's statement is a primary source, so Seeger and McCrae would have no reason to question his experience. Choice (C) is incorrect because while both authors accept death in battle as worthwhile, neither comments on what it is like to watch someone die.

3. **(A) Quality control for the Sportmax SUV is inadequate.** The testimonial from the Sportmax SUV owner is glowing in its praise for the manufacturer, expressing confidence that quality control ensures the safety of the vehicle. On the other hand, the newspaper story reports a Sportmax SUV recall on the grounds that the transmission is unsafe and implies, by citing the CEO's statement, that this defect may be due to poor quality control. The two authors would disagree on the adequacy of quality control, making choice **(A)** correct. Choice (B) is out of scope, because vehicles other than the Sportmax SUV are not mentioned. Neither statement compares SUVs and sedans, so choice (C) is incorrect. The difference of opinion is not about whether manufacturers try to make their cars safe but how successful they actually are in doing so, so (D) is incorrect.

## Lesson 2: Making Inferences About Fiction

1. **(D) a disorganized procrastinator.** As with all inference questions, the answer is not explicitly written in the passage, but the author provides enough clues to make a logical conclusion. Johnny gets a late start because he sets his alarm clock wrong and admits being late is his own fault. He needs to cram because "the day had slipped away from him without his notice, *just as it always did.*" He had to find his car keys, and in his rush to reach for his phone, spills his coffee. All this adds up to someone who is disorganized and procrastinates (puts off doing tasks until it's too late to do them well), as choice **(D)** describes. Choice (A) is opposite to what is implied: Johnny crams for his meeting, indicating that he's not lazy, and he is concerned about getting to work on time, so he is not apathetic. Choice (B) is not supported: though there is to be an important meeting, we do not know whether it will boost Johnny's career. Maybe doing well at the meeting is necessary to keep his job. Choice (C) runs counter to the evidence; Johnny seems to be less of a victim of hard luck than someone who is actually responsible for his own predicaments.

2. **(B) describe Johnny's arrival at the office and the upcoming meeting.** Consider what the author has already written in the beginning of the story and what logically comes next. The author has described Johnny through showing how he gets ready for an important meeting, so the author most likely doesn't need to add more examples, eliminating choice (A). Choice (C) wouldn't make sense, since the author will describe the meeting before relating Johnny's reaction to it. (D) completely skips the middle of the story and goes straight to the end. This leaves the correct choice, **(B)**. Since the author has

already heralded Johnny's rush to the office and the impending important meeting, it is likely that she will next get Johnny to the office and describe the meeting.

**3. (C) He is not fully aware of his actions and their consequences.** Johnny's plaintive question "Why do these things always happen to me?" shows his tendency to be unaware of what he has done to put himself in a predicament. It was his own fault that he set the alarm for the wrong time, that he failed to prepare before 1:00 AM, and that he spilled his coffee, but he still wonders why so much went wrong, indicating that he doesn't connect his own actions with their consequences, a match for choice **(C)**. Choice (A) is an opposite; the author writes that despite cramming, Johnny had developed a strong presentation. Choice (B) is unsupported; we're never told that he blames others. Choice (D) is an unfounded inference; the protagonist has had too little sleep, which "doesn't bode well for the rest of the day," but perhaps he can overcome his sleep deficit and in any event, there is no evidence he is usually too tired to perform well at work.

# Lesson 3: Evaluating an Argument

### Questions 1–4: Passage Map

Conclusion: Junk food in school lunches will cause obesity
Evidence: Examples of junk foods served
Assumption: There are no offsetting factors (e.g., healthier food at home, more exercise)

**1. (C) Home meals consist of similarly unhealthy choices.** Though the author is specific about school lunches and obesity, his conclusion is more generally about a future of obese children with poor eating habits. Providing support beyond the example of school lunches would bolster this conclusion, and **(C)**, extending poor food choices to the home, does just that. Choice (A) may be true but is out of scope; exercise is not part of the argument. Choice (B) is opposite to the author's statement and would actually weaken his conclusion. Choice (D) gives a reason why less healthy food might be served, but the author is not concerned with why but merely with the fact that this food is given to children.

**2. (A) example.** The author concludes that future generations will be obese based on the evidence of junk food being served at school lunches and the examples of a piece of chocolate as compared to an apple. This is a match for answer choice **(A)**. Choice (B) is incorrect because there is no reference to expert opinions on the subject, and choice (C) is incorrect because there is no opposing argument. An analogy, choice (D), would require the author to compare the situation with junk food to something else, using the words "like" or "as," which is not done.

**3. (D) School lunches are unhealthy and result in overweight children.** The author's claim is that junk food served in school lunches will produce a generation of obese people. This matches answer choice **(D)**. Choice (A) is extreme. It cannot be assumed that absolutely no healthy foods are offered; the argument only claims that unhealthy foods are served. The author states choice (B), but this is only a part of the evidence, not a restatement of the conclusion and evidence. Choice (C) is out of scope, since the author does not mention eating a variety of foods, only the difference between eating healthy and unhealthy foods.

**4. (B) most children bring healthy lunches from home.** The author's conclusion about obesity being caused by unhealthy school lunches depends on the assumption that children are eating those lunches. The conclusion would not follow from the evidence if children ate homemade healthier lunches instead. That statement, if true, would undermine the argument, making choice **(B)** correct. Choice (A) might make school lunches a bit less fattening, but it does not address pizza and chocolate. Even if choice (C) were true, it wouldn't mean that the chefs actually make healthier lunches. Choice (D) is incorrect because it makes an irrelevant comparison; even if the food in vending machines were worse, that wouldn't change the fact that school lunches are bad, which is the evidence on which the author's conclusion depends.

# Lesson 4: Integrating Data From Different Formats

1. **(A) Blood pressure monitor** The passage text states that the table includes instruments used in a medical setting. Of the three instruments listed, only one appears to be limited to use with a healthcare client, and that's the blood pressure monitor, used to monitor either pressure or pulse rate. Scales can be used for weighing either people or medication, and thermometers can be used to measure temperature of either people or the air in a room. Barometers, which are not used in a medical context but to determine outdoor air pressure to predict weather, are not mentioned in the stimulus.

2. **(A) 2%** The pie chart shows today's percentage of people in the overweight and obese categories as 33% and 20%, respectively, for a total of 53%. The passage explains that these numbers reflect the current population, while during the Dust Bowl, these categories "switched places" with the underweight category, making 2% the correct answer.

3. **(D) She turns left onto Main Street.** The diagram shows that Route 29 runs east into the town of Oak Ridge, and the text explains that Starries have to drive east to get into town. A Starry driving east on Route 29 would, once entering Oak Ridge, turn left on Main Street in order to reach the post office. There would be no need for an additional turn.

# Mathematics: Answers and Explanations

## Chapter 1: Arithmetic and Algebra

### Lesson 1: Arithmetic

1. **(C) $\frac{8}{25}$, 32%** You are asked to convert a decimal to a fraction and percent. To convert 0.32 to a fraction, note that the last digit, 2, is in the hundredths column, so write $\frac{32}{100}$. Reduce to lowest terms: $\frac{32}{100} = \frac{8}{25}$. To convert 0.32 to a percent, move the decimal point two places to the right and add a percent symbol: 32%. Check your work: confirm the simplification step and decimal placement.

2. **(C) 40.** You are asked for the least common multiple (LCM) of three integers. Some multiples of 4 are 4, 8, 12, 16, 20, 24, 28, 32, 36, 40, 44. Some multiples of 8 are 6, 16, 24, 36, 40, 48. Some multiples of 10 are 10, 20, 30, 40, 50. The LCM of 4, 8, and 10 is 40—that's the smallest multiple they have in common.

3. **(B) $\frac{1}{4}, \frac{3}{8}, \frac{2}{5}$** You are asked to order the given fractions from least to greatest. To order the fractions, compare them in pairs using the X method. Comparing $\frac{3}{8}$ and $\frac{2}{5}$, you get $3 \times 5 = 15$ and $2 \times 8 = 16$. So $\frac{3}{8} < \frac{2}{5}$. Eliminate choice (A).

Comparing $\frac{3}{8}$ and $\frac{1}{4}$, you get $3 \times 4 = 12$ and $1 \times 8 = 8$. So $\frac{3}{8} > \frac{1}{4}$. The correct order is $\frac{1}{4}, \frac{3}{8}, \frac{2}{5}$. Alternatively, you could have converted $\frac{1}{4}$ to $\frac{2}{8}$ to make that comparison.

Double-check that you ranked the fractions from least to greatest. Choice (D) ranks them from greatest to least.

4. **(B) $2\frac{5}{24}$** Convert the mixed number to an improper fraction: $1\frac{5}{8} = \frac{(1 \times 8) + 5}{8} = \frac{8 + 5}{8} = \frac{13}{8}$. Find a common denominator for $\frac{13}{8}$ and $\frac{7}{12}$. The LCM of 8 and 12 is 24. Once you have converted each fraction, you can add

$\frac{13}{8} + \frac{7}{12} = \frac{13 \times 3}{8 \times 3} + \frac{7 \times 2}{12 \times 2} = \frac{39}{24} + \frac{14}{24} = \frac{53}{24}$. Now convert $\frac{53}{24}$ to a mixed number. When you divide 53 by 24, you get 2 with a remainder of 5. So, $\frac{53}{24} = 2\frac{5}{24}$.

5. **(D) 279** You are asked the value of an expression. Solve using PEMDAS. Becaue there are no exponents or parentheses, take care of division and multiplication first:

Multiplication/division: $81 + 12 - 18 + 204$
Addition/subtraction: $93 - 18 + 204$
$\phantom{xxxxxxxx} 75 + 204$
$\phantom{xxxxxxxx} 279$

6. **(C) 50** You are asked the value of an expression. Solve using PEMDAS.

Parentheses: $8 + 7 \times 6$
Multiplication/division: $8 + 42$
Addition/subtraction: $50$

### Lesson 2: Algebra

1. **(A) 7** The question asks you to solve for $x$. Use inverse operations. First, subtract 16 from both sides to yield $2x = 14$. Next, divide both sides by 2 to yield $x = 7$.

2. **(C) $14y + 70$** The question asks you to simplify, so combine like terms. Note that when you add the variable terms $5y + 9y = 14y$, you can quickly eliminate two of the answer choices, (A) and (B). Next, add $-11 + 81 = 70$. Note that this is the same as subtracting 11 from 81: $81 - 11 = 70$. Finally, add the terms: $14y + 70$. These are unlike terms, so the expression cannot be further simplified.

3. **(C) 3** The question asks you to solve for $b$. First, add 21 to both sides to yield $10b = 30$. Next, divide both sides by 10 to yield $b = 3$.

4. **(D) $56x + 4$** The question asks you to add the expressions, so combine like terms. Note that when you add the variable terms $44x + 12x = 56x$, you can quickly eliminate two of the answer choices, (A) and (B). Next, add: $-1 + 5 = 4$. Finally, add the unlike terms: $56x + 4$.

**5. (D) 10** The question asks you to solve for $a$. First, to cancel the division on the left side, multiply both sides by 2 to yield $5a = 2(2a + 5)$. Next, simplify on the right side: $5a = 4a + 10$. Finally, subtract $4a$ from both sides to yield $a = 10$.

# Lesson 3: Solving Word Problems

**1. (C) $15.75** This question gives you information about the cost of different food items and asks for the total spent on lunch. To find a total, add the individual amounts. Because they "both" get a soda, first multiply the $1.50 for the soda by 2: $1.50 \times 2 = $3.00. Then add the sandwich and mac 'n' cheese: $3.00 + $8.00 + 4.75 = $15.75. You can check your work by subtracting each food item from the total: $15.75 − $8.00 − $4.75 − $1.50 − $1.50 = $0.

**2. (B) $257.50** You are given information about Jamal's monthly income and his expenses, and you're asked how much he will save each month. Find the money left over after expenses by subtracting from the total: $2,875 − $2,360 = $515. He will save only half of that, so divide by 2: $515 ÷ 2 = $257.50. Check your work by performing the calculations in reverse: double $257.50 and add it to $2,360 to get $2,875.

**3. (A) 5** This word problem presents information about the number of students who have chosen different art projects and the number of crayons available. It asks you to calculate how many crayons the teacher gives "each student" if she distributes them "equally." Divide the total number of crayons, 60, by the total number of students $(3 + 9 = 12)$: $60 ÷ 12 = 5$. Check your work by reversing the calculations: Does 12 students times 5 crayons each equal 60 crayons? Yes, it does.

**4. (D) 60** This word problem gives you information about Tyler's strawberry growing: how many bales of straw to grow a pallet of strawberries and how much profit he makes on six pallets. You need to find the number of bales of straw it takes to earn a $400 profit. First, divide Tyler's total profit by his profit per six pallets: $400 ÷ $80 = 5. He needs to sell six pallets five times to earn $400 profit; in other words, he needs to sell $6 \times 5 = 30$ pallets. Then he needs two bales of straw per pallet, so multiply 30 pallets by 2 bales to get the total bales needed: $30 \times 2 = 60$ bales of straw.

**5. (B) 35 minutes** You are told the distance Kaitlyn travels to work and her different speeds in the morning and the afternoon. The amount of distance traveled equals the speed of travel multiplied by the time spent traveling. Translate this into the formula distance = rate × time. To calculate her travel time, rearrange the formula: $\text{time} = \dfrac{\text{distance}}{\text{rate}}$. Because

she travels at different rates, perform the calculation twice.

Morning: $\dfrac{10 \text{ miles}}{40 \text{ mph}} = \dfrac{1}{4}$ hours = 15 minutes. Afternoon:

$\dfrac{10 \text{ miles}}{30 \text{ mph}} = \dfrac{1}{3}$ hours = 20 minutes. Then add the times to get

the total: 15 minutes + 20 minutes = 35 minutes.

**6. (B) 24** First, calculate how much money the therapist would earn at Clinic A. Translate "$25 per client treated" into $25 per client × 30 clients = $750. Then translate "plus a flat weekly salary of $200" into $750 + $200 = $950. This is the total weekly income at Clinic A. If the total weekly income at Clinic B equaled this amount, the equation would be $40 × B = $950, where $B$ is the number of clients seen. Find $B$: $950 ÷ $40 per client = 23.75 clients. You want the therapist's income at Clinic B to exceed that at Clinic A, so he needs to see more than 23.75 clients. Because there can't be partial clients (and all the answers, thankfully, are whole numbers), round up to the nearest whole number. The minimum number of clients at Clinic B necessary to earn more than $950 is 24.

**7. (D) $45 \leq n \leq 90$** This question presents a scenario about varying rates of cars passing through a light, and the answer choices are inequalities. You need to calculate the range of possible numbers of cars that can pass in 15 minutes. Start by calculating how many cars can pass in a minute at the minimum rate: 60 seconds ÷ 10 seconds per car = 6 cars per minute. Now calculate how many can pass at the maximum rate: 60 seconds ÷ 20 seconds per car = 3 cars per minute. (Note that the "in between" rate of one car every 15 seconds is irrelevant to your calculations, because you only need to find the minimum and maximum rates.) Once you've calculated the minimum and maximum number of cars per minute, multiply each quantity by 15 minutes: 3 cars per minute × 15 minutes = 45 cars; 6 cars per minute × 15 minutes 90 cars. Thus, 45 is the minimum number of cars that will pass, and 90 is the maximum. $n$ is greater than or equal to 45 and less than or equal to 90.

**8. (D) 40** Because the vegetable garden uses one-fourth of 36 gallons, translate that into $\dfrac{1}{4} \times 36 = 9$, so 9 gallons are applied to the vegetables. Thus, the filter processes 9 gallons of water per day. The question says the filter needs replacement after 360 gallons, so divide this amount by the gallons per day to find the number of days the filter will last before it has to be replaced: 360 gallons ÷ 9 gallons per day = 40 days.

# Lesson 4: Ratios, Percentages, and Proportions

1. **(C) 20% increase** The question states that the value of the investment first dropped by 20% but then increased by 50% from the lowered value and asks for the overall percent change. Because no specific values are given and this question is about percentages, pick 100 as the starting value of Juanita's investment. The 20% drop then would have been $\frac{20}{100} \times 100 = 20$. Subtract 20 from 100 to determine the reduced value of 80. The 50% increase was based on this reduced value: $\frac{50}{100} \times 80 = \frac{1}{2} \times 80 = 40$. Add this increase of 40 to 80 to obtain a final value of 120. At this point, you know the value of the investment went up (from 100 to 120), so eliminate choices (A) and (B). Finally, use the formula for percentage change, subtracting the starting value from the new value and setting that over 100: $\frac{120-100}{100} = \frac{20}{100} = 20\%$. Choice (D) is a trap answer because it equals $50 - 20$, but the 50% increase was based on a lower value. Check your logic and calculations.

2. **(B) 400** The question asks you to determine the amount that 60 would be 15% of. Percentage problems with an unknown value can be set up as a proportion: $\frac{15}{100} = \frac{60}{x}$. Cross multiply to obtain $15x = 6000$. To avoid more difficult long division, tackle this in two steps. Both sides of the equation are divisible by 3, so $5x = 2000$. Now divide both sides by 5 to get $x = 400$. Verify your logic in setting up the proportion and check your math.

3. **(A) 5 bandages and 4 swabs** The question lists the desired ratio of three items and the current inventory of those items, and it asks how many of what two types of supplies must be added to bring the inventory ratio into line. The requirement to add to the stock of only two items is a clue as to how to solve this problem. By comparing the current inventory of each item to the specified ratio, you can determine which of the three supplies will not need to be augmented. There are 6 units of ointment and its part of the ratio is 2, so the "multiplier" for that supply is $6 \div 2 = 3$. For the bandages, the multiplier is $10 \div 5 = 2$, so some bandages will need to be added. The multiplier for swabs is $20 \div 8 = 2.5$, so some swabs will need to be added as well. To bring the multiplier for bandages up to 3 to "match" the multiplier for ointment, there should be $3 \times 5 = 15$ in inventory, which would require adding 5 more to the current inventory of 10. There need to be $3 \times 8 = 24$ swabs, a quantity that is obtained by adding 4 swabs to the current inventory of 20. The correct answer is **(A)**. Another way to solve this problem would be to try each answer choice and calculate the resulting ratio until you find the correct answer. Check your answer to be certain it is correct: divide each term of 6:15:24 by 3 to get the desired inventory ratio, 2:5:8.

4. **(D) 8** The question provides the scale proportionality of a drawing and the measured length of a hallway on that plan. You are asked to determine how many 8-foot pieces of molding are needed for *both* sides of that hallway. To determine the actual length of the hallway, set up a proportion based on the scale of the drawing: $\frac{\frac{1}{4} \text{ in.}}{1 \text{ ft}} = \frac{7\frac{3}{4} \text{ in.}}{x \text{ ft}}$. (Its all right to mix inches and feet because both ratios have inches in the numerator and feet in the denominator.) Cross multiply to get $\frac{1}{4}x = 7\frac{3}{4}(1) = \frac{31}{4}$. Now you can multiply both sides of that equation by 4 to get $x = 31$ feet. The question states that the molding is being installed on *both* sides of the hallway, so $2 \times 31 = 62$ feet are needed. The molding is purchased in 8-foot pieces. Because 8 pieces total 64 feet in length and 7 pieces would leave you short, at only 56 feet in length, 8 is the number that must be bought. Choice (A), 4 pieces, is a trap answer because that is the number of pieces needed for *one* side of the hallway. Verify that you answered the question that was asked, that you set up the proportion properly, and that your calculations are accurate.

5. **(D) $\frac{0.2 \text{ cc}}{\text{minute}}$** The question provides the amounts of fluid in an IV bag at two different times. This particular solution has a concentration of 5% medication, and the question asks for the unit rate at which the medication is dispensed. First, determine the drip rate of the total solution: $\frac{780 \text{ cc} - 300 \text{ cc}}{(10-8) \text{ hours}} = \frac{480 \text{ cc}}{2 \text{ hours}} = 240 \frac{\text{cc}}{\text{hour}}$. Because only 5% of the solution is medication, that would be $0.05 \times 240 = 12$ cc of medication per hour. Unfortunately, none of the answer choices match that delivery rate. Choice (A) is a trap answer; this is the delivery rate of the solution rather than the medication. Also, be careful of choice (B): this is mathematically correct, but *unit* rates are stated with a denominator of 1. Both of the remaining choices are expressed as unit rates per minute, so divide the hourly rate by 60 to obtain the rate per minute: $12\frac{\text{cc}}{\text{hour}} \div \frac{60 \text{ minutes}}{1 \text{ hour}} = 12\frac{\text{cc}}{\text{hour}} \times \frac{1 \text{ hour}}{60 \text{ minutes}} = 0.2\frac{\text{cc}}{\text{minute}}$. Double-check that you used the correct values from the question and that your logic and calculations are correct.

## Lesson 5: Estimating and Rounding

1. **(B) 3** The question asks you to convert a measurement from cubic centimeters to the nearest liter. The answer choices are all displayed as whole numbers. Because a liter is defined as 1000 cubic centimeters, divide 2753 by 1000. Do this by moving the decimal point 3 places to the left to get 2.753. Round this result to the nearest liter by looking at the first digit to the right of the decimal point. Because this number is 7, round up to 3 liters.

2. **(B) 378** A quick glance at the answer choices reveals that they are far enough apart that estimating will be an efficient approach. Round the given numbers to get $(60 - 40) \times (40 - 20)$. So, $20 \times 20 = 400$. The answer choice closest to 400 is **(B)**, 378.

3. **(C) 1056 mL** The question provides the hourly rate of leakage from a faucet and asks how much water would be lost over 2 days. A quick glance at the answer choices shows that they are widely spaced, so you can estimate the correct answer. Convert days to hours to match the units in the drip rate:

$2 \text{ days} \times \dfrac{24 \text{ hrs}}{\text{day}} = 48 \text{ hrs}$. Round 48 up to 50 and the drip rate

down from 22 to 20. Because one number was rounded up and one down, it will be safe to multiply to get an estimate:

$20\dfrac{\text{mL}}{\text{hr}} \times 50 \text{ hrs} = 1000 \text{ mL}$. Scanning the answer choices, only

**(C)**, 1056 mL, is close to this estimate.

4. **(C) 12** The problem provides information about the number of cookies per case and the average breakage rate, and it asks for the expected number of broken cookies per case. This is a percentage rate problem that can be solved by estimating because the answer will be rounded to a whole number and the answer choices are quite spread out. The breakage rate is given as a percentage, so set up a proportion, with $30 \times 24$ representing the total number of cookies in a case:

$\dfrac{1.72}{100} = \dfrac{x}{30 \times 24}$. To simplify the calculations, round 24 down

to 20 and 1.72 up to 2: $\dfrac{2}{100} = \dfrac{x}{30 \times 20} = \dfrac{x}{600}$. Cross multiply

to get $100x = 1200$ and $x = 12$. The estimate of 12 exactly equals correct answer **(C)**.

Note that after cross multiplication, the 24, 30, and 1.72 were all multiplied together. Because the amount of rounding was significant (1.72 up to 2 accounts for just over a 15% increase, and 24 down to 20 is a little over a 15% decrease), it's important that they were rounded in opposite directions. In fact, even if there were 25 packages in a case, it would still be more accurate to round down than up, despite the "5 and up" rule. Consider the cumulative effect of rounding when adding or multiplying many numbers together and break the rules when necessary.

5. **(A) 1161** The question asks for the value of the product of two 2-digit numbers. The estimated value of this expression is $30 \times 40 = 1200$. Given the closely spaced answer choices, that estimate is of no value. However, there is another shortcut that can occasionally be used with multiplication questions: the last-digit test. If you were to actually multiply 27 by 43, you would start with $7 \times 3 = 21$, and the last digit of the product would be 1. Before plodding through the rest of the multiplication process, check the answer choices to see if this tidbit of information is helpful. Sure enough, only choice **(A)** ends with 1, so that has to be the correct answer.

# Chapter 2: Statistics, Geometry, and Measurements

## Lesson 1: Graphs and Tables

1. **(D) Demetria** The graph displays the numbers of ink cartridges and cases of paper purchased by four people. The question provides the prices of these items and asks which person spent the most money. To calculate the amounts spent by each person, determine the numbers of each item from the graph, multiply by the prices, and total the two amounts. Arthur bought 6 ink cartridges and 1 case of paper, so he spent $6 \times 15 + 1 \times 25 = 90 + 25 = \$115$. Beth purchased 3 and 3; her total was $3 \times 15 + 3 \times 25 = 45 + 75 = \$120$. Charles's purchases totaled $1 \times 15 + 4 \times 25 = 15 + 100 = \$115$. Finally, Demetria bought only paper: $5 \times 25 = \$125$, so her total was the greatest and **(D)** is correct.

2. **(B) There were as many sets smaller than 47″ sold as here were sets larger than 47″.** The graph shows the percentage distribution of TV sales by screen size and asks which of the answer choices could be true. Therefore, the three incorrect answers *must* be false and the correct answer might or might not be true. To evaluate choice (A), add the percentages of TVs with screens 39″ or smaller (2% + 7% + 22% = 31%) and compare this to the percentage of TVs sold with screens 50″ or larger (18% + 23% = 41%). Since the latter is greater, this statement is false and (A) is incorrect. Evaluating choice **(B)** will require some creative thinking. The calculations above showed that 41% were 50″ or larger and 31% were 39″ or smaller. Therefore, the size at which half the sets sold were larger and half were smaller must have been between 40″ and 49″, so it *could* have been 47″. This appears to be the correct answer, but check the remaining choices to be certain. Since 2% of sales had screen sizes 19″ or smaller, choice (C) cannot be true. To evaluate (D), add the two categories that comprise screen sizes between 40″ and 59″: 28% + 23% = 51%. Thus, sales in this range were greater than 50%, and (D) is incorrect. Answer choice **(B)** is correct.

3. **(A) There is a seasonal pattern for skateboarding.** The line graph shows the number of emergency room cases due to skateboard accidents for 12 months and asks what conclusion can be inferred from the information. Since the numbers of cases are the highest in the summer months (in the Northern Hemisphere), the data appear to show a seasonal pattern. The numbers on the chart are *injuries* and the correct answer refers to *skateboarding,* but it is reasonable to infer that increased skateboarding activity directly results in increased injuries. Check the other answer choices as well. The number of cases increased, then decreased, and ended up right about where it started. Thus, there is no clear trend, and both (B) and (C) are incorrect. Although it is a good idea to wear a helmet when skateboarding, the information presented does not provide any insight into whether the skateboarders seen in the emergency room wore helmets. Therefore, (D) is not a conclusion that can be inferred *from the graph*, even though you might make such an inference from real-world experience. Choice **(A)** is correct.

4. **(B) B, 2008, 2009** The bar graph shows the number of cases sold for each of three drugs for every year from 2007 to 2010. The question asks which drug had the greatest year-to-year sales increase and between which two years. Instead of immediately obtaining all 12 values represented in the answer choices from the graph and performing 9 subtractions, first simplify the task as much as possible. Visually evaluate the graph. Choice (A) can be eliminated because the increase for drug A between 2007 and 2008 is much smaller than several other increases in the lengths of the bars from year to year. The remaining answer choices do not mention 2007, so focus on the changes from 2008 to 2009 and from 2009 to 2010. Drug B had a large increase in sales between 2008 and 2009, greater than its increase between 2009 and 2010, so eliminate choice (C). Compare the two remaining choices. The increase for drug B between 2008 and 2009 was 1900 − 1400 = 500; the increase for drug C between 2009 and 2010 was 2400 − 2000 = 400. Choice **(B)** is correct.

## Lesson 2: Statistics

1. **(C) 2** The question lists six numbers and asks for their median. Start by rearranging the numbers in order from least to greatest: −6, −1, 1, 3, 4, 5. Since there is an even number of values in the group, 1 and 3 are both middle numbers. The median is the average of those two numbers, $\frac{1+3}{2} = 2$, which is choice **(C)**. If you calculated the mean instead of the median, you got 1, which is choice (B).

2. **(B) 420 miles** The question shows the gallons of fuel remaining on the vertical axis and the miles driven on the horizontal axis. The line connecting data points slopes downward to the right. This makes sense since the more miles Ruby drives, the less fuel remains in her tank. The question asks how many miles Ruby will have driven when she has 2 gallons left in her tank if the same trend continues. The graph shows that when Ruby drove 300 miles, her fuel remaining dropped from 16 gallons to 6 gallons, so it took 10 gallons to drive those 300 miles. Thus, the rate (trend) is 30 miles/gallon. Since there are 6 gallons left and Ruby wants to refuel with

2 gallons left, she can drive enough more miles to use 4 gallons. Calculate: $4 \text{ gal} \times 30\dfrac{\text{miles}}{\text{gal}} = 120$ miles. Added to the 300 miles already traveled, that is 420 total miles. Choice **(B)** is correct.

3. **(A) Bimodal** The chart shows the number of arrivals at a major airport in each of 24 one-hour intervals. The numbers of arrivals are minimal in the early morning, then rise to a peak between 9:01 AM and 10:00 AM. After that, the arrivals per hour diminish somewhat, then rise to another peak between 6:01 PM and 7:00 PM before falling off later at night. With two peaks in the data values, the graph of the data is bimodal.

## Lesson 3: Covariance and Causality

1. **(A) There is a positive covariation between wolf populations and stream water quality.** The question stem states that increased wolf populations are associated with higher water quality and lower wolf populations are associated with lower water quality. This describes positive covariation. Choice (B) describes describes causality. Choice (C) incorrectly identifies the relationship between variables as inverse. Choice (D) is contradicted by the information in the question stem.

2. **(C) Positive covariation; number of asthma attacks is the dependent variable; pollen count is the independent variable.** The scenario describes an increase in the number of asthma attacks in association with a higher pollen count and a decrease in the number of asthma attacks in association with a lower pollen count. This is an example of positive covariation. The hypothesis being tested states that pollen count is the independent variable and number of asthma attacks is the dependent variable (asthma attacks depend on pollen). Choice (D) describes causality, which cannot be determined from a single study.

3. **(B) The more a person works, the more fatigued he or she becomes.** This answer describes positive rather than negative covariance, since both values (amount of work and fatigue) increase together. All the other answer choices describe negative covariance.

## Lesson 4: Geometry

1. **(C) $18 + 2\pi$** The question presents an irregular shape with two dimensions provided, and it asks you to find the perimeter. Break the figure into familiar shapes and use your knowledge of these shapes to solve. The lower section of the figure is a rectangle with dimensions $w = 4$ and $l = 7$, and the upper section is half of a circle with a diameter of 4. Start with the rectangle: the formula for the perimeter of a rectangle is $2l + 2w$, which equals $14 + 8 = 22$—but be careful! You have to subtract the "missing" side of the rectangle (the side that connects to the circle). In other words, only three sides of the rectangular portion of the shape are part of the perimeter, so subtract 4 from 22 to yield 18, which is the combined length of the three straight sides. Now calculate the circumference of the semicircle: circumference of a circle is $2\pi r$ or $\pi d$. In this case, the diameter is 4, so the circumference is $4\pi$. Again, you have to be careful; the perimeter of the shape here includes only half of the circle, so that portion is half of $4\pi$, or $2\pi$. Now combine this length with the length of the three straight sides: $2\pi + 18$, which is equivalent to answer choice **(C)**.

2. **(C) 48** The diagram shows one rectangle inside another and the dimensions of the larger rectangle. The question says this is a picture in a frame and gives the dimensions of the smaller rectangle (the picture). You need to find the area of the frame. The area of the frame is the area of the larger rectangle minus the area of the smaller rectangle: $(8 \times 10) - (4 \times 8) = 80 - 32 = 48$.

3. **(D) 8 inches** The question provides the area of a circle and asks you to determine the circle's diameter. Use your knowledge of the area formula to find the diameter. The area of a circle is $\pi \times$ radius squared $= \pi r^2$, so in this case, $16\pi$ square inches $= \pi r^2$. Divide both sides by $\pi$ to yield $16 \text{ in}^2 = r^2$. Take the square root of both sides to yield $4 \text{ in} = r$. Since diameter equals 2 times radius, diameter $= 2 \times 4$ inches $= 8$ inches, and choice **(D)** is correct.

# Lesson 5: Converting Measurements

1. **(C) 0.45 L** You are asked to convert between two units: fluid ounces and liters. Use the conversion ratios $\dfrac{30\text{ mL}}{1\text{ fl oz}}$ and $\dfrac{1\text{ L}}{1000\text{ mL}}$. To solve, multiply by the conversion ratios: $15\text{ fl oz} \times \dfrac{30\text{ mL}}{1\text{ fl oz}} \times \dfrac{1\text{ L}}{1000\text{ mL}}$ and cancel the common units: $15 \times \dfrac{30}{1} \times \dfrac{1\text{ L}}{1000}$, leaving liters in the final calculation. Simplify to 0.45 L. To check your work, make sure the denominator of the appropriate conversion ratio has the same unit as the measurement you are converting from. The common units will cancel, leaving you with the unit you set out to convert to. When you have multiple conversion rates, double-check each one.

2. **(D) 116 oz** You are asked to convert between two units: kilograms and ounces. Use the conversion ratios $\dfrac{2.2\text{ lb}}{1\text{ kg}}$ and $\dfrac{16\text{ oz}}{1\text{ lb}}$. Set up the conversion ratios so units will cancel out: $3.3\text{ kg} \times \dfrac{2.2\text{ lb}}{1\text{ kg}} \times \dfrac{16\text{ oz}}{1\text{ lb}} \rightarrow 3.3 \times \dfrac{2.2}{1} \times \dfrac{16\text{ oz}}{1}$, leaving ounces as the unit in the final calculation. Simplify to 116.16 oz. So, 3.3 kg is 116.16 oz, which is closest to **(D)**, 116 oz. To double-check your work, confirm that the conversion ratios are set up so the common units cancel out, leaving the unit you want to convert to.

3. **(C) 0.14 L** You are asked to convert between two units, teaspoons and liters, and to calculate the amount in liters needed for 14 days. You have to convert in two steps—teaspoons to mL and then mL to L—and multiply by the number of days to determine the total amount requested. The conversion ratios are $\dfrac{5\text{ mL}}{1\text{ t}}$ and $\dfrac{1\text{ L}}{1000\text{ mL}}$. Set up the equation so that common units cancel out: $2\text{ t} \times \dfrac{5\text{ mL}}{1\text{ t}} \times \dfrac{1\text{ L}}{1000\text{ mL}}$, leaving liters as the unit in the final calculation. Simplify to $2 \times \dfrac{5}{1} \times \dfrac{1\text{ L}}{1000} = 0.01\text{ L}$. Multiply by 14 to get the total amount requested, 0.14 L, **(C)**. Check that you set up the conversion correctly and your arithmetic is correct. Notice that (A) is the daily dose, which you may have gotten if you forgot to multiply by 14 days.

# Science: Answers and Explanations

## Chapter 1: Human Anatomy and Physiology

### Lesson 1: Human Anatomy and Physiology: An Overview

1. **(B) Lysosomes** Macrophages will need extra organelles whose primary function is to break down cellular waste, so macrophages will have more lysosomes.

2. **(A) Urinary** The function of the urinary system is to filter the blood and eliminate waste products. Urine is named after its main component, urea, which is produced in the liver.

3. **(D) transverse** The transverse plane divides the body into top (superior) and bottom (inferior) halves.

### Lesson 2: The Skeletal System

1. **(A) Osteoblast** Osteoporosis is caused by a demineralization of bone. Treatment would increase the activity, or *upregulate*, the activity of bone-building cells, osteoblasts.

2. **(B) Humerus** The humerus is a long bone found in the upper arm. Carpals, located in the wrist, are short bones. The vertebrae are irregular bones, and the pelvis is a flat bone.

### Lesson 3: The Neuromuscular System

1. **(A) an afferent neuron.** Messages transmitted to the brain are sent via sensory neurons, also called afferent neurons. Efferent neurons and motor neurons refer to the same type of nerve, which relays messages from the brain back to the musculature. The brain stem sends and receives messages related to critical involuntary functions.

2. **(B) difficulty walking.** The cerebellum is the part of the brain involved in motor control and muscle coordination. Speech and short-term memory would be affected by damage to the frontal lobe of the cerebrum, whereas damage to the brain stem would result in life-threatening injuries to critical body functions such as heartbeat and respiration.

3. **(D) Muscle fibers contract in an all-or-none fashion.** Even when a person is at rest, vital muscular contractions involving smooth muscle are still occurring. Muscle contraction is activated by actin and myosin; myelin is the insulation surrounding axons. Sensory neurons carry signals from the muscle to the brain; motor neurons stimulate muscle tissue to contract.

### Lesson 4: The Cardiovascular System

1. **(D) Tricuspid** The tricuspid valve separates the right atrium from the right ventricle. The aortic valve prevents blood from backflowing from the aorta into the left ventricle. The terms *bicuspid valve* and *mitral valve* both refer to the valve that separates the left atrium from the left ventricle.

2. **(C) Left ventricle - aorta - capillaries - vena cava - right ventricle** From the left ventricle, blood flows through the circuit system to the aorta, then through the arteries, arterioles, and capillaries, and then returns to the heart via venules, veins, and the vena cava, where it enters the right atrium. It flows through the pulmonary circuit from the right atrium to the right ventricle, then through the pulmonary artery to the lungs, returning to the left atrium via the pulmonary vein.

3. **(A) Platelets** Hemoglobin is responsible for binding oxygen in the red blood cell. Lymph is the fluid of the open circulatory system that removes waste products from the tissues. Antibodies are plasma proteins that work with the immune system to remove foreign pathogens.

# Lesson 5: The Respiratory System

1. **(B) Residual volume** This question is asking which lung volume prevents lung collapse. Recall that the total lung capacity is the sum of the vital capacity and residual volume. The residual volume, choice **(B)**, is the volume of air always remaining in the lungs. It functions to prevent lung collapse. The tidal volume, (A), is the air exchanged during normal breathing. The vital capacity, (C), is the total volume of air that can be inhaled and exhaled. The total lung capacity, (D), is the sum of the vital capacity and residual volume and represents the maximum volume of air that can reside in the lungs.

2. **(C) The pH of the blood is decreased** This question is asking what leads to an increase in ventilation rate. Recall that the medulla oblongata senses changes in blood carbon dioxide concentration and blood pH. When carbon dioxide concentration increases, the pH of the blood decreases, triggering an increase in ventilation rate. The medulla oblongata does not sense changes in oxygen level, so choice (A) can be eliminated. A decrease in blood carbon dioxide concentration, (D), would lead to an increase in blood pH, (B), both of which would cause a decrease in ventilation rate.

3. **(C) Tuberculosis** This question is asking about lung infections. Recall that tuberculosis is caused by a mycobacterium infection. Influenza, (A), is caused by a coronavirus infection. Pneumonia, (B), is caused by a mycoplasma infection. Asthma, (D), is caused by environmental and genetic factors, not infection.

# Lesson 6: The Gastrointestinal System

1. **(D) Vitamin K** This question is asking about the vitamin absorption that takes place in the colon. Recall that the colon is part of the large intestine and is the site of water and electrolyte absorption. Vitamins that are produced by colonic bacteria—specifically vitamin K—are absorbed, even though vitamin K is also absorbed elsewhere in the intestines. This prediction matches answer choice **(D)**. Vitamins $B_6$, C, and D are only absorbed in the small intestine.

2. **(A) Acidic and partially digested** This question is asking about the state of digested food just after it passes through the pyloric sphincter. Recall that the pyloric sphincter separates the stomach from the duodenum. The pH of the stomach is acidic due to gastric secretions. The acid also converts pepsinogen to pepsin, which begins protein digestion. This prediction matches answer choice **(A)**. Pancreatic bicarbonate released into the duodenum turns the chyme alkaline, and protein digestion continues in the small intestine with the secretion of trypsin and brush border enzymes.

3. **(C) Leptin** This question is asking about hormonal regulation of hunger. Recall that ghrelin and leptin act antagonistically in response to hunger and satiety. Ghrelin, (B), is triggered by an empty stomach, signaling hunger, and leptin is triggered by adipose cells signaling the hypothalamus that the body is full. Answer choice **(C)** matches the prediction. Gastrin, (A), stimulates the release of gastric acid in the stomach, and secretin, (D), stimulates the pancreas to release bicarbonate and other enzymes.

# Lesson 7: The Genitourinary System

1. **(C) Ureter** This question is asking about the flow of urine. Recall that urine is produced in the collecting ducts of the kidneys. From there, it flows into the renal pelvis before moving into the ureters. This matches choice **(C)**. The ureters transport the urine to the urinary bladder, (A), for storing until it is expelled from the body by traveling through the urethra, (D).

2. **(A) Afferent arteriole** This question is asking about the flow of blood into the glomerulus. Recall that blood leaves the heart and travels to the kidneys through the renal arteries, (D). These branch into the smaller afferent arterioles that form the glomerulus. This matches choice **(A)**. The glomerulus filters the blood into Bowman's capsule, (B), part of the nephron. Blood components that are not filtered into the nephron, such as blood cells and large proteins, return to circulation through the efferent arterioles, (C).

3. **(C) Angiotensin and aldosterone** This question is asking about sodium reabsorption in the renal tubule. Recall that sodium reabsorption in the renal tubule increases the osmolality of blood, causing more water to be reabsorbed into the blood by osmosis. Predict that the correct hormones will cause an increase in blood pressure and act directly on the renal tubule. This matches choice **(C)**. Both angiotensin and aldosterone increase the reabsorption of sodium from the renal tubule. Epinephrine, (B), does increase the blood pressure, but it does so by vasoconstriction and does not act on the renal tubule. While the adrenal glands, (A), are located on the kidneys, "adrenal" is not the name of a hormone. Renin, in choices (A) and (D), activates angiotensin. ADH, (D), acts on the collecting duct.

## Lesson 8: The Endocrine System

1. **(C) Adrenal cortex** This question is essentially asking which endocrine gland releases aldosterone. Recall that the adrenal cortex produces steroid hormones that regulate salt and sugar balance. Thus, a tumor in the adrenal cortex, choice **(C)**, would cause an overproduction of aldosterone. Tumors in the hypothalamus, (A), and anterior pituitary, (B), would lead to many hormones being overproduced, not just aldosterone, while the adrenal medulla, (D), produces epinephrine.

2. **(C) Blood glucose rises, triggering a release of insulin and causing blood glucose to decrease.** This question is asking what happens following a meal high in glucose. Recall that the pancreas releases glucagon and insulin to regulate blood glucose levels. Following a meal high in sugar, blood glucose levels rise, so choices (B) and (D) can be eliminated. Following a spike in blood glucose, the pancreas releases insulin, which induces the storage of glucose, so blood glucose levels would then drop. This is a match to choice **(C)**. Choice (A) is incorrect because blood glucose would decrease, not increase, following insulin release.

## Lesson 9: The Reproductive System

1. **(B) A decrease in progesterone** This question is asking what triggers menstruation. Recall that after the corpus luteum atrophies, progesterone levels drop as in choice **(B)**, and since progesterone maintains the uterine lining, the lining breaks down, triggering menses. LH, choice (A), is responsible for driving ovulation. FSH, (B), induces the maturation of the ovarian follicle, and an increase in progesterone, (D), would lead to maintenance of the uterine wall, not shedding.

2. **(C) Urethra** This question is asking which component of the male reproductive system is also found in females. Recall that the male system is composed of the seminiferous tubules, epididymis, vas deferens, ejaculatory duct, urethra, and penis. Of these six structures, only the urethra, choice **(C)**, is found in females, as part of the urinary system. The vas deferens, (A), and epididymis, (B), are exclusively found in males, and the cervix, (D), is exclusively found in females.

3. **(A) Testes** This question is asking for the site of testosterone production. Recall that the testes, choice **(A)**, produce testosterone in males. The uterus, (B), and penis, (D), do not produce any hormones, and the ovaries, (C), produce estrogen in females.

## Lesson 10: The Immune System

1. **(B) Cytotoxic T cells kill beta cells that display the antigen.** This question is asking what immune cell would specifically target and kill beta cells in the pancreas. Recall that the cellular immune system can be broken down into the innate and adaptive immune system. The innate immune system recognizes common patterns on pathogens and kills them by phagocytosis and is not antigen-specific. Both macrophages (A) and neutrophils (D) are components of the innate immune system and would not specifically target an antigen; eliminate. The adaptive immune system is antigen-specific and includes both B and T cells. Helper T cells activate other immune cells but do not directly kill cells, so choice (C) can be eliminated. Cytotoxic T cells directly kill any cell that displays a particular antigen, as described in choice **(B)**.

2. **(A) T cell** This question is asking which of the immune cells listed is not a component of the innate immune system. The correct answer will be a component of the adaptive immune system. Recall that the adaptive immune system is composed of T and B cells, making choice **(A)** correct. Macrophages, (B); dendritic cells, (C); and neutrophils, (D), are all components of the innate immune system and can be eliminated.

3. **(A) Macrophage** This question is asking for an immune cell that phagocytoses pathogens without specifically targeting them. Recall that the innate immune system is not antigen-specific and includes natural killer cells, granulocytes, and monocytes. The monocytes, including macrophages and dendritic cells, are phagocytes. Macrophages, choice **(A)**, phagocytose pathogens displaying common patterns but are not antigen-specific. Natural killer cells, (C), are innate immune cells that are not phagocytic. B cells, (D), produce antibodies and do not directly kill cells. Helper T cells, (B), activate other adaptive immune cells.

## Lesson 11: The Integumentary System

1. **(B) Keratin** This question is asking about the composition of hair and nails. Recall that hair and nails are produced by follicles in the dermis that contain high concentrations of keratin-producing cells. Therefore, predict that hair and nails are comprised mainly of keratin. This matches choice **(B)**. Collagen, (A), and elastin, (D), are proteins found in the skin that allow it to maintain its firmness and elasticity. Melanin, (C), is a pigment that gives skin and hair their color.

2. **(A) Sweating** This question is asking about the body's regulation of heat loss. Recall that the body increases heat loss by increasing blood flow to the skin and increasing evaporative cooling. Answer choice **(A)** matches the prediction that the correct answer will involve one of those processes. Sweating increases evaporative cooling as the water absorbs body heat.

Vasoconstriction, (B), reduces blood flow to the skin, and shivering, (C), generates heat; both would reduce heat loss. Panting, (D), is how animals that lack numerous sweat glands cool their bodies via evaporation.

3. **(D) Adipose tissue** This question is asking about the anatomic features present in the hypodermis. Recall that the hypodermis is the deepest layer of the skin and contains fat (adipose) tissue, blood vessels, and connective tissue. This matches choice **(D)**. Apocrine glands, (A), are a type of sebaceous gland, found in the dermis. Hair follicles, (B), are also located in the dermis. Pores, (D), are the openings in the epidermis through which glands release their secretions.

# Chapter 2: Biology and Chemistry

## Lesson 1: Macromolecules

1. **(D) Glycogen** This question is asking about the carbohydrate form of energy stored in the liver. Recall that the liver stores glycogen, which is a branched polysaccharide composed of glucose molecules. This matches choice **(D)**. Plants store energy in the form of amylose, (A). Cellulose, (B), is also found in plants and provides cell structure. Glycerol, (C), is a component of a triglyceride, which is a lipid used in long-term energy storage.

2. **(C) Uracil** This question is asking about the nitrogenous bases of RNA. Recall that there are four nitrogenous bases for DNA: guanine, adenine, cytosine, and thymine. Predict that the correct answer will not be one of those four. Answer choice **(C)** matches your prediction; uracil replaces thymine in RNA.

3. **(A) Enzymes are proteins that increase the rate of biological reactions.** This question is asking about enzymes. Recall that enzymes are proteins that decrease the amount of energy needed for a reaction to take place, thus increasing the rate of that reaction. This matches answer choice **(A)**. Choice (B) is incorrect because enzymes are formed by joining two amino acids, not nitrogenous bases, with a peptide bond. Choice (C) is incorrect because enzymes only bind to one specific molecule, called the enzyme's substrate. Choice (D) is incorrect because enzymes are globular proteins, not fibrous proteins. Fibrous proteins are not water soluble and include collagen and keratin.

## Lesson 2: Heredity

1. **(A) genotype: Dd; phenotype: dark hair** The question asks for the correct heterozygous genotype and phenotype of dark versus light hair. The term *heterozygous* indicates the alleles will be different, so look for Dd. Given the dominance of the dark hair trait, offspring will have dark hair if the D allele is present. Choice **(A)** meets both criteria.

2. **(B) The black male is heterozygous.** A rabbit with a dominant phenotype is crossed with a rabbit with a recessive phenotype for fur, and one offspring shows the recessive phenotype. The question asks what fact would account for this result. The answer choices all relate to genotypes. Recall that if even one dominant allele is present, the dominant trait will be expressed. Thus, the mother must be homozygous for

white fur—eliminate (A)—and the baby must be homozygous for white fur—eliminate (C). The offspring must have received a recessive allele from both parents, meaning that dad must be heterozygous and choice **(B)** is correct. The genotype of one offspring is independent of that of other offspring, so choice (D) is incorrect.

3. **(C) Four cells, each with 23 chromosomes** This question is testing your knowledge of meiosis. Recall that during meiosis, which creates gametes (sperm and ova), the original cell divides twice, creating four cells. Each of the four daughter cells contains half the original number of chromosomes. Humans have 46 chromosomes, so their gametes have 23 chromosomes each. Choice **(C)** is correct. Choice (B) is the result of mitosis.

## Lesson 3: Atoms and the Periodic Table

1. **(A) Eighty percent of boron isotopes have 6 neutrons.** The question provides the atomic number and mass for boron and asks which of the answer statements *could* be true. The information given means that boron has 5 protons and 5 electrons and an average of $(10.8 - 5) = 5.8$ neutrons. Examine answer choice (A). If 80% of the isotopes have 6 neutrons and 20% have 5 neutrons, the weighted average is $(6 \times 0.8 + 5 \times 0.2 = 4.8 + 1.0)$ 5.8 neutrons. This is not necessarily the only combination of neutrons that would result in an average of 5.8, but it *could* be. Choice (B) is incorrect because for boron to have an average of 5.8 neutrons, at least some isotopes would have more than 5. The periodic table contains many masses that are not whole numbers in order to account for isotopes, so choice (C) is wrong. There is no such thing as a "partial" neutron; eliminate (D). Even if you were not comfortable calculating the weighted average, you could have selected **(A)** by eliminating all the other choices.

2. **(C) its group in the periodic table.** The question asks which of the answer choices has the strongest influence on an element's chemical characteristics. Since the topic is *chemical* characteristics, you could predict that the correct answer will have something to do with the electrons in the element's outermost orbit. The amount of the element has nothing to do with its chemical characteristics; eliminate choice (A). Similarly, physical appearance is entirely different than chemical properties, so choice (B) is incorrect. Groups in the periodic table correspond to the number of electrons needed to fill the outermost orbit; this matches the prediction, so choice **(C)** is correct. The periods in the periodic table, choice (D), correlate with the number of energy levels, which is not as big a factor as the number of electrons in the outermost orbital.

## Lesson 4: Properties of Substances

1. **(A) mixture.** The question describes how sand behaves in water and asks for the proper categorization of that combination of materials. Recall that because the sand falls to the bottom, Ricardo has not created anything more than a mixture of sand and water, choice **(A)**. A substance, (B), is defined as being uniform. The sand does not dissolve in the water, so it cannot be a solution, (C), nor can it be a solute, so choice (D) is also incorrect.

2. **(C) 1.10 g/mL** This question provides volume and mass measurements of a liquid and asks for the density of that liquid. The volume of the liquid is 80% of a 50 ml container: $0.80 \times 50 = 40$ mL. The mass of the container plus the liquid is 74 g, but the container alone has a mass of 30 g. Therefore, the mass of the liquid is $74 \text{ g} - 30 \text{ g} = 44$ g. Density is $\dfrac{\text{mass}}{\text{volume}}$, so the density of this liquid is $\dfrac{44 \text{ g}}{40 \text{ mL}} = \dfrac{1.1 \text{ g}}{1 \text{ mL}}$.

3. **(B) Gasoline is made up primarily of nonpolar molecules.** The question asks why gasoline does not dissolve in water. Recall that water is a good solvent because its polar molecules attract ions or polar molecules of other substances. Predict that since gasoline does not dissolve in water, it is made up of substances with nonpolar molecules. This matches answer choice **(B)**. Choice (A) addresses boiling points. Since Lucretia's observations were based on liquids, this does not apply. Choice (C) is the opposite of the prediction. Choice (D) merely states that water is a good solvent but, since the gasoline did not dissolve in the water, this choice does not explain the phenomenon that was observed.

## Lesson 5: States of Matter

1. **(D) Low pressure and decreasing temperature** Deposition of water occurs when water vapor is cooled quickly in a low pressure environment and turns directly into solid ice. Choice **(D)** contains the two necessary conditions for this process: low pressure and decreasing temperature.

2. **(C) 1080 calories** Because the hydrogen is changing from liquid to gas, the heat energy will be increasing. You can eliminate choices (A) and (B) on that basis. No energy is necessary to bring the substance to the temperature where it begins phase change, because it is already at its boiling point. The answer can be calculated using the following formula: heat change = mass × latent heat of vaporization. Thus, $H = (10 \text{ g})(108 \text{ cal/g}) = 1080$ cal.

3. **(C) Triple point** The triple point, choice **(C)**, is a point of thermodynamic equilibrium at which temperature and pressure allow for all three states of a substance to coexist with one another.

## Lesson 6: Chemical Reactions

1. **(A) Zn + 2 HCl → ZnCl$_2$ + H2** The question asks which of the answer choices outlines a chemical reaction between a metal and an acid to produce a salt and a gas. Recall that an acid is a compound that will release H+ ions in solution and a salt is an ionic bond molecule that usually contains elements from opposite sides of the periodic table. In choice **(A)**, the reactants are a metal (Zn) and an acid (HCl), and the products are the salt ZnCl$_2$ and hydrogen gas, H$_2$. This matches the criteria given. Choice (B) is the reverse of (A) and is incorrect. Choice (C) is a double displacement reaction between the metals aluminum and magnesium. Choice (D) depicts a simple substitution reaction between metals. Even if you were not able to identify all the components in the answer choices, you could have eliminated choices (C) and (D) because neither has any hydrogen, a necessity to form an acid. You might also have observed that choice (B) has the hydrogen-containing acid as a product rather than a reactant.

2. **(D) Covalent** The question states that when MgCO$_3$ is dissolved in water it separates into Mg$^{2+}$ and CO$_3^{2-}$ ions and asks what type of bond exists between C and O. Notice that these particular ions carry charges of +2 and −2 rather than the single charges in previous examples. Recall that atoms that are ionically bonded will separate into ions in water. Since the carbon and oxygen bonds remain in place, producing the polyatomic CO$_3^{2-}$ rather than individual C or O ions, it can be reasonably assumed that the bonds between C and O are covalent, making choice **(D)** correct. Note that choices (A) and (C) are parts of atoms and not types of bonds.

3. **(B) MgSO$_4$** The question asks which of the answer choices is *not* an organic substance. Recall that organic substances contain both carbon and hydrogen and are related to living things. Predict that the correct answer will be a substance that does not contain both carbon and hydrogen. Choice (A), glucose, contains both carbon and hydrogen and is an organic molecule. Choice **(B)**, magnesium sulfate, which features in Epsom salts, does not have any carbon atoms and is therefore correct. Choices (C), the formula for ethanol, and (D), the formula for sucrose, are organic substances.

# Chapter 3: Scientific Procedures and Reasoning

## Lesson 1: Scientific Measurements and Relationships

1. **(C) 3 grams** The abbreviation *cg* means centigrams, so the cube weighs 300 centigrams. A centigram is 1/100th of a gram, so 100 centigrams = 1 gram, Thus, the 300 centigram cube weighs 3 grams, **(C)**. (A), 3 milligrams, is equivalent to 0.3 centigrams, while (D), 3 decagrams, is 30 grams or 3000 centigrams. (B), 3 centimeters, is a unit of distance and not applicable.

2. **(B) She will have some difficulty seeing or hearing, even though she might be in a good mood.** Since .08 falls between .07 and .09, look at the row in the table for those values. According to the table, a BAC of .08 results in impaired motor coordination, hearing, and vision, as well as feelings of elation or depression. These changes are correctly described in choice **(B)**.

3. **(A) Measuring tape** The volume of solid forms is calculated by multiplying length, width, and height, which can be determined with a measuring tape, **(A)**. Both an electronic balance and a triple-beam balance measure mass, so (B) and (C) can be rejected. (D) can also be rejected: a volumetric pipette is used to measure small volumes of liquids.

4. **(A) Beaker** Don't be misled by the different shapes of the vessels. If you look closely at the measuring lines, the beaker, **(A)**, contains about 2500 mL of liquid; that is more than the test tube, (B), with 1000 mL; the graduated cylinder, (C), 2000 mL; or the globe, (D), almost 2000 mL.

## Lesson 2: Designing and Evaluating an Experiment

1. **(C) Recruit more men for the experiment.** This question describes an experimental design and asks how it can be improved. Recall that all experiments should include a control group and that study participants should be evenly divided between the control and experimental group. Because equal numbers of individuals receive the placebo and vitamin drink, it is not necessary to redistribute the participants, so choices (A) and (B) can be eliminated. However, in the experiment, there is a disproportionately large number of females, making the sample unrepresentative. To improve the design of the experiment, more men should be enrolled, as in choice

**(C)**. Enrolling more women would further skew the sample, so choice (D) can be eliminated.

2. **(D) Measure the resistance of the new and old conductors 50 times each under the same conditions and compare the two results.** This question is asking for the best experimental design to compare a new resistor to one that is commonly used. A quick glance at the answers shows that there are two things to consider: the number of trials and whether to include the commonly used resistor in the experiment. Recall that strong experiments have a large sample size and use a control group. To have the best design, the commonly used resistor should be directly compared to the new one using the largest possible number of trials, as described in choice **(D)**.

3. **(B) Heart rate** This question describes an experimental design and asks for the dependent variable. Recall that the dependent variable is the parameter that is measured. In this experiment, the researcher is measuring heart rate, so choice **(B)** is correct. Caffeine, (A), is the independent variable, whereas sugar, (C), and age, (D), are control variables since they are held constant between the control and experimental groups.

4. **(A) Erythromycin can shrink a population of *Staphylococcus aureus*.** This question provides a graph of growth rate of *Staphylococcus aureus* over varying concentrations of erythromycin and asks what conclusion is best supported. Recall that strong conclusions are directly supported by experimental evidence and do not go beyond the scope of the experiment. Based on the data, you can conclude that treatment of *Staphylococcus aureus* with erythromycin decreases the population of the bacteria, **(A)**, since the growth rate becomes negative above a certain concentration. However, since this experiment did not test other antibiotics, you cannot conclude that any antibiotic will decrease the population of *Staphylococcus aureus*; eliminate choices (C) and (D). Furthermore, this experiment did not test erythromycin efficacy on other bacterial strains, so you cannot conclude that it will decrease the population of any bacteria, (B).

# English and Language Usage: Answers and Explanations

## Chapter 1: Spelling, Punctuation, and Sentence Structure

### Lesson 1: Spelling

1. **(C) Wierd** "Weird" is an exception to the "*i* before *e*" rule.

2. **(D) injurious** The root word, "injury," ends in a *y* that is preceded by a consonant, so the REBS rule to follow is "Change the *y* to *i* and add the suffix."

3. **(A) frolicked** The root word, "frolic," ends in a *c*, so the REBS rule to follow is "Add a *k* when adding a suffix beginning with *e, i,* or *y.*"

4. **(B) principal/principles** "Principal," used here as an adjective modifying "reason," means "primary," and "principle" is a noun that means "guiding rule." Note that when *principal* is used as a noun, it refers either to the leader of a school or to an amount of money that is invested to earn interest.

### Lesson 2: Punctuation

1. **(C) Although I am an experienced hiker, I was not prepared for the rocky terrain.** Choice (A) is a simple sentence, and a comma is missing after the introductory prepositional phrase. Choice (B) is an incorrectly punctuated compound sentence—a semicolon is missing before "however." Because it is both the wrong sentence structure and incorrectly punctuated, eliminate. Choice (D) is a complex sentence, but it incorrectly offsets the subordinate clause with a comma. In this choice, the comma is incorrect since the subordinate clause appears after the independent clause. Choice **(C)** is a correctly punctuated complex sentence.

2. **(B) "We must all do our part," she said, "even when doing so is difficult."** When a direct quote is interrupted by a reference to the speaker, the first half of the quote should end in a comma, and the second half should be introduced with a comma.

3. **(D) Because the weather forecast predicted storms, we decided to postpone our vacation until next month.** "Because the weather forecast predicted storms" is a subordinate clause and must be followed by a comma.

4. **(B) ;** The sentence is made up of two independent clauses. When two independent clauses need to be connected in a sentence and no conjunction is present, a semicolon should be placed between the two clauses.

### Lesson 3: Sentence Structure

1. **(A) Working** The independent clause is "Working hard is important," because this could stand alone as a complete sentence. "Working" is the subject—the thing that "is important." This is an example of a verb form having -*ing* added and being used as a noun (it's called a *gerund*). "Important" is a complement. The other words are in the dependent clause. Note that in a complex sentence like this one, the subject of the independent clause is also the subject of the sentence.

2. **(C) his** A pronoun is a word that is used instead of a noun. "His" is the pronoun that refers back to the noun "Bob."

3. **(A) Because the book was confusing, Sarah stopped reading it, so now she needs something new to read.** This is the only sentence to incorporate two independent clauses and one or more dependent clauses. The independent clauses are "Sarah stopped reading the book" and "so now she needs something new to read."

4. **(D) story** The direct object is a person or thing that receives the action of the verb. The story (the direct object) is being told to me (the indirect object).

# Chapter 2: Grammar, Style, and the Writing Process

## Lesson 1: Grammar

1. **(A) Run-on sentence; Before 1906, postcards had space for a message on one side and the recipient's address on the other. It was illegal to write a message on the address side.** The sentence contains two independent clauses and should be split into separate sentences. Choice **(A)** breaks the original sentence into two shorter, and correct, sentences.

2. **(C) Inappropriate transition word choice** This sentence contains two related independent clauses. The second clause provides a reason for the first, so "despite" is not appropriate. An appropriate transition would be *due to*.

3. **(A) The client will be late to her appointment.** "Client" is a singular noun and requires a singular verb and a singular pronoun; "will be late" and "her" are both singular. In choice (B), "people" is plural, but "has asked" is singular. The error in choice (C) is that the pronoun "she" has no antecedent; "she" likely refers to Dana, but "Dana's" is possessive and functions as an adjective. The noun preceding "she" is "insurance," which isn't what the pronoun represents. In choice (D), the noun "physician" is singular but is represented by the plural pronoun "they."

4. **(D) Some detergents have prevented colors from bleeding in the wash if you forget to sort by colors.** The verbs in this sentence are not in the same tense, which results in the sentence not making sense. "[H]ave prevented" is past perfect tense, and "forget" is present tense. Both verbs should be in present tense to convey a general truth: *Some detergents prevent colors from bleeding in the wash if you forget to sort by colors.* All other answer choices contain grammatically correct sentences.

## Lesson 2: Formal and Informal Style

1. **(B) Giving your young children access to books encourages them to read early and often and prepares them for a lifetime of learning.** A message from a principal to parents with young children would be formal but not overly academic. Choices (A) and (C) are too technical and impersonal, while (D) is too casual and colloquial. Choice **(B)** strikes a professional tone but also speaks directly to the parents in a warm and engaging manner.

2. **(D) A physician's note on a medical chart** The sentence in the stimulus outlines the specific condition of one client, a description that would likely appear on a medical chart. It does not include the technical language that one would expect in a medical journal, and the content focuses on a client rather

on than a medication or procedure. Choice **(D)** is the most likely medium in which the sentence would appear.

3. **(C) Anna knew that the long winter days would soon be upon them, so each day she helped her father and mother gather firewood, salt meat, and stow away the few vegetables they were able to grow that first year.** Each answer choice offers context clues that indicate the time period and location in which it is set. Choice (A) references a train, but trains had not yet been invented in colonial America. Similarly, the radio mentioned in (B) did not exist during colonial times. Choice (D) is set near an ancient city, none of which existed near colonial American settlements. Only the context clues in choice **(C)** point to life in the early American colonies, where families had few resources and had to make many preparations to survive the elements. The reference to "first year" also indicates that Anna's family was new to the property, as colonists might be.

## Lesson 3: The Writing Process

1. **(A) The word *nightmare* is derived from an Old English word for a mythological creature that torments people with scary dreams.** This is information taken directly from a research source—perhaps a dictionary that includes etymological information, a book on the influence of Old English on contemporary English, or an encyclopedia entry on mythological monsters. Therefore, the source must be cited. Choice (B) draws entirely on personal knowledge. (C) draws on personal observation and/or commonsense knowledge. Choice (D) is an idea that cannot be attributed to a specific person or group, so it does not need a citation.

2. **(C) I, IV, III, II** A logical paragraph begins with a topic sentence that states the main idea and is followed by sentences with supporting details. Only answer choice **(C)** logically orders the sentences, beginning with a topic sentence that is followed by additional details. Choices (A), (B), and (D) are all incorrect, as they suggest beginning the paragraph with a supporting detail rather than a topic sentence.

3. **(B) Rereading the first draft to find errors and make improvements** This is part of proofreading, not planning. Choices (A), brainstorming; (C), researching; and (D), establishing writing habits are all parts of the planning stage.

4. **(C) One way to gain more experience in the field is to volunteer.** Because this sentence refers to one specific way to achieve an objective, this is an example of a supporting detail, not a topic sentence. The topic sentence of this paragraph might address the need to gain experience to advance in one's career. Choices (A), (B), and (D) are all examples of topic sentences that introduce the main idea of a paragraph that could be further developed by supporting details.

# Chapter 3: Vocabulary

## Lesson 1: Using the Correct Word

1. **(D) The new budget will help to check government spending in the coming year.** The word *check* has several meanings as both a noun and a verb. The question stem indicates that the correct answer choice uses *check* as a verb meaning "to restrain or slow down." In choice (A), "check" means to select a particular item on a list by adding a check mark. "Check" in choice (B) means to evaluate something against a standard. In (C), "check" means to turn one's baggage over to someone else's care during a journey. Only choice **(D)** has the definition of *check* required in the question stem. To "check government spending" means to restrain or slow down the rate at which money is being spent, and a budget would logically help achieve this goal.

2. **(A) Antepartum** In choices (A) and (C), the root word *partum* comes from the Latin word for "giving birth," just as the root word *natal* in choices (B) and (D) comes from the Latin term for "being born." Since all four choices have root words that have to do with birth, examine each word's prefix to locate the correct answer. The prefix *peri-* in (B) means "around or about," so "perinatal" indicates the time before, during, and after birth. In (C), the prefix *post-* means "after," which is opposite of the correct answer's meaning. The prefix *neo-* in (D) comes from the Greek word for "new," so *neonatal* means "having to do with a newborn." The prefix *ante-* in choice **(A)** means "before," and "antepartum" is therefore the correct answer.

3. **(C) Patch** The context clues in this sentence indicate that "plot" means a small portion, or patch, of land. Choice **(C)** is correct.

4. **(B) Abnormality** To determine the meaning of "aberration" in the sentence, use the context clues. The contrast word "otherwise" indicates that the student's failing grade on the test was the only failing grade he has received. In other words, receiving a failing grade was an unusual occurrence. "Abnormality" in choice **(B)** is the correct match for this meaning.

5. **(A) Auxocardia** If the terms in the answer choices are unfamiliar, use the word parts to determine the general meaning of each. The question is asking for a term that means "an enlarged heart," so look for a choice or choices that have a heart-related root word. Choices (A) and (D) both include the root *cardia*, which means "heart" or "having to do with the heart." When comparing these two choices, evaluate their prefixes. In correct choice **(A)**, *auxo-* means "to become greater," while *tachy-* in (D) means "rapid."

6. **(B) To participate in something** To "engage in . . . activities" is to join in or to participate in the activities, which matches choice **(B)**. *Engage* can also mean to give one's attention to an activity, so choice (A) might have been tempting. In this case, use the remaining context clues for help. Merely giving one's attention to an activity would not likely put further strain on an injured hand, while participating in an activity would.

# Appendix—Glossaries

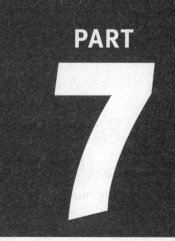

Here in the appendix you will find four glossaries of key terms and their definitions, one for each content area of the TEAS:

- *Reading*
- *Mathematics*
- *Science*
- *English and language usage*

Reviewing these terms—whether in these pages, by making flashcards, or by having a friend quiz you—can be an excellent way to make sure you know the concepts that you will see on Test Day.

# Reading Glossary

| Term | Definition |
| --- | --- |
| **argument** | A statement of an author's claim (conclusion) and evidence used to support it |
| **assumption** | Implicit (unstated) evidence that connects the author's evidence to the conclusion based on that evidence |
| **bold print** | A print feature intended to emphasize certain words in a text. In this book, terms included in the glossary are set in bold print. |
| **conclusion** | An opinion that the author holds and supports with evidence, or an opinion that someone else holds with which the author may or may not agree. Another word for conclusion is *claim*. |
| **connotative** | Referring to a secondary or associative meaning of a word, invoking an idea or a feeling, related to the way the word is customarily used |
| **context** | Words that are used with a certain phrase or word that help the reader determine its meaning |
| **denotative** | Referring to the direct or explicit meaning of a word, such as that found in a dictionary |
| **dictionary** | A book or website that contains a selection of words with their meanings and often other information such as pronunciations, origins, and forms |
| **evidence** | Explicit support the author provides for a claim (conclusion) that does not have to be inferred or assumed |
| **expository** | A mode of writing in which the author intends to explain or inform |
| **figurative** | Involving a figure of speech (e.g., *a loud shirt* is brightly and perhaps unfashionably colorful, not literally loud) |
| **figure of speech** | An expressive use of language in which words are used in other than their literal sense to suggest an image or picture |
| **flowchart** | A diagram that, with shapes and lines, shows the steps in a procedure |
| **footnote** | An explanatory note or comment at the bottom of a page, referring to a specific part of text on that page. May include a reference to another source and/or further detail that would interrupt the flow of the main text if placed there. |
| **graph** | A diagram that visually represents the values of two or more variables |
| **heading** | A title or caption at the beginning of a chapter, page, or other section of text that typically summarizes what follows |
| **illustration caption** | Title or brief explanation of a picture or illustration |
| **index** | In a book, a detailed alphabetical listing of names, places, events, and other important topics in the text along with the number(s) of the page(s) on which they are mentioned. Located near the end of the book. |
| **inference** | An unstated fact or conclusion that follows logically from an explicit statement or statements in a stimulus |
| **inform** | A purpose for writing that involves communicating facts about the topic |

| Term | Definition |
|---|---|
| italics | A print feature used to set off specific words in a text. May be done for emphasis or because the words are the title of a book, film, newspaper, or magazine; are in a foreign language; or are being used as a word (e.g., the words *and* and *but* are three letters long). |
| key word or phrase | A word or phrase the author uses to signal an idea of particular importance, the author's opinion about an idea, or the relationship of one idea to another in a piece of writing |
| map | Short notes about the topic, scope, and purpose of a stimulus (or the author's conclusion, evidence, and assumptions if the stimulus is an argument) and the key ideas of each paragraph or graphic |
| map legend | A small box or table on a map that explains what the symbols found on the map mean |
| metaphor | A figure of speech in which a word or phrase is applied to an object or action to which it is not literally applicable in order to suggest a resemblance |
| mode | The type of text (e.g., narrative, descriptive, argumentative, or expository) |
| narrative | A mode of writing in which the author intends to tell a story |
| personification | A figure of speech in which human characteristics are attributed to animals, inanimate objects, or abstract concepts |
| persuade | A purpose for writing that involves arguing for a particular point of view |
| persuasive | A mode of writing in which the author intends to convince or compel |
| point of view | The author's perspective or opinion on a topic |
| prediction | A reader's statement or an expectation about will happen, based on information given in the stimulus |
| primary source | A work produced by the person who actually experienced or witnessed an event |
| purpose | The author's reason for writing a text or presenting a graphic (e.g., to inform, to persuade, to narrate, to entertain) |
| quotation | Text that is copied word for word (not paraphrased) from work by another author, such as a speech, book, or article |
| scope | The specific aspect of the topic on which the author focuses |
| secondary source | A work produced by a person at least one step removed from the actual experience or event that is the topic |
| sidebar | A distinct section of a page that comments on or supplements the main text |
| simile | A figure of speech in which two dissimilar things are explicitly compared, frequently using *like* or *as* |
| strategic | With a plan of action. When you read strategically, you plan to note the author's topic, scope, and purpose as well as key ideas. |
| synonym | A word having the same or nearly the same meaning as another; opposite of *antonym* |
| table | Values arranged into rows and columns |

| Term | Definition |
|---|---|
| **table of contents** | In a book, the list of divisions (e.g., chapters or articles) and the pages on which they start. Located near the beginning of the book. |
| **theme** | The subject or central idea of a piece of work. Different text or graphic works may share the same theme. |
| **thesaurus** | A dictionary of synonyms and antonyms |
| **title** | Distinguishing name of a book, story, piece of music, work of art, etc. |
| **tone** | The emotional content of a stimulus. May be neutral, as when the author is relating facts to inform the reader; or it may be happy or sad, as when the author is telling a story; or it may be urgent or angry, as when the author is seeking to persuade the reader. |
| **topic** | The author's overall subject matter |

# Mathematics Glossary

| Term | Definition |
|------|------------|
| acute angle | An angle less than 90 degrees |
| area | A measure of the surface space taken up by a two-dimensional shape |
| arithmetic average | *See* mean. |
| bar graph | A graph that displays values of different categories in columns and can accommodate multiple variables |
| bimodal | Data whose distribution is characterized by two peaks |
| bivariate | Consisting of two variable values, such as a point on a Cartesian coordinate graph |
| Cartesian coordinates | A system of graphing paired values using an $x$-axis and $y$-axis |
| causality | When changes to one variable or factor (the independent variable) cause changes to another (the dependent variable) |
| chart | A table or graph |
| circle | A curved shape with all points equally distant from the center |
| circle graph (pie chart) | A graph that displays parts of a whole as sectors of a circle |
| circumference | The perimeter of a circle, or the distance once around the circle |
| common denominator | A denominator shared by two or more fractions (e.g., $\frac{3}{10}$ and $\frac{5}{10}$ have the common denominator of 10 and can be added or subtracted) |
| constant | A value that doesn't change, typically a number |
| constant of proportionality | The fixed ratio between two quantities, often represented by $k$ (e.g., if the cost for a gallon of gasoline is \$2, $k = 2$) |
| constant term | A term containing only a number |
| conversion ratio | The ratio of one unit of measure to another (e.g., to convert seconds to minutes, multiply the number of seconds by a conversion ratio of 1 minute to 60 seconds) |
| coordinate grid | A way of displaying quantities in two dimensions with perpendicular axes representing the $x$ and $y$ values |
| covariation | The change in the values of two related variables; also called *covariance* |
| cross multiply | A method of solving proportions by multiplying each numerator by the denominator of the other ratio |
| decimal | A number that uses place value to show amounts less than 1 (e.g., 0.3 or 2.4) |
| denominator | The bottom number of a fraction |
| dependent variable | The variable that is caused to change by another variable (e.g., if clients report less pain when they take more of a certain medication, pain is the dependent variable). This is the value that is observed in a scientific experiment. |
| dimensional analysis | A series of steps used to convert a measurement in one unit to an equivalent measurement in another unit (e.g., from ounces to pounds) |

| Term | Definition |
|------|------------|
| **estimating** | Calculating an approximate value for a numeric expression |
| **expected value** | The most likely value or range of values of one variable given the value of the other variable |
| **fraction** | Two numbers used to represent a part and a whole, respectively, or one number divided by the other (e.g., $\frac{2}{3}$ is two parts out of three or 2 divided by 3) |
| **gram** | The standard unit of weight or mass in the metric system |
| **graph** | A diagram that visually represents the values of two or more variables |
| **histogram** | A bar graph with one variable in which the bars of different heights display the frequency of occurrence of each value or range of values |
| **hypotenuse** | The longest side of a right triangle, opposite the right angle |
| **improper fraction** | A fraction representing a value greater than 1 so that the numerator is greater than the denominator |
| **independent variable** | The variable that causes change in another variable (e.g., if gum disease increases as people floss less often, frequency of flossing is the independent variable). This is the value that is manipulated in a scientific experiment. |
| **inverse operations** | Arithmetic operations that are used to cancel or "undo" each other (e.g., subtraction is the inverse operation of addition) |
| **least common multiple (LCM)** | The smallest number that is a multiple of two given numbers (e.g., the LCM of 3 and 5 is 15) |
| **legend (key)** | A reference section of a chart that explains conventions and symbols used |
| **like terms** | Terms that have the same form and can be combined (e.g., $3x$ and $2x$ are like terms) |
| **line graph** | A graph that connects the data points with lines, often used to show trends |
| **liter** | A measurement unit of volume equal to 1000 cubic centimeters |
| **mean (arithmetic average)** | The midpoint of a set of values that equals the sum of the values divided by the number of values in the group |
| **measures of central tendency** | Measures such as mean, median, and mode that quantify the middle values in a data set |
| **median** | The middle value of a data set when the numbers are arranged in order. In an even number of values, the median is the average of the middle two values. |
| **meter** | The standard unit of length in the metric system, a little longer than a yard |
| **mixed number** | A fraction greater than 1 that is written as a whole number and a proper fraction |
| **mode** | The value in a group of numbers that appears the most times (e.g., in the data set {1, 2, 2, 3, 3}, there are two modes, 2 and 3) |
| **negative covariance** | When two variables move in opposite directions in relation to each other (e.g., as the price of apples rises, people buy fewer apples; as the price of apples falls, people buy more apples) |

| Term | Definition |
|------|-----------|
| **number line** | A line representing all real numbers. Numbers to the left of zero are negative, and those to the right of zero are positive. |
| **numerator** | The upper part of a fraction |
| **obtuse angle** | An angle greater than 90 degrees |
| **operation** | Any calculation used to combine two numbers (e.g., addition, subtraction, multiplication, division) |
| **order of operations** | The rule governing the order in which to apply operations while evaluating any expression: parentheses, exponents, multiplication and division, addition and subtraction |
| **ordered pair** | The $x$ and $y$ values of a point on a graph, usually written in parentheses separated by a comma (e.g., if $x$ is 3 and $y$ is 2, the ordered pair is (3, 2)) |
| **origin** | The point where the axes of a graph cross. On a Cartesian coordinate graph, this is (0, 0). |
| **outlier** | A data point that is distinctly different from others, or an unexpected value |
| **parallel lines** | Lines that never touch or intersect. When graphed on the coordinate plane, parallel lines have the same slope. |
| **part-to-part ratio** | The numerical relationship of two parts of a whole to one another |
| **part-to-whole ratio** | The numerical relationship of one part of a whole to the entire whole |
| **percent, percentage** | "Per hundred" or "out of one hundred." This is a ratio expressed in parts per 100, represented with the % symbol (e.g., 32% equals 32 out of 100). |
| **perimeter** | The length around the outside of a two-dimensional shape |
| **perpendicular lines** | Lines that intersect to form a 90-degree angle |
| **place value** | The values expressed by a given decimal place (e.g., tenths, ones, and tens) |
| **positive covariance** | When two variables rise or fall together (e.g., as the price of corn rises, farmers plant more corn; as the price of corn falls, farmers plant less corn) |
| **proper fraction** | A fraction representing a value less than 1 so that the numerator is less than the denominator |
| **proportion** | An equation that sets two ratios equal to each other |
| **range** | The absolute difference between the highest and lowest values in a group of numbers |
| **rate** | A ratio with units in the numerator and denominator that have a fixed relationship to each other |
| **ratio** | A representation of the numerical relationship of one quantity to another |
| **reciprocal** | The fraction that results from switching the numerator and denominator of a given fraction (e.g., the reciprocal of $\frac{3}{5}$ is $\frac{5}{3}$) |
| **rectangle** | A four-sided shape that is made up of two pairs of parallel lines and that has four right angles |
| **right angle** | An angle equal to 90 degrees |
| **right triangle** | A triangle that contains a right angle |

| Term | Definition |
|------|------------|
| rounding | Approximating the value of a number in order to simplify calculations |
| scale | The ratio of values in a graphic representation to actual values (e.g., a floorplan might be drawn to a scale such that 1 inch represents 1 meter in the actual building) |
| scatterplot | A graph with all individual data points plotted |
| shape | The visually observable characteristics of graphs, including symmetry, number of modes, and skewness |
| signed number | A number with a positive (+) or negative (−) sign |
| skewness | A directional (left or right) characteristic of graphed data that describes which side has more data points |
| slope (of a line) | The change in the value of $y$ per unit change in $x$ |
| spread | A characteristic that describes how centralized or dispersed certain data are |
| square | A type of rectangle with four sides of equal length |
| square units | A measurement of area, such as square inches ($in^2$), square feet ($ft^2$), or square centimeters ($cm^2$) |
| standard (customary) system | System of everyday measurements in the United States (e.g., inches, miles, cups, gallons, pounds, and tons) |
| standard deviation | A statistical calculation of the amount of dispersion in data |
| symmetry | Balance between the right and left sides of a graph |
| table | Values arranged into rows and columns |
| term | A variable, constant, or product of a constant and a variable |
| transversal | A line that crosses two or more other distinct lines in a plane. When a transversal crosses two or more parallel lines, all obtuse angles created are equal, and all acute angles created are equal. |
| trend | The general relationship of data points (e.g., there could be a trend for prices to rise over time); also called *data trend* |
| trendline | A plotted or calculated line on a graph that shows the relationship between the two variables, often described by referring to the slope of the line |
| triangle | A three-sided shape that is made up of three straight lines |
| unimodal | Data whose distribution is characterized by a single peak |
| unit rate | The ratio between two related quantities with the denominator equal to 1 |
| variable | A letter used to represent a numerical value that is unknown |
| vertical angles | Angles that are directly across from each other when two or more lines intersect. They are always equal to each other. |
| $x$-axis | The horizontal axis of a graph |
| $y$-axis | The vertical axis of a graph |

# Science Glossary

| Term | Definition |
| --- | --- |
| absorption | Movement of a substance such as nutrients from the intestine into the bloodstream |
| acetylcholine (ACh) | A neurotransmitter that triggers the contraction of skeletal muscle |
| acidity | The property of having excess $H^+$ ions |
| acidosis | A decrease in blood pH |
| acquired immunodeficiency syndrome (AIDS) | A disease caused by human immunodeficiency virus (HIV) in which the body's immune system is compromised, leading to infections and tumors |
| actin | The thin filament protein of muscle tissue |
| action potentials | A rapid polarization of a nerve cell that generates a nerve impulse |
| activation energy | The energy required for a chemical reaction to take place |
| active immunity | The production of antibodies by plasma cells |
| active site | The part of an enzyme that is especially suited to bond with a substrate |
| adaptive arm | The part of the immune system that is slower to activate in response to pathogens but specifically targets a pathogen and forms memory cells |
| adenosine triphosphate (ATP) | The form in which nucleotides function as a source of energy |
| adhesion | The property of polar molecules to attract other substances |
| adipose | Fat tissues |
| adrenal glands | Endocrine glands located above the kidneys that secrete hormones, including several that regulate blood pressure and fluid balance |
| adrenocorticotropic hormone (ACTH) | Hormone released by the anterior pituitary that acts on the adrenal glands to stimulate hormone release |
| afferent arteriole | The blood vessel that enters the glomerulus |
| afferent (sensory) neurons | The neurons that carry sensory information from the body toward the central nervous system |
| aldosterone | A hormone released by the adrenal cortex that induces sodium reabsorption at the distal convoluted tubule of the nephron |
| alimentary canal | The pathway in the body through which food travels while being digested and absorbed |
| alkalinity (basicity) | The property of having excess $OH^-$ ions |
| alkalosis | Increased blood pH |
| allele | One of two or more variations of a single gene |
| alveoli | Small sacs in the lungs that are the site of gas exchange, facilitated by walls only one cell layer thick |
| amino acid | A protein monomer consisting of an amino group ($NH_3^+$), a carboxyl group ($COO^-$), hydrogen (H), and a side chain (R group) |

| Term | Definition |
|------|-----------|
| amylopectin | A glucose polymer that is part of starch |
| amylose | A glucose polymer that is part of starch |
| anal sphincter | A ring-shaped muscle that tightens to control the excretion of solid waste from the digestive tract |
| anatomical planes | Divisions of the body into distinct halves. The three main planes are the coronal, sagittal, and transverse. |
| anemia | A condition characterized by low levels of hemoglobin in the blood |
| anion | A negatively charged ion |
| anterior pituitary | The endocrine gland that releases hormones that control other glands or act directly on a target |
| antibody | A protein that specifically binds to a viral antigen |
| antidiuretic hormone (ADH) | *See* vasopressin. |
| antigen | A microbial protein |
| antimicrobial peptides | Broad-spectrum antimicrobials secreted by cells that target and kill many bacterial, viral, and fungal pathogens to prevent infection |
| anus | The terminal end of the alimentary canal and the site of solid waste excretion |
| aorta | The artery that carries blood pumped from the left ventricle of the heart into systemic circulation. This is the largest blood vessel in the body. |
| apocrine glands | Sweat glands that are not active until puberty and are found in the armpits, nipples, and groin |
| appendicular skeleton | Movable parts of the skeleton (e.g., limb bones) |
| aqueous solution | A substance dissolved in water |
| arteries | Vessels that carry blood under relatively high pressure from the heart |
| arterioles | Branches of the arteries |
| arthritis | A disease of the joints caused by the breakdown of cartilage |
| asthma | A disease caused by inflammation and narrowing of the airway |
| atherosclerosis | A narrowing of the arteries due to plaque buildup |
| atom | The smallest component of an element that retains the properties of that element |
| atomic mass unit | A unit used to delineate the mass of an atom |
| atomic number | The number of protons in the nucleus of an element |
| atria | The chambers of the heart that receive blood returning to the heart |
| atrioventricular valves | Valves that separate the atria and ventricles in the heart |
| atrophy | The shrinkage of myofibrils resulting from disuse of a muscle |
| autoimmune disease | A disease (e.g., type 1 diabetes and lupus) in which the adaptive immune system targets healthy body cells |

| Term | Definition |
|------|------------|
| autonomic nervous system | The part of the nervous system that sends and receives signals from smooth and cardiac muscle |
| axial skeleton | The part of the skeletal system that provides the general framework of the body (e.g., the skull, vertebrae, and rib cage) |
| axon | The part of the nerve cell that carries messages away from the cell body |
| B cell | An adaptive immune system cell that develops into a plasma cell and secretes one specific type of antibody |
| basophils | Granulocytes responsible for releasing histamine and mediating allergic reactions |
| bias | Intentional or unintentional skewing of experimental results to favor a particular outcome |
| bicuspid | *See* mitral valve. |
| bile | Product of the liver that emulsifies fats |
| blood pressure | Pressure of blood in the circulatory system consisting of two measurements, one at systole and one at diastole |
| boiling point | The temperature at which a liquid boils, or bubbles up and turns into a vapor |
| bolus | Chewed food |
| bone marrow | The site of red blood cell (i.e., erythrocyte) and lymphocyte production |
| Bowman's capsule | The part of the nephron that surrounds the glomerulus |
| brain | The organ that coordinates the nervous system |
| brain stem | The part of the nervous system that connects the cerebrum to the spinal cord and controls critical involuntary body functions |
| bronchi | Originating where the trachea splits, passages that carry air to the left and right lungs (singular: *bronchus*) |
| bronchioles | The smaller passages formed from branching of the bronchi that carry air to the alveoli |
| bulbourethral glands | Glands that secrete a viscous fluid that lubricates the male reproductive tract |
| calcitonin | The hormone released by the thyroid gland that decreases blood calcium |
| calories | The energy needed to increase the temperature of 1 gram of water by 1 degree Celsius |
| canaliculi | Microscopic channels connecting the lacunae |
| capillaries | Blood vessels, the smallest in the body, that receive blood from the arterioles and return it to the venules |
| carbohydrate | A macromolecule that is a sugar or starch containing carbon, oxygen, and hydrogen |
| cardiac cycle | The period between the start of one heartbeat and the beginning of the next |
| cardiac muscle | Muscle tissue located in the heart and under involuntary contraction |

| Term | Definition |
|---|---|
| cartilaginous joints | The meeting of bones at a connection made of cartilage that is partly movable |
| catalyst | A substance that enhances a chemical reaction but remains unchanged upon completion of the reaction |
| cation | A positively charged ion |
| causality | The relationship between two events or states such that one brings about the other, with the independent variable being the cause and the dependent variable being the effect |
| cecum | A pouch at the junction of the small and large intestines |
| cellulose | A polysaccharide composed of glucose polymers and found in the structural material of plants |
| central nervous system (CNS) | The part of the nervous system consisting of the brain and spinal cord |
| centrosome | The organelle that organizes all of the microtubules in a cell |
| cerebellum | The part of the brain that coordinates movement and balance |
| cerebrum | The part of the brain that coordinates voluntary movement |
| cervix | The opening that connects the vagina and uterus |
| chemical digestion | The breaking down of food at the molecular level by means of enzymes or acid |
| chemical equation | A symbolic representation of the reactants and products in a chemical reaction |
| chemical properties | The characteristics of substances that affect how a substance interacts with other matter |
| chitin | A polysaccharide containing glucose and amino acids that forms the exoskeleton of arthropods |
| chromosomes | Large strands of DNA in the nucleus that each contain several genes |
| chyme | The contents of the stomach as they exit that organ |
| cilia (of a cell) | Membranous protrusions used for cellular movement or to increase surface area |
| cilia (respiratory tract) | Hair-like structures found on the cells of the respiratory tract that beat to move mucus and other particles up and out of the lungs |
| circulatory system | The system of organs responsible for moving blood throughout the body to enable nutrient delivery and waste removal |
| closed circulatory system | The double-loop path of the blood throughout the human body |
| codominance | A form of inheritance in which both alleles are independently expressed |
| codon | A sequence of three nucleotides that together form a unit of genetic code in a DNA molecule |
| cohesion | The property of polar molecules to attract other molecules of the same substance |

| Term | Definition |
|---|---|
| colon | The large intestine |
| combustion | A type of oxidation reaction |
| common bile duct | A tube that conveys bile from the gallbladder to the duodenum |
| compact bone | Denser tissue that comprises the shaft of long bones, supporting the body and storing calcium |
| complement system | A system composed of multiple proteins in the blood that can be recruited by antibodies to cause cell lysis |
| compound | A substance composed of molecules containing atoms of different elements |
| condensation | The process of vapor or gas converting into a liquid |
| congestive heart failure | The condition in which the heart can no longer pump blood effectively |
| connective tissue | The tissue that connects and supports different structures of the body |
| control | Changing only one variable in an experiment at a time so differences between groups can be conclusively linked to that variable. Including a control group in an experiment helps with this. |
| control group | A group that is identical to the experimental group in all respects except that the independent variable is not changed (e.g., group of study participants who receive a placebo instead of the medication being tested) |
| controlled variables | Parameters that are held constant in an experiment so that the effect of the independent variable can be clearly observed |
| corpus callosum | The band of nerve fibers that connects the right and left hemispheres of the cerebrum |
| corpus luteum | A structure that develops from the ruptured follicle and secretes progesterone |
| covalent bond | A bond created by the sharing of electrons |
| cranial nerves | Nerves that reach the interior of the brain, with each set of cranial nerves having a specific function |
| cranium | The part of the skull that houses the brain |
| critical point | The point on a phase diagram at which the gas and liquid phases of a substance have the same density due to the effects of temperature and pressure and are therefore indistinguishable |
| crystal | A solid with a high degree of molecular order |
| cystic fibrosis | A genetic disorder characterized by thick mucus, difficulty breathing, and chronic lung infections |
| cytoplasm | An aqueous mixture of proteins and other biological molecules that surrounds the organelles in a cell |
| cytotoxic T cell | An antigen-specific killer T cell that circulates in the blood and lymph systems |
| decomposition reaction | A chemical reaction in which a molecule is broken down into its component parts |
| dehydration synthesis | The removal of water to create a covalent bond. This is the type of bond present in polymers. |

| Term | Definition |
|---|---|
| dendrites | Treelike extensions of the neuron's cell body that receive electrochemical stimulation from other neurons |
| dendritic cell | A phagocytic cell that kills extracellular pathogens |
| density | An intensive property that equals mass per unit volume |
| deoxyribonucleic acid (DNA) | The primary genetic material inside human cells that stores genetic information |
| dependent variable | Parameter that is thought to be affected by the independent variable and is measured in an experiment |
| deposition | The process by which gas undergoes a phase transition into a solid without first passing through the liquid phase |
| dermis | The middle layer of skin, which contains nerve endings, capillaries, glands, hair follicles, and other structures |
| diabetes | Disease caused by either a lack of insulin production or a dysregulation of blood glucose |
| diaphysis | The cylindrical shaft of a long bone |
| diastole | The phase of the cardiac cycle when the heart muscle relaxes |
| diffusion | The process by which substances and gases are exchanged across a membrane. Substances in solution tend to diffuse from areas of higher concentration to areas of lower concentration. |
| diffusion rate | The speed of movement down a concentration gradient |
| digestion | The chemical and mechanical breakdown of foods into smaller compounds that can be used by the body |
| digestive system | The system of organs that breaks down foods into nutrients the body can use |
| dihybrid cross | A mating between two individuals with different alleles of each of two genes |
| diploid | Description of a cell containing two complete sets of chromosomes, one from each parent |
| direct hormones | Hormones that function directly on a target to initiate a response |
| directional terminology | A set of terms used to describe the location of different parts of the body |
| disaccharide | The polymer that results when two monosaccharides undergo dehydration synthesis |
| dominant | Description of an allele that hides the expression of the recessive allele in the phenotype of the offspring |
| double displacement reaction | A chemical reaction in which two elements or molecular ions switch places |
| duodenum | The first part of the small intestine |
| eccrine glands | The primary sweat glands of the body |
| efferent arteriole | The blood vessel that exits the glomerulus |
| efferent (motor) neurons | The neurons that carry sensory information from the central nervous system toward the muscles of the body |

| Term | Definition |
|---|---|
| ejaculatory duct | The site where secretions from different glands are mixed with sperm to produce semen |
| electron configuration | A description of the shells and subshells of all the electrons of an atom |
| electronic balance | A device used to make very precise measurements of weight |
| electrons | Particles orbiting the nucleus of an atom that have a negative electric charge |
| element | A pure type of matter that cannot be separated into different types of matter by ordinary chemical means |
| emphysema | A breakdown of the alveoli, leading to increased difficulty breathing |
| endocrine system | The system of organs that produces and releases hormones that control many bodily functions |
| endometrium | Highly vascularized lining of the uterus |
| endorphins | Hormones released by the anterior pituitary that inhibit the perception of pain |
| endothermic | Description of a reaction that consumes heat |
| enzyme | A protein that catalyzes chemical reactions in the body by lowering the activation energy |
| eosinophils | Granulocytes responsible for killing parasites |
| epidermis | The outermost layer of skin, which serves as a barrier to infections from the environment and regulates water loss |
| epididymis | Site in the testes where sperm mature and are stored |
| epiglottis | Flap of cartilage in the pharynx that prevents food from entering the trachea |
| epinephrine | Hormone released by the adrenal medulla that induces the "fight or flight" response |
| epiphyseal plate | Site of new bone growth |
| epiphyses | Ends of a long bone |
| epithelial tissue | Covers the body (e.g., skin tissue) and produces secretions (e.g., glandular tissue) |
| erythrocytes | Red blood cells |
| esophageal sphincter | A ring-shaped muscle that tightens to separate the stomach and esophagus |
| esophagus | The portion of the alimentary canal between the pharynx and the stomach |
| estrogen | Hormone released by the ovaries that induces the thickening of the endometrium |
| eukaryotic | A type of cell that has a nucleus and membrane-bound organelles |
| evaporation | The process by which a liquid changes into a gas due to an increase in temperature and/or pressure |
| exothermic | Description of a reaction that gives off heat |
| experiment | Carefully designed procedure used to test a hypothesis |

| Term | Definition |
|---|---|
| experimental group | Group in a scientific study for which the independent variable is changed (e.g., group of study participants who receive a medication as opposed to a placebo) |
| expiratory reserve volume | The quantity of air that can be additionally exhaled following normal exhalation |
| extensive properties | Physical properties that depend upon the amount of matter being measured |
| fallopian tubes | Tubes that connect the ovaries to the uterus. A fallopian tube is the site of fertilization. |
| fascicle (muscle) | A bundle of muscle fibers that is surrounded by connective tissue |
| fatty acid | A hydrocarbon chain that ends in a carboxyl group |
| fibrous joints | Joints held together only by ligaments and not movable |
| fibrous protein | A non-water-soluble protein (e.g., keratin and collagen) |
| flat bones | Bones that provide protection to internal organs |
| flora | Nonpathogenic microbes that compete for resources with pathogenic organisms, thereby inhibiting the pathogens' occupancy |
| follicle-stimulating hormone (FSH) | The hormone released by the anterior pituitary that triggers the ovaries to produce estrogen and the testes to produce testosterone |
| follicular phase | The phase in the menstrual cycle in which the ovarian follicle matures |
| freezing | The process by which a substance in a liquid transitions into a solid due to the removal of heat |
| gametes | Reproductive cells (i.e., sperm or ova) |
| gas | A substance with weak intermolecular forces that does not have definite shape or volume |
| gastric juice | Liquid in the stomach containing hydrochloric acid and enzymes |
| gastrointestinal system | The system of organs that converts food into nutrients that the body can use; also called the *digestive system* or *GI system* |
| gene | A short segment of DNA that codes for a single protein or trait |
| genitourinary system | The system of organs responsible for removing toxins and waste and maintaining water balance, blood pressure, and blood pH. Includes parts of the urinary, renal, and excretory systems. |
| genotype | The genetic makeup of an individual, including both dominant and recessive alleles |
| globular protein | A water-soluble protein (e.g., hemoglobin) |
| glomerulus | A cluster of porous capillaries through which blood components are filtered into the nephron |
| glucagon | A hormone produced by alpha cells in the pancreas that increases blood glucose |
| glycogen | A polysaccharide composed of glucose and stored as a form of energy |
| goiter | Enlargement of the thyroid gland caused by insufficient iodine intake |

| Term | Definition |
|---|---|
| Golgi apparatus | The organelle that is responsible for the sorting and packing of cellular proteins |
| graduated cylinder | A narrow vessel used to quickly measure liquid volume |
| granulocytes | Cells of the innate immune system (e.g., basophils, eosinophils, and neutrophils) containing reactive oxygen compounds and cytokines in their cytoplasm |
| group | A column in the periodic table |
| growth hormone | The hormone released by the anterior pituitary that induces growth of the organism |
| hair follicles | Columns in the skin that have a large concentration of keratin-producing cells |
| haploid | Description of a cell having a single set of unpaired chromosomes |
| Haversian canal | A hollow tube running down the length of osteons that contains blood vessels |
| heart | The organ that propels blood through the circulatory system |
| helper T cell | A cell that activates other adaptive immune cells (e.g., cytotoxic T and B cells) |
| hematuria | The presence of blood in the urine, indicating damage to the urinary tract or kidney |
| hemoglobin | Protein in erythrocytes that facilitates gas exchange by binding to oxygen or carbon dioxide |
| hepatic portal vein | The vein that carries blood from the gastrointestinal tract to the liver |
| heredity | The passing of traits or characteristics from parents to offspring through the inheritance of genes |
| heterozygous | Having two different alleles for a trait |
| homeostasis | The status achieved when all of the systems in the body are in balance |
| homozygous | Having two of the same alleles for a trait |
| hormone | A signaling molecule that travels through the blood to enact a change when bound to its receptor on the target |
| human immunodeficiency virus (HIV) | The virus responsible for acquired immunodeficiency syndrome (AIDS) |
| hyaline cartilage | Strong, flexible tissue that covers the articulating surfaces of bones to cushion them at joints |
| hydrocarbon chain | A long strand of hydrogen and carbon atoms in a lipid |
| hydrolysis | The addition of water to break a covalent bond. It releases energy in a polymer. |
| hydrophilic | Dissolving in water |
| hydrophobic | Not dissolving in water. This is a characteristic of hydrocarbon chains. |
| hypertension | Chronic high blood pressure |

| Term | Definition |
|------|------------|
| hyperthermia | Body temperature elevated above normal |
| hyperthyroidism | Thyroid disease caused by overproduction of thyroid hormones that may result in weight loss and hyperactivity |
| hypodermis | The deepest layer of the skin, which contains blood vessels and fat tissues |
| hypothalamus | Master regulatory gland of the endocrine system |
| hypothermia | Body temperature that is below normal |
| hypothesis | Testable statement investigated in an experiment |
| hypothyroidism | Thyroid disease caused by insufficient production of thyroid hormones that may result in weight gain and fatigue |
| ileum | The terminal part of the small intestine and the location of $B_{12}$ absorption |
| immune system | Protects the body from foreign pathogens |
| incomplete dominance | A form of inheritance in which both heterozygous alleles are expressed |
| independent variable | A parameter that is thought to affect the dependent variable and is changed between groups in an experiment to study its effect |
| inferior vena cava | The vein that carries deoxygenated blood to the heart. This is the largest vein in the body. |
| inflammation | Process that leads to swelling, produces fever, and recruits immune cells |
| innate arm | The part of the immune system that responds quickly to pathogens but is not specific to individual pathogens and does not form memory cells |
| inspiratory reserve volume | The quantity of air that can be additionally inhaled following normal inhalation |
| insulin | Hormone produced by beta cells in the pancreas that induces glucose storage |
| integument | The skin |
| integumentary system | The system of organs comprised of skin, hair, nails, and accessory glands |
| intensive properties | Physical properties that are independent of the amount of matter being measured |
| interferon | A chemical messenger that signals to nearby cells the presence of a foreign pathogen and activates innate defenses in those cells |
| intermolecular forces | Forces that cause particles to be attracted to one another or to repulse one another |
| intramolecular forces | The bonds that hold a molecule together |
| ion | A positively or negatively charged atom or combination of atoms |
| ionic bond | A bond created by the transfer of electrons |
| irregular bones | Bones that vary in shape and structure (e.g., vertebrae, sacrum) |
| ischemia | Damage to muscle tissue due to inadequate blood flow |
| isotopes | Atoms of the same element that have different numbers of neutrons |
| jejunum | The middle part of the small intestine where most nutrient absorption occurs |
| kidneys | Organs that filter blood to remove excess waste and water from the body |

| Term | Definition |
|---|---|
| lactic acid | Substance produced by muscular contractions and changes muscle tissue pH, potentially resulting in muscle fatigue |
| lacunae | Spaces in the lamellae where bone cells reside |
| lamellae | Concentric rings of the mineralized matrix that makes up the osteon |
| larynx | The voice box |
| latent heat | The heat required for a substance to undergo a phase transition at a constant temperature |
| latent heat of fusion | The heat required for a substance to transition from a solid to a liquid at a constant temperature |
| latent heat of vaporization | The heat required for a substance to transition from a liquid to a gas at a constant temperature |
| leukocytes | White blood cells, which are part of the body's immune response system |
| ligaments | These attach bone to bone at joints |
| lipid | A macromolecule containing hydrocarbon chains; also called a *fat* |
| liquid | A type of matter with a defined volume but no defined shape. It is able to flow and change shape depending on the surface upon which it rests or the container in which it is held. |
| long bones | Bones that support the weight of the body and enable movement. They are hollow, filled with marrow, and longer than they are wide. |
| luteal phase | Phase in the menstrual cycle that starts following ovulation in which the corpus luteum produces progesterone in preparation for fertilization of the ovum |
| luteinizing hormone (LH) | Hormone released by the anterior pituitary that triggers ovulation in females |
| lymph | Clear fluid that absorbs waste products |
| lymph nodes | Small glands that filter lymph and contain high concentrations of lymphocytes |
| lymphatic system | Network of capillaries that drains toxins and wastes away from body tissue into the blood |
| lymphocyte | Type of white blood cell that releases antibodies in response to disease |
| lysosome | Organelle that is responsible for the breakdown of cellular waste products |
| lysozyme | The enzyme that degrades bacterial cell walls and causes them to lyse, or burst. It is found in saliva, tears, and mucus. |
| macromolecules | The carbohydrates, lipids, proteins, and nucleic acids that make up living organisms |
| macrophage | A cell that digests dying cells, especially in the spleen where red blood cells die |
| malleability | The capacity of a material to be manipulated into different shapes |
| measuring wheel | A device consisting of a single wheel attached to a handle and meant to be pushed or pulled along to measure length; also called a *surveyor's wheel* |

| Term | Definition |
|------|-----------|
| mechanical digestion | The physical breaking down of food into smaller pieces |
| medulla | The part of the brain that regulates involuntary functions such as breathing, swallowing, and beating of the heart |
| meiosis | A process of cell division in which the original cell divides twice and the four resulting cells (haploid cells) each contain a single copy of each chromosome |
| melatonin | Hormone released by the pineal gland to regulate sleep |
| melting | The process by which a solid substance liquefies due to the introduction of heat |
| melting point | The temperature at which a substance changes from solid to liquid |
| memory | In the body's immune system, the ability to remember a pathogen that has been previously encountered |
| menstruation | Process during which the endometrium is shed |
| metal | A general descriptive term for elements on the left side of the periodic table, which are malleable and ductile and conduct heat and electricity readily |
| metric system | The decimal measuring system based on the meter, liter, and gram as units of length, volume, and weight or mass, respectively |
| microvilli | Microscopic protrusions in the membrane of the intestine that increase surface area for absorption |
| mitochondria | Organelle with a double-membrane structure responsible for the production of ATP, which is the cell's source of energy |
| mitosis | A process of cell division that results in two identical daughter cells (diploid cells) from a single parent |
| mitral valve | Valve that separates the left atrium and ventricle; also called the *bicuspid valve* |
| mixture | Matter that is composed of more than one substance |
| molecular (polyatomic) ion | A molecule with an unbalanced charge due to loss or gain of electrons |
| molecule | A group of two or more atoms bonded together |
| monohybrid cross | A mating between two individuals with different alleles of one gene |
| monomers | Building blocks of macromolecules |
| monosaccharide | A carbohydrate monomer with the chemical formula $C_nH_{2n}O_n$ |
| motor unit | A group of muscle fibers enervated by a single motor neuron |
| multiple sclerosis | A demyelinating disorder that results in uncoordinated muscle movement |
| muscle fatigue | The result of exerting a muscle strenuously over a long period |
| muscle strain | The overstretching or tearing of muscle fibers |
| muscular system | The system of skeletal, smooth, and cardiac muscle that permits movement and circulates blood |
| muscular tissue | Tissue that provides movement. There are three kinds of muscular tissue: skeletal, cardiac, and smooth. |

| Term | Definition |
|---|---|
| myelin | A protein and phospholipid coating that insulates nerve fibers and increases the speed at which electrical impulses are transmitted |
| myofibril | The basic unit of a muscle cell that extends the length of the muscle |
| myosin | The thick filament protein of muscle tissue |
| natural killer (NK) cell | Attacks and kills cells (e.g., tumor cells) that contain intracellular pathogens or display abnormal surface antigens |
| negative feedback | A signaling loop in which the end product leads to the production of less product. This is the more common kind of feedback loop in the human body. |
| negative pressure breathing | Inhalation of air due to a decreased pressure in the lungs |
| nephron | The functional unit of the kidney and the site of blood filtration |
| nervous system | System of nervous tissue that transmits and coordinates signals between different parts of the body, allowing the body to sense and respond to external and internal environmental changes |
| nervous tissue | Tissue that provides the structure for the brain, spinal cord, and nerves and transmits electrical impulses to control bodily processes |
| neuromuscular junction | A synapse between a motor neuron and muscle fiber |
| neuron | A cell that conducts electrical impulses, allowing the transmittance of information from one part of the body to another |
| neuropathy | Peripheral nerve damage that leads to muscle weakness and even paralysis |
| neurotransmitters | Chemical messengers that carry the nerve impulse across a synapse |
| neutral atom | An atom that has the same number of protons and electrons |
| neutrons | Particles in the nucleus of an atom that have no electric charge |
| neutrophils | Granulocytes responsible for phagocytosing bacteria and mediating inflammatory responses |
| noble gas | An element in the group farthest to the right on the periodic table. Noble gases do not react readily with other elements. |
| non-metal | An element on the right side of the periodic table, in group 5, 6, or 7 |
| nucleic acid | A macromolecule that supplies genetic material (e.g., DNA and RNA) |
| nucleolus | The substructure within the nucleus where ribosomes are assembled |
| nucleotide | The monomer for nucleic acids |
| nucleus (of an atom) | The central core of an atom, consisting of a proton and neutron |
| nucleus (of a cell) | Site of DNA storage, as well as DNA replication and RNA transcription, within a cell |
| null hypothesis | Statement that assumes there is no causal relationship between the independent variable (e.g., "Physical therapy has no effect on length of nursing home stays"). If statistically significant evidence is found that the null hypothesis is not true, then it is rejected, and the research hypothesis is supported. |
| octet rule | The principle that most atoms will seek to have eight valence electrons |

| Term | Definition |
|------|-----------|
| oogenesis | Process by which ova are produced by meiotic division |
| optic nerve | A cranial nerve that transmits visual stimuli from the eye to the brain |
| orbital | A description of the potential path of an electron |
| organ | A group of tissues working together to perform a common function |
| organ system | A group of organs working together to perform a larger function |
| organelle | A membrane-bound compartment in a cell that performs a specific function |
| organic molecule | A molecule containing carbon (and usually hydrogen) that is found in living things |
| osmosis | A particular type of diffusion in which an imbalance is corrected by means of migration of the solvent |
| osteoarthritis | Degenerative joint disease characterized by a loss of cartilage in the joint |
| osteoblast | Bone cell that builds bone |
| osteoclast | Bone cell that breaks down bone |
| osteocyte | Bone cell that senses mechanical stress and regulates osteoblasts and osteoclasts |
| osteogenesis imperfecta | Genetic disorder that results in bones that are easily broken |
| osteon | Functional unit of bone |
| osteoporosis | Disease of bone characterized by loss of bone mineral density |
| ovarian follicle | Structure in the ovaries that contains a developing ovum |
| ovulation | Process that releases an ovum from the ovarian follicle |
| ovum (ova) | Female gamete, or egg; *ova* is the plural |
| oxidation reaction | A chemical reaction in which a reactant combines with oxygen |
| oxytocin | Hormone released by the posterior pituitary that stimulates uterine contractions to initiate labor in pregnant females |
| parasympathetic | The division of the autonomic nervous system that returns the body to a resting state |
| parathyroid hormone | Hormone released by the parathyroid gland that increases blood calcium levels |
| passive immunity | The introduction of antibodies from an external source (e.g., breastfeeding) |
| pathogen | Foreign infectious agent |
| pathogen-associated molecular patterns (PAMPs) | Common proteins and carbohydrates found on the surface of pathogens that are not specific to one microbial protein |
| penis | Male reproductive organ |
| peptide bond | The bond linking amino groups in proteins formed by removing water from the carboxyl and amino groups |
| peptide hormone | A signaling molecule composed of amino acids that binds to surface receptors and initiates a signaling cascade |

| Term | Definition |
|---|---|
| period | A row of the periodic table |
| periodic table | A table of all the elements ordered in specific rows and columns |
| periosteum | Fibrous sheath that surrounds and protects a bone |
| peripheral nervous system | The nerves outside the brain and spinal cord, divided into the somatic and autonomic nervous systems and functioning in sympathetic or parasympathetic mode |
| peristalsis | Wavelike contraction of muscles that moves material along the digestive tract |
| pH | A measure of acidity (pH less than 7) or alkalinity (pH greater than 7) |
| phagocytose | To engulf and destroy a pathogen |
| pharynx | Dividing point between the trachea and esophagus, where the throat senses the presence of food and triggers swallowing |
| phase diagram | A graph that depicts the pressure and temperature necessary for a substance to undergo a phase change from one state to another |
| phase transition | The transition of a substance from one state of matter into another |
| phenotype | The visible characteristics of an individual, determined by genotype |
| phospholipid | A type of lipid that contains two fatty acids bound to a hydrophilic phosphate group |
| physical properties | The characteristics of substances that can be observed or measured and are unrelated to chemical changes |
| placenta | A structure that develops from the endometrium during pregnancy to facilitate gas and nutrient exchange between the mother's body and the developing fetus |
| plasma | The liquid component of blood in which other components are suspended |
| plasma cell | A mature B cell that secretes a pathogen-specific antibody |
| plasma membrane | The semipermeable lipid bilayer that surrounds a cell and controls the movement of solutes into and out of the cell |
| platelets | The cell fragments that mitigate bleeding by forming blood clots |
| pleura | Each of a pair of tough membranes surrounding the lungs |
| pleural fluid | The fluid found between the pleural membranes (pleurae) |
| polar molecules | Molecules that have slight asymmetrical positive and negative charges |
| polarization | An influx of positive charge inside a nerve cell that triggers an action potential |
| polymers | Multiple monomers joined together |
| polypeptide chain | Multiple amino acids linked by peptide bonds and a protein's primary structure |
| polysaccharide | A long chain of carbohydrate monomers |
| positive feedback | A signaling loop in which the end product leads to the production of more product. This less common kind of feedback loop tends to lead to dramatic changes in the human body. |

| Term | Definition |
| --- | --- |
| posterior pituitary | Endocrine gland that releases hormones that act directly on a target |
| products | The substances that are the outputs of chemical reactions |
| progesterone | Hormone released by the corpus luteum that maintains the endometrium |
| prolactin | Hormone released by the anterior pituitary that acts on the mammary glands of females to induce milk production |
| prostate gland | A gland that secretes an alkaline fluid to enable sperm to survive in the acidic reproductive tract of females |
| protein | A macromolecule composed of amino acids |
| protons | Particles in the nucleus of an atom that have a positive electric charge. The number of protons is the element's atomic number. |
| pulmonary circuit | The part of the circulatory system that carries blood to and from the lungs |
| pulmonary veins | Veins that return oxygenated blood from the lungs to the heart |
| Punnett square | A graphical tool used to calculate the probabilities of inheritance |
| pyloric sphincter | A ring-shaped muscle that tightens to separate the stomach from the small intestine |
| random error | Uncertainty introduced into an experiment due to imprecision in measurement |
| reactants | The substances that are the inputs to chemical reactions |
| receptor | A protein in cells that recognizes a specific signaling molecule |
| recessive | Description of an allele that expressed in the phenotype of the offspring only if the offspring has two copies of that trait |
| rectum | The final portion of the large intestine |
| renal arteries | Vessels that carry blood from the heart to the kidneys |
| renal corpuscle | The blood-filtering portion of the nephron comprised of the glomerulus and Bowman's capsule |
| renal tubule | The part of the nephron where blood components are reabsorbed into the bloodstream |
| reproducibility | The ability to produce the same results from independent experiments |
| reproductive system | The system of organs that produce gametes and facilitate fertilization |
| residual volume | The quantity of air remaining in the lungs at all times to prevent lung collapse |
| respiratory system | The system of organs that oxygenate blood and release carbon dioxide |
| rheumatoid arthritis | An autoimmune disease in which immune cells attack the cartilage in joints |
| ribonucleic acid (RNA) | A macromolecule that translates DNA into a form that can be read to create proteins |
| ribosome | Cellular structure composed of both RNA and a protein that translates messenger RNA into proteins |
| rough ER | Organelle that is studded with ribosomes and is responsible for the translation of proteins that are either membrane bound or secreted |
| salivary glands | Glands that release enzymes to initiate the digestive process in the mouth |

| Term | Definition |
|---|---|
| sarcomere | The contractile component of the myofibril, composed of actin and myosin |
| saturated | Description of a lipid in which every carbon molecule is bound to two hydrogens |
| sciatic nerve | A spinal nerve that enervates the leg |
| scientific method | The stepwise process used by researchers to design and execute an experiment |
| scrotum | The sac that hangs outside the male body and contains the testes |
| sebaceous glands | Oil glands that secrete sebum, a mixture of fats and proteins that prevents the skin and hair from drying out |
| self-tolerant | A description of the fact that a healthy adaptive immune system does not respond to normal cellular antigens |
| seminal vesicles | Glands that secrete a fructose-containing liquid to nourish sperm |
| seminiferous tubules | The site in the testes where sperm are produced |
| shell | The electron subshells that share the same principle energy level |
| short bones | Bones that provide stability and some movement and are wider than they are flat |
| SI system | A complete system of units of measure with base units of meter (length), liter (volume), gram (weight or mass), second (time), ampere (electric current), kelvin (temperature), mole (amount of matter), and candela (luminous intensity) |
| sickle-cell trait | A genetic blood condition that causes irregularly shaped red blood cells |
| simple diffusion | The movement of membrane-permeable solutes down a concentration gradient |
| single displacement (substitution) reaction | A chemical reaction in which one element or molecular ion in a molecule is replaced by a different element or molecular ion |
| skeletal muscle | The muscles composed of fascicles and involved in voluntary movement |
| skeletal system | The system of bones and other tissues that protects organs, creates blood cells, and provides a framework for muscle |
| small intestine | The part of the alimentary canal below the stomach in which digestion is completed and absorption of nutrients into the bloodstream occurs |
| smooth ER | The organelle responsible for lipid synthesis and detoxification of cellular waste products and drugs |
| smooth muscle | A type of muscle tissue located in the hollow organs (e.g., GI tract) and blood vessels and responsible for involuntary muscle contraction |
| solid | A substance with a defined shape and volume |
| solute | A substance that is dissolved in another substance |
| solution | One substance that is dissolved in another |
| solvent | A substance in which another substance is dissolved |
| soma | The cell body of a neuron |

| Term | Definition |
|---|---|
| **somatic nervous system** | The part of the nervous system that sends and receives signals from skeletal muscle |
| **specific heat capacity** | The amount of energy needed to change the temperature of 1 gram of a substance by 1 degree Celsius |
| **sperm** | A male gamete |
| **spermatogenesis** | The process by which sperm are produced through meiotic division |
| **spinal cord** | A cylindrical column of nerves that runs through the center of the spine |
| **spinal nerves** | Nerves that transmit sensory and motor signals between the spinal cord and the body |
| **spongy bone** | Less dense tissue located at the ends of bones that contains bone marrow |
| **starch** | A polysaccharide composed of glucose polymers and stored as energy in plants |
| **state (of matter)** | The distinct form assumed by matter (e.g., solid, liquid, or gas) |
| **steroid** | A type of lipid that does not contain fatty acids (e.g., cholesterol and sex hormones) |
| **steroid hormone** | A signaling molecule derived from cholesterol. It binds to receptors inside the cell and initiates changes in host cell transcription and protein translation. |
| **stomach** | The hollow organ below the esophagus where mechanical and chemical digestion occur |
| **sublimation** | The process through which a solid substance transitions directly into a gas without first going through the liquid phase. This occurs when temperature and pressure are below the substance's triple point. |
| **subshell** | The designation of a group of orbitals that has a maximum capacity for electrons |
| **substance** | Physical matter that has uniform properties |
| **sudoriferous glands** | Sweat glands |
| **surfactant** | The detergent in the lungs responsible for reducing surface tension to prevent lung collapse |
| **surfactant insufficiency** | A genetic disorder caused by a mutation in one of the surfactant proteins that makes breathing difficult |
| **sympathetic** | The division of the autonomic nervous system that manages the "fight or flight" response |
| **synapse** | The junction between the axon of one neuron and the dendrite of another |
| **synovial fluid** | Lubricating fluid found in synovial joints |
| **synovial joints** | Most common joints in the body and capable of movement |
| **synthesis (direct combination) reaction** | A chemical reaction in which more than one reactant component combines to form the product |
| **systemic circuit** | The part of the circulatory system that carries oxygenated blood away from the left ventricle and returns deoxygenated blood to the right atrium |

| Term | Definition |
|------|------------|
| systole | The phase of the cardiac cycle in which muscular contraction propels blood |
| T cell | An adaptive immune system cell, born in the bone marrow and matured in the thymus |
| T (transverse) tubules | Tunnel-like extensions of the muscle membrane found in skeletal and cardiac muscle cells that allow for the conduction of electrical impulses |
| tendons | Fibrous connective tissue that joins muscle to bone |
| testes | The structure in which male gametes are produced |
| testosterone | Hormone released by the testes that induces spermatogenesis in males |
| thrombocytopenia | Condition of having too few platelets that can cause excessive bleeding |
| thymus | A glandular lymphoid organ in which T cells mature |
| thyroid hormones | Hormones released by the thyroid that regulate metabolism |
| thyroid-stimulating hormone (TSH) | Hormone released by the anterior pituitary that acts on the thyroid to stimulate hormone release |
| tidal volume | The quantity of air that moves during normal breathing |
| tissue | Cells working together for a common function |
| total lung capacity | The maximum volume of air that can reside in the lungs |
| trachea | The tube that carries air from the mouth and nasal cavities to the lungs (i.e., the windpipe) |
| transcription | The first step of gene expression, in which a particular segment of DNA is copied into mRNA |
| translation | The decoding of mRNA by a ribosome to produce a specific amino acid chain |
| tricuspid valve | The valve that separates the right atrium and ventricle |
| triglyceride | A type of lipid that contains three fatty-acid chains bound to a glycerol molecule |
| triple beam balance | A device used to make precise measurements of weight. It is somewhat less precise than an electronic balance. |
| triple point | The point at which temperature and pressure allow a substance to coexist in its solid, liquid, and gas states |
| tropic hormones | Hormones that function on targets to stimulate hormone release |
| unsaturated | Describing a lipid in which some carbon molecules are bound to one hydrogen and double-bonded to the adjacent carbon |
| urea | The metabolic waste product excreted in urine |
| ureters | Ducts by which urine passes from the kidney to the bladder |
| urethra | The duct through which urine is expelled and, in males, semen flows to exit the body |
| urinary bladder | The hollow muscular organ that stores urine prior to its being expelled from the body |

| Term | Definition |
|------|------------|
| urinary system | The system of organs that filters blood and eliminates waste products through urine |
| urine | The fluid made by the kidneys that is expelled from the body. It contains water and urea. |
| vaccination | The introduction of harmless organisms into the body to spur the formation of memory cells and produce immunity (e.g., to polio) |
| vagina | The passage between the cervix and the external genitalia in females |
| vagus nerve | A cranial nerve that transmits signals from the abdominal organs to the brain and helps regulate parasympathetic responses |
| valence electrons | Electrons in the outermost orbital of an atom |
| vapor | A substance that has been diffused into the air as a gas at a temperature below its boiling point |
| vas deferens | The channel that connects the epididymis to the ejaculatory duct |
| vasopressin | A hormone released by the posterior pituitary in response to high blood osmolality. It functions at the collection duct of the nephron to increase water reabsorption. |
| veins | Vessels that return blood to the heart and contain valves to prevent the backflow of blood |
| ventilation rate | The rate of inhalation and exhalation per unit of time |
| ventricles | Chambers of the heart that collect and expel blood from the heart |
| venules | Vessels that receive blood from the capillaries and merge to form veins |
| villi | Fingerlike projections that extend into the small intestine |
| vital capacity | The sum of the tidal, inspiratory reserve, and expiratory reserve volumes of air in the lungs |
| Volkmann canal | A hollow channel in bone that contains blood vessels, allowing nutrient exchange between osteons |
| volumetric flask | A piece of laboratory glassware calibrated to contain a precise volume at a particular temperature |
| volumetric pipette | A piece of laboratory glassware, smaller than a volumetric flask, calibrated to contain a small and precise volume at a particular temperature; also called a *bulb pipette* |
| zymogen | An inactive substance that is converted into an active enzyme in the presence of a third substance |

# English and Language Usage Glossary

| Term | Definition |
|---|---|
| adjective | A word (e.g., *funny*, *breakable*, or *round*) that describes a noun or a pronoun |
| adverb | A word (e.g., *quickly*, *cheerfully*, or *very*) used to modify a verb, an adjective, or another adverb |
| affix | A letter or letters that attach to a word or word root at either its beginning or end, changing its meaning (i.e., a prefix or a suffix) |
| agreement | The appropriate pairing of singular nouns with singular verbs or pronouns, or of plural nouns with plural verbs or pronouns |
| ambiguity | Refers to uncertainty of meaning or a lack of clarity |
| antecedent | The noun that a pronoun is used to represent. A pronoun must agree in number and kind with its antecedent. |
| apostrophe | Punctuation mark that indicates possessive case or the omission of numbers or letters (e.g., "Shirley's study group can't meet today") |
| article | A word (e.g., *a, an,* or *the*) used with a noun to limit it or make it clearer |
| brainstorming | Thinking creatively, without self-censorship, of a list of ideas for approaching a task, problem, or project |
| citation | Formally formatted bibliographic information about the source of an idea or quoted text |
| clarity | How readily understandable a text is |
| cliché | A phrase or expression that is overused and has therefore lost its novelty |
| colloquialism | The use of informal words or phrases that may be appropriate in casual writing or familiar conversation but are inappropriate in business, academic, or formal social writing |
| colon | Punctuation mark used to introduce a series or quote (e.g., "He bought these groceries: milk, bread, and butter"; At the end of the meeting, he said this: "That was the most unproductive hour I have ever spent"). A colon is also used in the expression of times and ratios (e.g., 6:00 PM; the ratio 4:3). |
| comma | Punctuation mark used to indicate a pause in a sentence, to separate parts of a sentence, or to separate items in a list |
| complement | A word or group of words added to a sentence to make it complete |
| complex sentence | A sentence containing an independent clause and one or more dependent clauses |
| compound sentence | A sentence that has at least two independent clauses joined by either a comma and a coordinating conjunction (i.e., *for, and, nor, but, or, yet,* or *so*) or a semicolon. This sentence structure gives the ideas in the two clauses equal weight. |
| compound-complex sentence | A sentence that incorporates two independent clauses and one or more dependent clauses |
| conjunction | A word used to connect independent or dependent clauses (such as *and, but,* or *if*) |

| Term | Definition |
|---|---|
| connotation | The sense or image associated with a word, in addition to the denotation given by its dictionary definition. Positive and negative senses are connotations, as are formal and informal usage. |
| context clues | Words or phrases in a sentence that help the reader understand the meanings of unfamiliar words |
| dependent clause | Contains a subject and verb but does not express a complete thought |
| derivational morpheme | A prefix or suffix that changes a word's part of speech or meaning |
| end punctuation marks | The punctuation marks that end sentences (e.g., period, question mark, and exclamation point) |
| formal style | A style of writing that fits particular conventions and is appropriate to business or academic writing. Such writing may include jargon if the intended audience will understand such terms. |
| homographs | Words that are spelled the same as each other but have different meanings (e.g., *bear* can mean "to carry" or "a large, omnivorous mammal with a shaggy coat") |
| homonyms | Words that share the same spelling (homographs) or pronunciation (homophones) but have different meanings |
| homophones | Words that sound the same as each other but have different meanings (e.g., *beer* is a beverage, while a *bier* is a platform used at a funeral) |
| independent clause | A part of a sentence that contains a subject and verb and expresses a complete thought |
| indirect object | A person or thing to whom/which or for whom/which something is done |
| inflectional morpheme | A suffix that does not change the basic meaning or part of speech of a word but rather adapts it appropriately for changes in number and tense or to express comparison or possession |
| informal style | A style of writing that is familiar and conversational. Such writing may include slang, colloquialisms, or broken syntax. |
| interjection | A word or phrase that expresses sudden or strong feeling (e.g., "Hooray!" or "Oh!") |
| jargon | Specialized words or expressions that are particular to a group and may be difficult for others to understand |
| modifier | A word (e.g., an adjective or adverb) or phrase that describes another word or group of words |
| morpheme | The smallest unit of grammar that has meaning |
| noun | A person, place, or thing |
| object | A person or thing that receives the action of the verb |
| outline | A general description or plan that organizes material into a logical framework. Writers may use an outline to plan their work. |
| paragraph | A group of related sentences |
| parentheses | Punctuation marks that offset a word, phrase, or clause that provides an additional explanation or afterthought in a sentence |

| Term | Definition |
|---|---|
| **predicate** | Part of a sentence that expresses what a subject does and includes the verb |
| **prefix** | An affix that attaches to the beginning of a word, typically changing the word's meaning |
| **preposition** | A word expressing a relationship to other words (e.g., "the drawing *on* the page" and "she arrived *after* the play") |
| **pronoun** | A word (e.g., *I, he, she, you, it, we,* or *they*) that is used instead of a noun |
| **proofreading** | Correcting mistakes in a piece of writing |
| **quotation marks** | Punctuation marks that indicate spoken dialogue or a direct quotation from another written source |
| **root word (root)** | The simplest form of a word, with no prefixes or suffixes, that provides the foundation of its meaning |
| **run-on sentence** | Occurs when two or more independent clauses are incorrectly joined |
| **semicolon** | Punctuation mark used in lieu of a conjunction to separate two independent clauses or to separate items in a list that themselves are series (e.g., "Ravi studied nouns, verbs, and modifiers; ratios, rates, and proportions; and bones, muscles, and skin") |
| **sentence fragment** | A "sentence" that lacks a subject and/or a verb and/or does not express a complete thought |
| **simple sentence** | A sentence containing only one clause. It must have at least one subject and one verb and express a complete thought. |
| **slang** | A type of language that is very informal and typically used in a context in which people know one another well |
| **subject** | The person or thing that is performing the action or being described |
| **suffix** | An affix that attaches to the end of a word and may change the word's meaning or part of speech |
| **supporting details** | Facts or ideas that provide more information about the topic introduced in the topic sentence of a paragraph, thereby helping to develop the passage's main idea |
| **thesis** | The main idea of a paragraph or passage |
| **topic sentence** | Summarizes the main idea of a paragraph |
| **transition words** | Words that establish the relationship between paragraphs, sentences, and parts of sentences, creating clarity and flow of text |
| **verb** | A word (e.g., *jump, think, happen,* or *exist*) that expresses an action or state of being |
| **verb tense** | Expresses the time at which the action takes place. A verb's tense must make sense given the context and the logical relationship of any other actions in the sentence. |